Hand Functional Anatomy and Therapy

Grégory Mesplié
Editor

Hand Functional Anatomy and Therapy

Springer

Editor
Grégory Mesplié
Institut Sud Aquitain de la Main et du
Membre Supérieur (ISAMMS)
Biarritz, France

ISBN 978-3-031-92504-7 ISBN 978-3-031-92505-4 (eBook)
https://doi.org/10.1007/978-3-031-92505-4

English translation of the original French edition published by Sauramps Médical, Montpellier, 2024

Translation from the French language edition: "Therapie de la Main" by Grégory Mesplié, © Sauramps Medical 2024. Published by Sauramps Medical. All Rights Reserved.

This Springer imprint is published by the registered company Springer Nature Switzerland AG
The registered company address is: Gewerbestrasse 11, 6330 Cham, Switzerland

To my mother, the illustrator, for her incredible work and kindness.

To my family and closed ones for their support, this book is also yours.

To the whole team at the Institut Sud Aquitain de la Main et du Membre Supérieur, without whom these books wouldn't exist.

Foreword

It is with the utmost respect and great pleasure that I write the foreword for the textbook titled *Hand Functional Anatomy and Therapy*, authored by Grégory Mesplié, an esteemed hand and wrist therapist from France. Mesplié has contributed extensively to this field through his numerous publications, and this latest work promises to continue that legacy. His previous books have been prefaced by renowned experts such as Dr. Mark Garcia-Elias, Dr. Elizabeth Haggert, and Judith Colditz, luminaries in the fields of hand surgery and therapy.

As I entered the fifth decade of my clinical practice in 2021, I continue to learn and refine new clinical insights and therapeutic techniques that enable the restoration of functionality in injured hands. This textbook offers the most up-to-date knowledge on functional hand anatomy and presents cutting-edge therapeutic interventions. It is an essential resource for clinicians, researchers, and students who are seeking to make informed decisions in hand surgery and therapy.

I have long admired Mesplié's dedication to his craft and his relentless efforts in compiling valuable resources for the professional community. Having read his previous works, I am confident that this upcoming textbook will present innovative, simplified, and effective therapeutic approaches that will further enhance clinical reasoning and problem-solving skills.

As a clinician, educator, and researcher, I have seen the profound evolution in clinical practice over the past five decades. With improved understanding and ongoing research, we, as practitioners, have been able to better equip the next generation with the knowledge and skills needed for excellence in the field.

This textbook provides comprehensive descriptions of a wide range of diagnoses and incorporates clinical reasoning from multiple perspectives, all aimed at restoring and optimizing extremity function. I believe this book will be invaluable to clinicians and healthcare professionals working with hand injuries, as it offers thorough, practical insights that support sound clinical judgment in both diagnosis and treatment. This new edition, in particular, introduces several well-conceived features, making it an indispensable resource for practitioners at all levels of expertise.

I am confident that the work presented by Mesplié will not only improve current clinical practices but also serve as a foundation for future generations of healthcare professionals.

With deep respect and best wishes,

Advanced Clinical Education Inc.
Mississauga, ON, Canada
Shrikant J. Chinchalkar

Contents

Part VII Complications of Hand Pathologies

Contributors

Jean-François Chauvet Institut Sud Aquitain de la Main et du Membre Supérieur (ISAMMS), Biarritz, France

Nicolas Christiaens Institut Sud Aquitain de la Main et du Membre Supérieur (ISAMMS), Biarritz, France

Alexandra Forli Unité Chir Plastique, Chirurgie de la Main, Hôpital Michallon, Grenoble, France

Denis Gerlac IUD Hand Rehabilitation and Orthopaedic Devices, Echirolles, France

Vincent Grelet Institut Sud Aquitain de la Main et du Membre Supérieur (ISAMMS), Biarritz, France

Olivier Léger Institut Sud Aquitain de la Main et du Membre Supérieur (ISAMMS), Biarritz, France

Grégory Mesplié Institut Sud Aquitain de la Main et du Membre Supérieur (ISAMMS), Biarritz, France

Alexandra Perret Centre Épaule Main, Voiron, France

Amélie-Anne Vienne Service Ergothérapie Appareillage, CHU Sud Réunion, Saint-Pierre, France

Part I

Functional Anatomy of the Hand

1 Functional Anatomy of the Hand

Grégory Mesplié

Bone Anatomy

The morphology of the hand is adapted to its function. The modification of its architecture that can happen after many types of injuries can have important functional consequences.

Hand Architecture

The hand's function is complex and depends on its architecture, which allows an adaptation to the different grips.

When grabbing voluminous objects, the hand has various arches (transverse, longitudinal, and oblique), anteriorly concave, which give the hand the shape of a cup, facilitating the grips (Fig. 1.1).

When the hand is pressed against a support, it can flatten and increase its support surface on a plane. The second and third metacarpals are relatively fixed, while the fourth and fifth are mobile, which allows an important adaptability of the ulnar side

The length of each osseous segment is essential for a harmonious winding of the fingers, as well as in maintaining the clamping force [1]. Even if this theory seems to be debated, finger winding seems to describe an equiangular spiral described by Fibonacci [2], according to his numerical series [0, 1, 1, 2, 3, 5, 8, 13, 21, 34] (Fig. 1.2).

When flexing the fingers, we can observe that the fingers converge towards the scaphoid tubercle, mainly because of the obliquity of the meta-

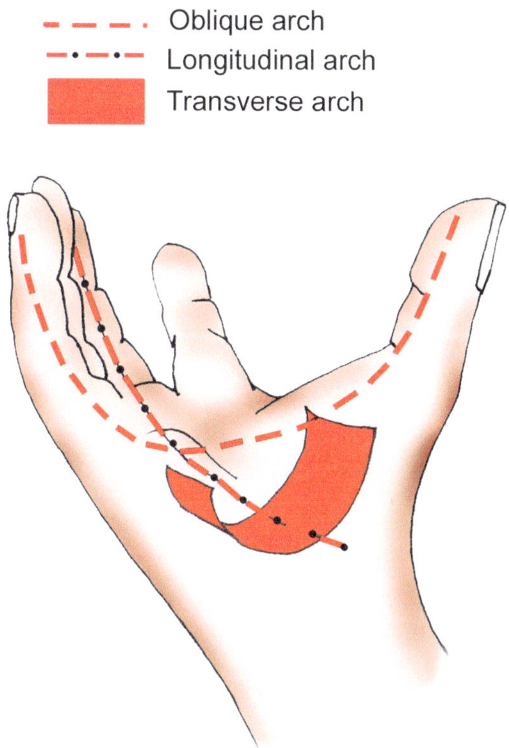

Fig. 1.1 The arches of the hand give it a cup shape, favoring the grips

G. Mesplié (✉)
Institut Sud Aquitain de la Main et du Membre Supérieur (ISAMMS), Biarritz, France

G. Mesplié (ed.), *Hand Functional Anatomy and Therapy*,
https://doi.org/10.1007/978-3-031-92505-4_1

carpophalangeal and interphalangeal joints (in a downward and outward direction).

When opening the fingers, the axis of the fingers converges towards the capitate. The axis of the third finger stays still (Fig. 1.3).

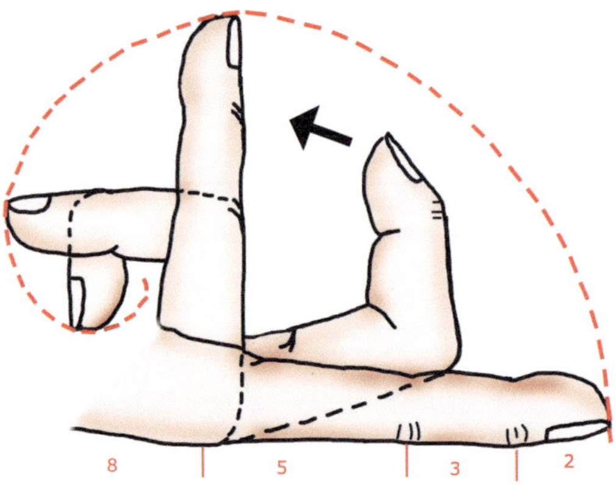

Fig. 1.2 The winding movement of the fingers describes an equiangular spiral because the lengths of the osseous segments follow the numeric series of Fibonacci, defined by the gold number (1.618, the "divine proportion")

Thumb Opposition

Thumb

The mobility of the thumb depends on the scapho-trapezium, trapezo-metacarpal, metacarpophalangeal, and interphalangeal joints.

These four joints, mobilized by the synergic action of the intrinsic and extrinsic muscles of the hand, contribute to the mobility of the thumb in the three planes of space according to a validated international nomenclature (Fig. 1.4). The thumb opposition is composed of various actions: a flexion, an abduction, and an automatic pronation, allowing the thumb to oppose its pulp to the fingers.

This automatic pronation of the thumb is related to osseous (topography of the trapezo-metacarpal joint surfaces, radial part of the metacarpophalangeal and interphalangeal joints larger than the ulnar part), ligamentous (radial ligaments longer than the ulnar ones), and muscular (external thenar muscles stronger than the internal the-

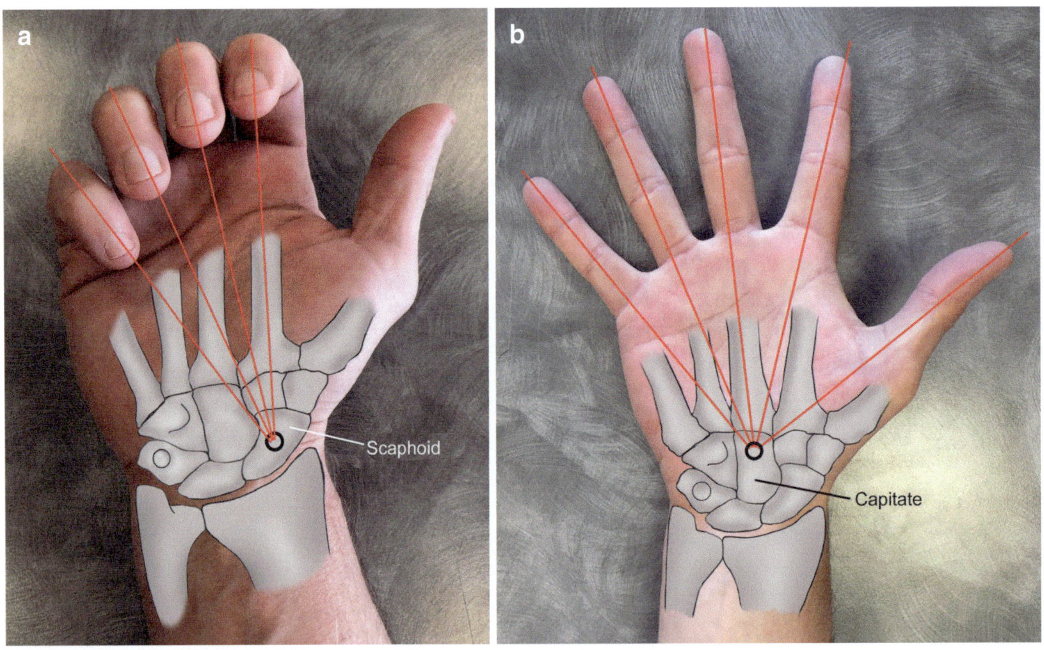

Fig. 1.3 (**a**) When flexing the fingers with the distal interphalangeal joints extended, there is a convergence of the fingers towards the tubercle of the scaphoid. (**b**) When the fingers are spread, the third finger remains fixed, and the finger axis converges towards the capitate.

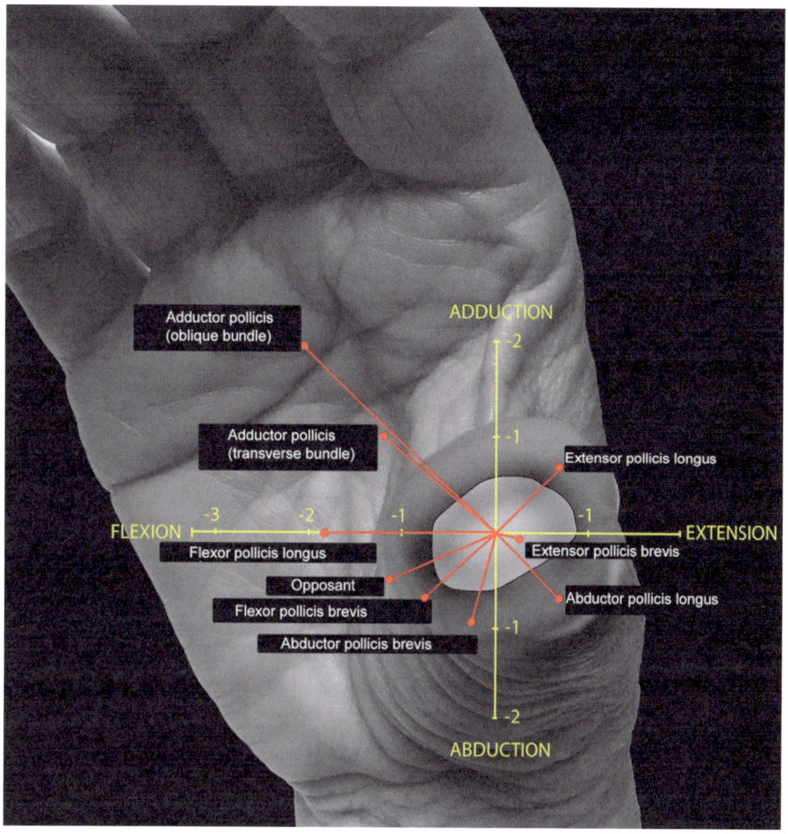

Fig. 1.4 International standard defining the movements of the trapezio-metacarpal joint

nar muscles during the opposition) factors (Fig. 1.5).

Fingers

In the fingers, the opposition between the pulps is allowed by an automatic rotation in supination during the flexion. It is related to the obliquity of the metacarpophalangeal and interphalangeal joints, the length of the ulnar collateral ligaments that are longer than the radial ones, and the predominant action of the ulnar interosseous muscle (Fig. 1.6).

This automatic rotation (and the important anatomical particularities previously described) decreases from the fifth to the second finger, as the segmental movement is more important in the fifth than in the second finger (the automatic supination is in fact being debated for the second finger).

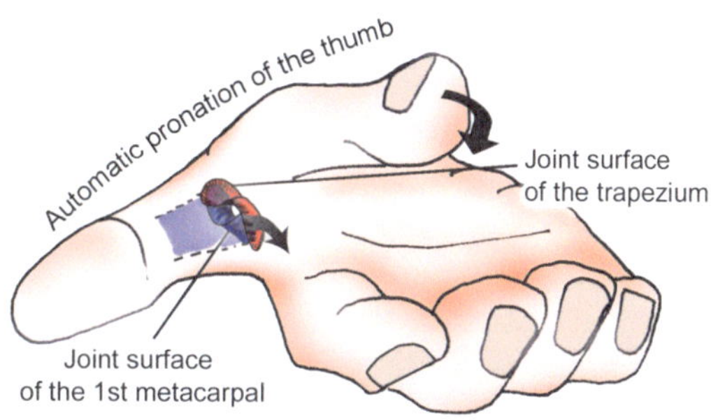

Fig. 1.5 Thanks to its bony (Kapandji's scoliotic horse) and ligamentous conformation, the trapezio-metacarpal joint automatically pronates during the oppositions between the thumb and the fingers, for a contact between the thumb's pulp and the fingers' pulps. The metacarpophalangeal and interphalangeal joints also participate in this automatic rotation phenomenon, but to a lesser extent.

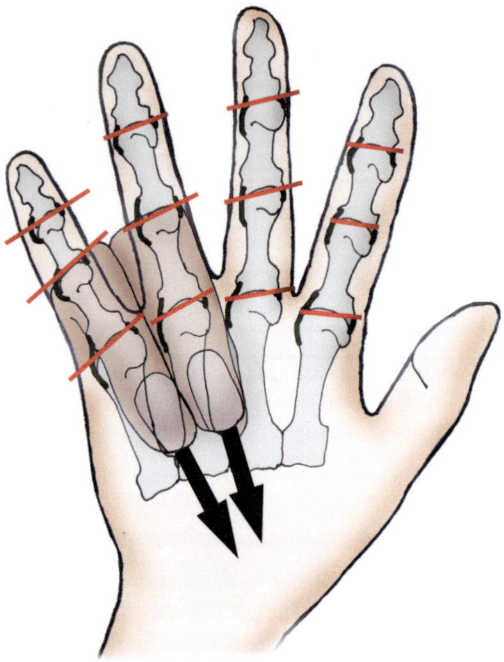

Fig. 1.6 In the fingers, flexion is automatically associated with supination, to promote the opposition between the pulps. For the index finger, some authors describe an automatic pronation.

Capsulo-Ligament Anatomy

Metacarpophalangeal Joints of the Fingers

The metacarpophalangeal joint is a condylar joint with two degrees of freedom, allowing flexion/extension and lateral tilting movements.

Although there is a great deal of variability between subjects, the amplitude of the metacarpophalangeal joints is usually 90° in flexion for the index finger, with increasing amplitude up to the fifth finger. Their passive extension is usually 30° to 40° and they allow varus/valgus movements in extension, where the collateral ligaments are relaxed [3].

Stability is ensured by several anatomical elements (Fig. 1.7):

- The collateral ligaments are divided into three bundles, of which the two posterior bundles are tensioned in full flexion. At 60°, the three bundles are tensioned, but all are relaxed in full extension, allowing varus/valgus movements. The tension of the collateral ligaments

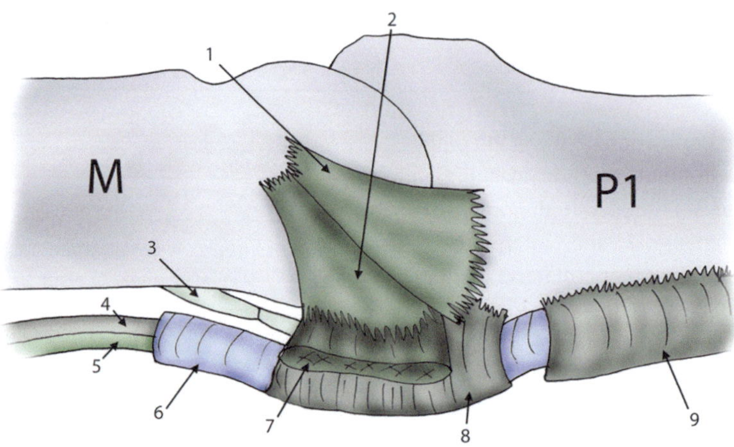

Fig. 1.7 Ligament system of the metacarpophalangeal joints of the fingers. 1—Posterior bundles of the collateral ligament. 2—Anterior bundle of the collateral ligament. 3—Volar plate. 4—Flexor digitorum profundus. 5—Flexor digitorum superficialis. 6—Digital sheath of the flexor tendons. 7—Inter-glenoid (or intermetacarpal) ligament. 8—A1 pulley. 9—A2 pulley

in flexion is linked to their dorsal location in relation to the articular center of the joint, and to the anterior part of the head of the metacarpals, which is wider anteriorly than posteriorly. At 90° of flexion, the most anterior bundles of the collateral ligaments tilt in front of the wider part of the metacarpal head, causing them to relax [4].

- The volar plate is not a fibrocartilage but a connective structure that is both extensible and elastic. It is put under tension when the joint is extended but often allows non-pathological hyper-extension movements. This elasticity and extensibility differentiate it from the volar plate of the proximal interphalangeal joints that are neither extensible nor elastic (Fig. 1.8).
- The intermetacarpal (or inter-glenoid) ligament is stretched between the volar plates of the metacarpophalangeal joints and therefore ensures the stability and cohesion of the transverse metacarpal arch.
- The active stability of the joint is ensured mainly by the interosseous muscles, whose neuromuscular abilities enable them to effectively protect the collateral ligaments in varus/valgus movements (anti-spreading effect of the palmar interosseous muscles and anti-overlapping effect of the dorsal interosseous muscles) and the volar plate in extension movements (anti-extension effect through the back of the interosseous muscles). Their contraction also plays a fundamental role in the rotational stability of the metacarpophalangeal joints.

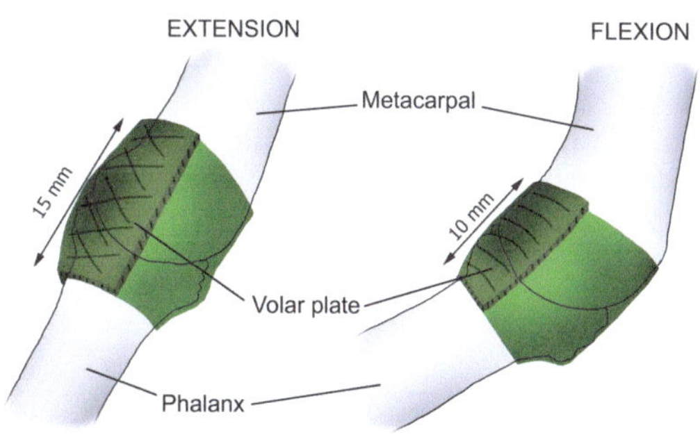

Fig. 1.8 Volar plate of the metacarpophalangeal joint, extensible and elastic

Proximal Interphalangeal Joints

The proximal interphalangeal joint is a trochlear joint with one degree of freedom. The flexion axis is evolutionary: perpendicular in extension, it becomes oblique in flexion to create a supination allowing the opposition between the pulp of the thumb and the pulp of the fingers. This obliquity is more important in the ulnar fingers, as the supination needed for the pulp opposition is more important (Fig. 1.9).

This automatic rotation is anatomically related to the asymmetry of the joint surface and a differential tensioning of the collateral ligaments.

The amplitude of the interphalangeal joints in flexion is approximately 90° (depending on the individual) [5]. This amplitude increases from the second finger to the fifth finger.

There is 0° of extension, even though there may be a tendency to recurvatum in the laxest patients.

The stability of the joint is related to various anatomical elements (Fig. 1.10):

- The collateral ligaments, spreading from the head of the first phalanx to the base of the second phalanx, the volar plate, and the flexor sheath [6]. The main fascicle is tensioned between the head of the first phalanx and the base of the second phalanx. The accessory fascicle is tensioned between the head of the first phalanx to the volar plate and the flexor sheath. Both fascicles are tensioned in extension. In 45° of flexion, the main fascicle stays tensioned but the accessory fascicle is less tensed. Both bundles are relatively relaxed in 90° of flexion [6, 7].
- The volar plate is a very resistant fibrocartilage, anchored between the first and second phalanges on the palmar side by the "check reins" [8–10]. It is tensioned in extension and slides over the anterior surface of the first phalanx in flexion (hinge system) to avoid an early abutment with the anterior surface of the head of the first phalanx (Fig. 1.11). Some authors [8] have described a sliding sequence during the first degrees of flexion, followed by a chronological elevation and rolling of the volar plate during the flexion of the proximal interphalangeal joint [11] (Fig. 1.12).

Fig. 1.9 Obliquity of the interphalangeal joints, for the opposition between the thumb's pulp and the fingers' pulps

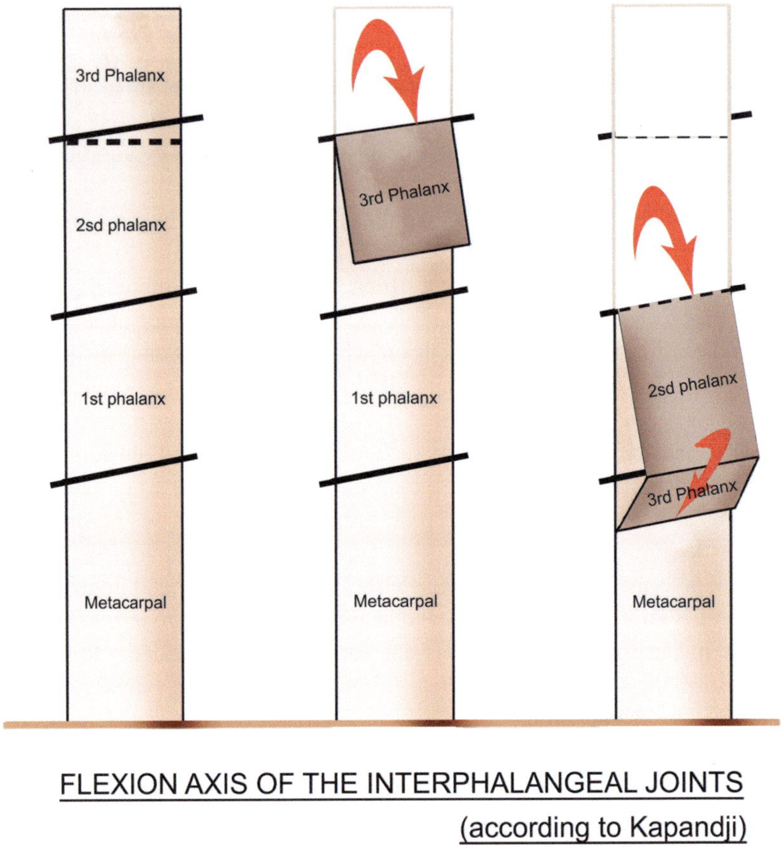

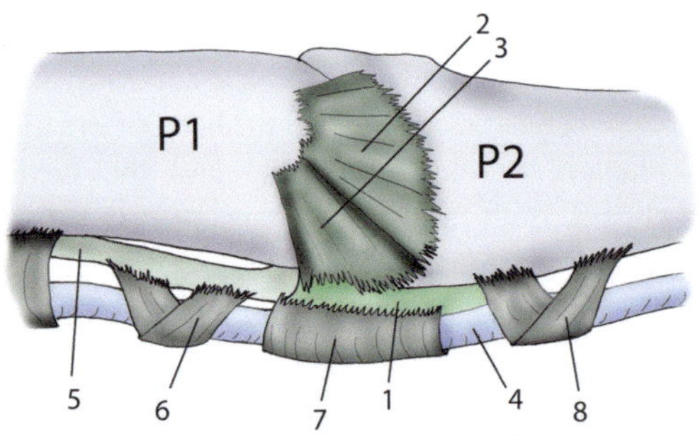

Fig. 1.10 Ligament system of the proximal interphalangeal joints of the fingers. 1—Volar plate. 2—Main bundle of the collateral ligament. 3—Accessory bundle of the collateral ligament. 4—Digital sheath of the flexor tendons. 5—Check-rein ligaments. 6—C1 pulley. 7—A3 pulley. 8—C2 pulley

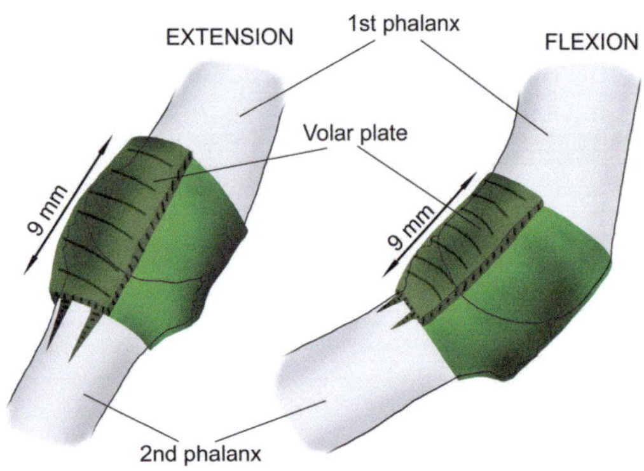

Fig. 1.11 In extension (tension position), the volar plate glides along the first phalanx, flexing the proximal interphalangeal joint to allow a larger range of motion

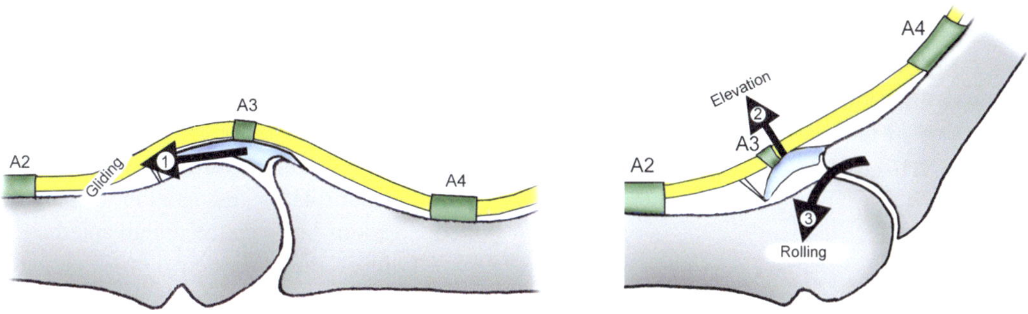

Fig. 1.12 Detailed movement of the volar plate during flexion in three stages: proximal gliding (1), elevation (2), and rolling (3)

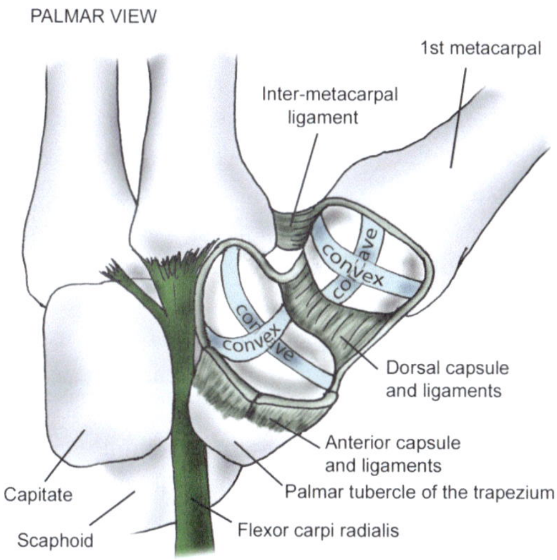

Fig. 1.13 Configuration of inverted double saddle of the trapezio-metacarpal joint

Trapezo-Metacarpal Joint

The trapezo-metacarpal joint is a toroid joint in the shape of the saddle of a scoliotic horse [3] (Fig. 1.13), which allows two degrees of mobility (flexion/extension and abduction/adduction) and an automatic rotation (pronation during flexion/abduction and supination during extension/adduction) allowing the opposition between the pulp of the fingers and the pulp of the thumb (Fig. 1.14).

The stability of the joint is linked to several ligaments [12, 13]:

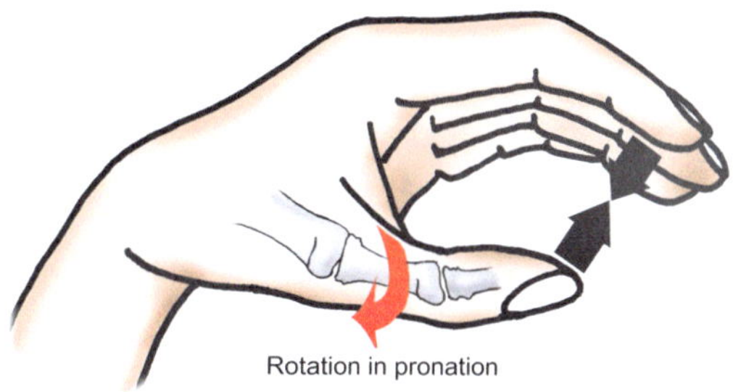

Fig. 1.14 The automatic rotation of the metacarpophalangeal joint of the thumb in pronation during the opposition between the thumb and the fingers is related to ligamentous (ulnar collateral ligament shorter than radial collateral ligament), muscular (external thenar muscles more active), and osseous (external part of the first metacarpal head longer than the internal one) factors.

- The palmar ligaments (anterior oblique ligament or anterior beak ligament and ulnar collateral ligament) that oppose the extension of the joint.
- The dorsal ligaments (dorso-radial ligament, central dorsal ligament, and posterior oblique ligament) that are put under tension at the end of the opposition. The end of the opposition is the position of stability of this joint due to the tensioning of the dorsal ligament system and the engagement of the beak of the first metacarpal in the trapezial recess, which "locks" the position.

The overall active stability of the joint is ensured by the thenar muscles and by the first dorsal interosseous muscle, which is the primary active element in preventing the dorso-radial gliding of the base of the first metacarpal (Fig. 1.15), whereas the opponens pollicis muscle increases this radial gliding during an isometric contraction in the resting position of the joint [14] (Fig. 1.16).

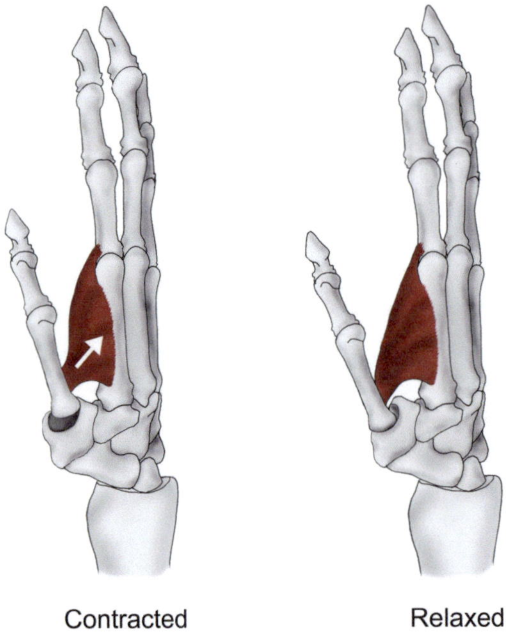

Fig. 1.15 Effect of the contraction of the first dorsal interosseous muscle on the base of the first metacarpal in a closed kinetic chain

Metacarpophalangeal Joint of the Thumb

It is a condyloid joint, which means it has two degrees of freedom (flexion/extension and varus/valgus), to which must be added a third one: the automatic axial rotation, essential in the pulp-to-pulp oppositions between the thumb and the fingers (with the participation of the trapezo-metacarpal joint and the interphalangeal joints).

This automatic rotation in pronation during the flexion is related to the combined action of several anatomical elements:

- Capsulo-ligamentous, because the ulnar collateral ligament (UCL) is shorter than the radial collateral ligament (RCL). During the flexion, the UCL slows the movement of the ulnar part of the first phalanx before the RCL holds the radial part back, which creates an automatic pronation of the phalanx on the metacarpal. The same mechanism occurs in extension, leading to a supination of the metacarpophalangeal joint.
- Muscular, as the external thenar muscles are more active in flexion than the internal thenar muscles and provide a combined movement of flexion-pronation-radial inclination.

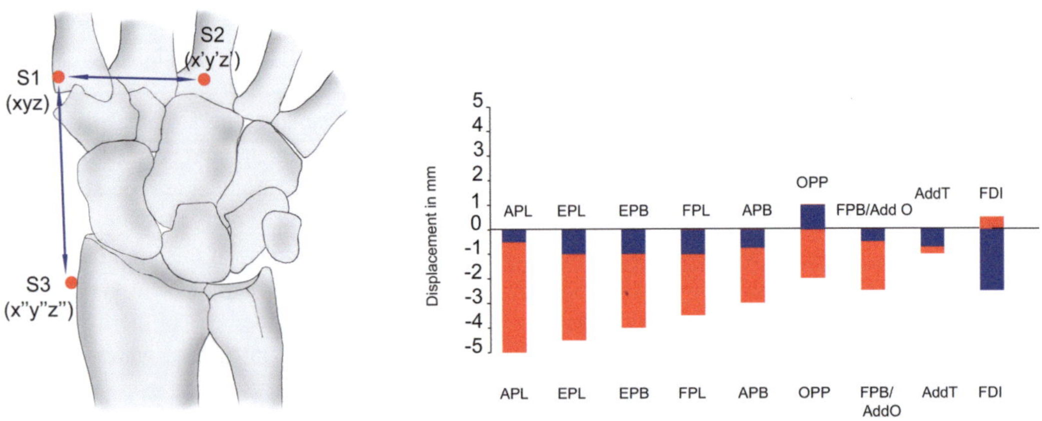

	APL	EPL	EPB	FPL	APB	OPP	FPB/AddO	AddT	FDI
ΔS1-S3 Vertical movement (in mm)	-4,973	-3,217	-3,045	-2,55	-2,543	-1,995	-1,98	-0,414	0,525
ΔS1-S2 Radio-ulnar migration (in mm)	-0,549	-1,164	-0,953	-1,056	-0,779	1,148	-0,591	-0,856	-2,096

Fig. 1.16 Effects of the isometric contraction of the thumb muscles on the stability of the trapezio-metacarpal joint. 1—The first dorsal interosseous muscle creates an ulnar recentering and decoaptation. 2—The opponens pollicis creates a radial displacement and compression. 3—The other muscles create an ulnar recentering and compression

It allows 60–70° of active flexion and up to 80° of passive flexion. The passive extension can be up to 10° in the laxest individuals.

Its position as an intermediate joint in the thumb column gives it the main role of ensuring the stability of the pollici-digital and cylindrical full palm grips.

The passive stability of the joint is mainly ensured by the collateral ligaments and the longitudinal ligaments (Fig. 1.17).

The collateral ligaments are made of two fascicles:

- The main fascicle goes from the head of the first metacarpal to the base of the first phalanx, slightly dorsal to the joint axis in flexion/extension. In flexion, it is tensioned, ensuring the lateral stability.
- The accessory fascicle is oblique at the palmar and distal level, it goes from the head of the first metacarpal to the corresponding sesamoid, thus creating a common structure with the longitudinal ligaments. It is tensed in extension, ensuring the lateral stability in this position.

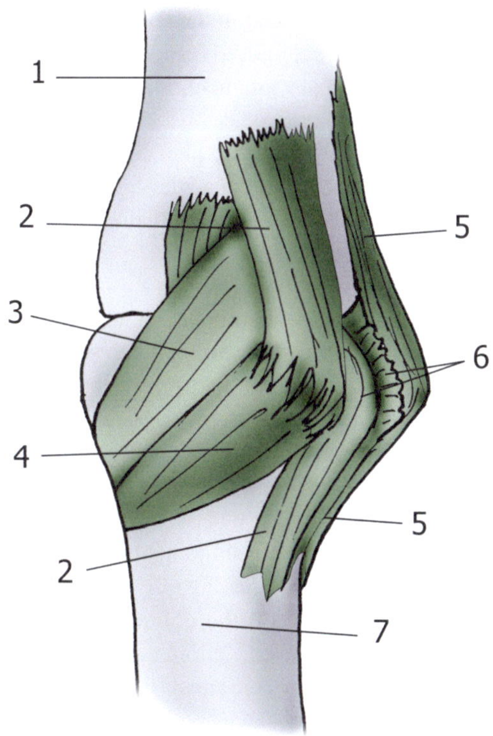

Fig. 1.17 Ligament system of the metacarpophalangeal joint of the thumb (radial view). 1—First phalanx. 2—Radial longitudinal ligament. 3—Main bundle of the collateral ligament. 4—Accessory bundle of the collateral ligament. 5—Ulnar longitudinal ligament. 6—Sesamoid bones. 7—First metacarpal

The ulnar and radial longitudinal volar ligaments are very resistant and contain the two sesamoid bones. They go from the anterior part of the first metacarpal to the anterior part of the first phalanx and oppose the metacarpophalangeal extension.

When the joint is in extension, the longitudinal volar ligaments and the accessory fascicle of the collateral ligaments are tensioned, but the main fascicle of the collateral ligaments is relaxed. Therefore, the most unstable joint position is the flexion, as the collateral ligaments and the longitudinal palmar ligaments are relaxed.

The active joint stability is ensured by the internal (adductor pollicis, inconstant first palmar interosseous) and external (abductor brevis and flexor brevis) sesamoid muscles (Fig. 1.18).

The combined movement of flexion-radial inclination-pronation made by the external and internal thenar muscles allows optimizing the cylindrical grips with a full palm, increasing the contact surface.

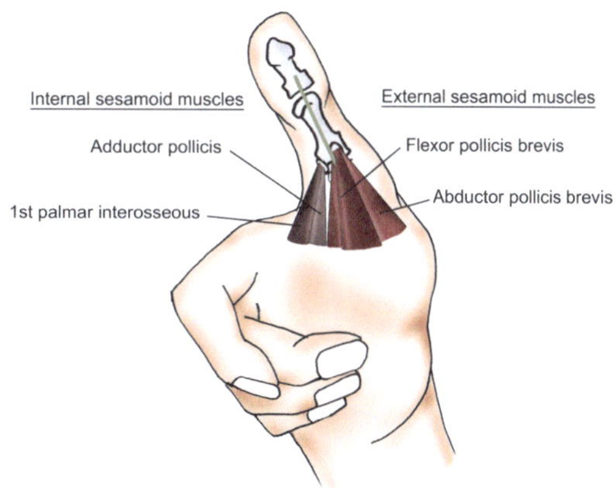

Fig. 1.18 Active stability of the metacarpophalangeal joint of the thumb, depending mainly on the internal and external sesamoid muscles

The opponens pollicis, which ends on the palmar side of the first metacarpal, does not play a role in the stability of the metacarpophalangeal joint, and the extrinsic muscles only have a moderate action.

Aponeurosis and Fascia Anatomy

Medium Palmar Aponeurosis (Fig. 1.19)

It spreads between the thenar and hypothenar aponeuroses, following the palmaris longus.

It is divided into four pre-tendinous strips that change direction at the level of the distal palmar crease to form various fibrous planes:

- Superficial, attaching to the dermis between the distal palmar crease and the proximal digital flexion crease (the crease of the metacarpophalangeal flexion).
- Medium that extends along each of the sides of the metacarpophalangeal joints to participate in the formation of the digital aponeurosis of the corresponding finger.
- Deep, attaching to the palmar side of the metacarpophalangeal joint and more distally on the flexors sheath (at the level of the C1 pulley).

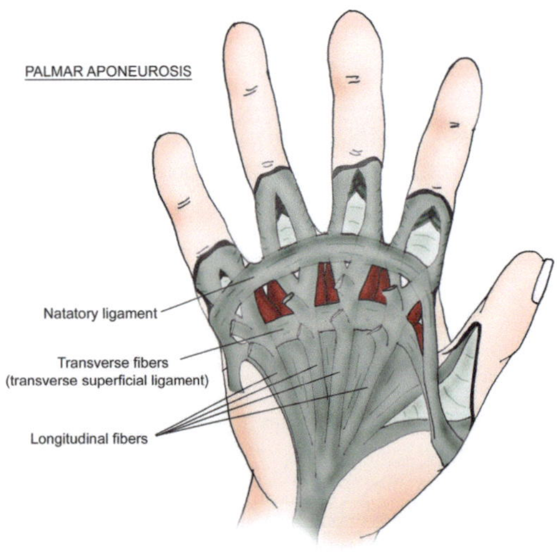

Fig. 1.19 Medium palmar aponeurosis

There are also some vertical partitions at the level of the proximal palmar crease, the partitions of Legueu and Juvara, connecting the medium and deep palmar aponeurosis.

These partitions delimit seven areas that contain alternatively the flexor system and the neurovascular pedicles with the corresponding lumbrical (Fig. 1.20).

Digital Aponeurosis

The medium plane of the pre-tendinous strips forms two bundles laterally prolonging towards the corresponding finger to form the sagittal strips of the finger.

These sagittal strips receive expansions from the natatory ligament to form the digital blade that protects the digital neurovascular system and fixes the cutaneous coating (Fig. 1.21).

This blade emits fibers at the level of the proximal interphalangeal joint to form the retrovascular strip, the Cleland ligament, and the Grayson ligament.

At the level of the second phalanx, its anterior fibers form the oblique retinacular ligament.

We should, however, individualize some of the elements of this aponeurosis:

- The oblique retinacular ligament, anchored on the flexors sheath next to the diaphysis of the first phalanx. It passes in front of the flexion axis of the proximal interphalangeal joint and joins the extensor system at the level of the distal interphalangeal joint. This ligament allows the coordination between the distal and proximal interphalangeal joints in flexion and extension. During the flexion of the distal interphalangeal joint, the oblique retinacular ligament gets tensed, automatically causing the flexion of the proximal interphalangeal joint. During the extension of the proximal interphalangeal joint, the oblique retinacular ligament gets tensed, automatically causing the extension of the distal interphalangeal joint [15, 16] (Fig. 1.22).
- The transverse retinacular ligament: its proximal half is anchored on the A3 pulley and its

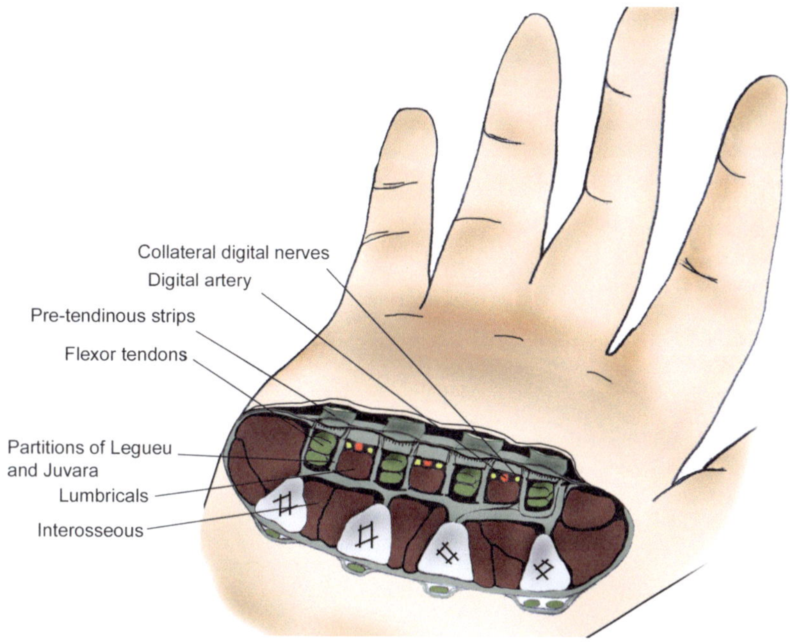

Fig. 1.20 Partitions of Legueu and Juvara

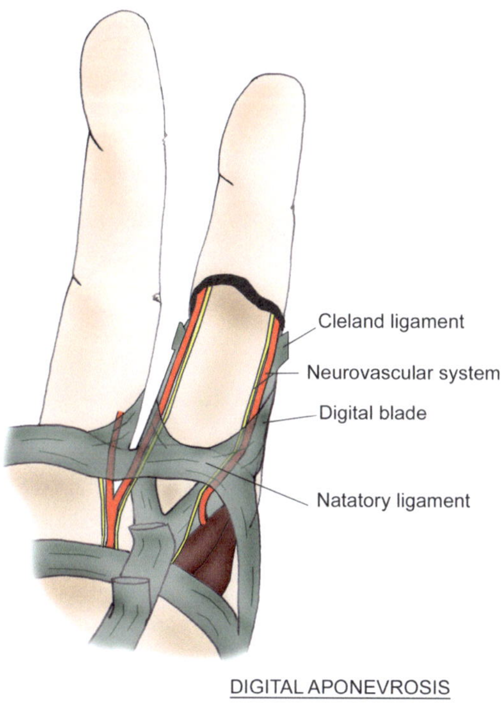

Fig. 1.21 Digital blade

distal half on the volar plate and the capsule of the proximal interphalangeal joint. It goes vertically towards the corresponding lateral strip of the extensor system. It favors the palmar movement of the lateral strips during the flexion of the proximal interphalangeal joint (Fig. 1.23). With the oblique retinacular ligament, it forms the lateral retinacular ligament.

- The dorsal retinacular ligament: composed of the median strip and the arch-shaped fibers, it is tensioned between the two strips of the extensor system. It favors the dorsal movement of the lateral strips during the extension of the proximal interphalangeal joint and limits their palmar gliding during flexion (Fig. 1.24).
- The Cleland ligament: laterally tensed between the osseous skeleton and the dermis, it creates a frontal partition behind the neurovascular pedicle. In addition to its role of protecting the neurovascular pedicle, it fixes the

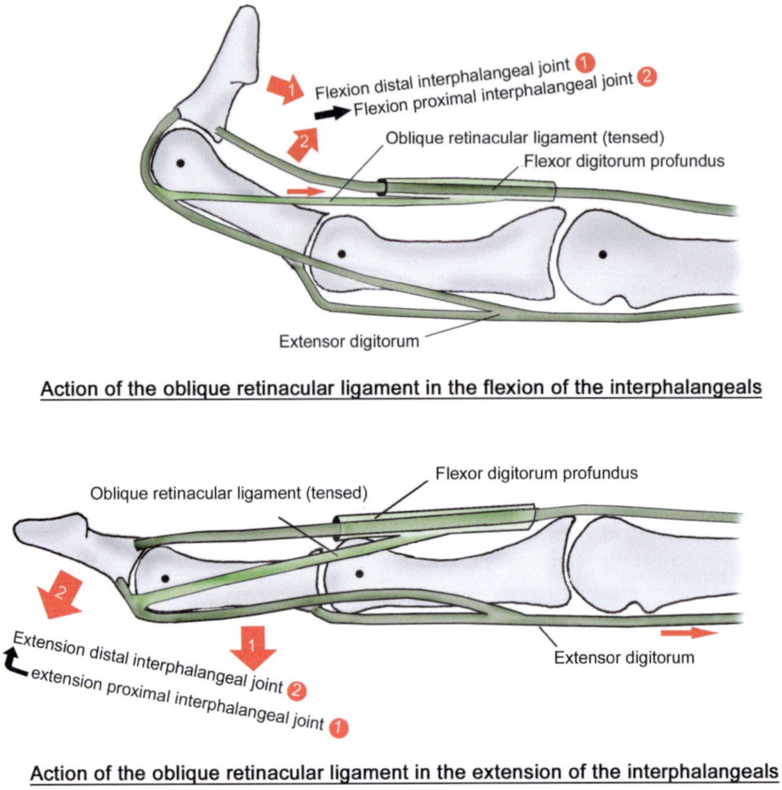

Fig. 1.22 The oblique retinacular ligament favors the functional coordination between the distal and proximal interphalangeal joints. The extension of the proximal interphalangeal joint puts it in tension, which leads to the extension of the distal interphalangeal joint. Meanwhile, the flexion of the distal interphalangeal joint is only possible if the proximal interphalangeal joint is flexed (relaxation of the oblique retinacular ligament)

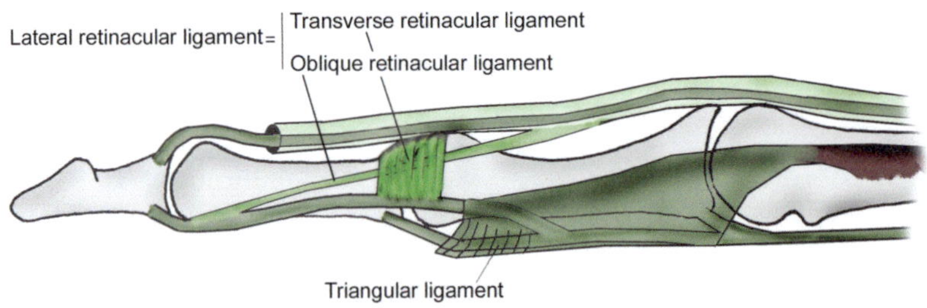

Fig. 1.23 The transverse retinacular ligament participates in the stabilization of the lateral strips of the extensor system, opposing their dorsalization

dermis to the fibrous skeleton. Some authors don't differentiate it from the retrovascular strip [17].

- The retrovascular strip: from the digital blade at the level of the proximal interphalangeal joint, it partitions the neurovascular pedicle from the back.
- The Grayson ligament: from the digital blade at the level of the proximal interphalangeal joint, it partitions the neurovascular pedicle from the front (Fig. 1.25).
- The longitudinal fibers: next to the flexion creases of the fingers (between the fat pads), they fix the dermis to the fibrous skeleton, allowing an efficient grip.
- The aponeurotic system of the first finger (Fig. 1.26).

Although the digital structures of the thumb are comparable to those of the fingers, there are some differences.

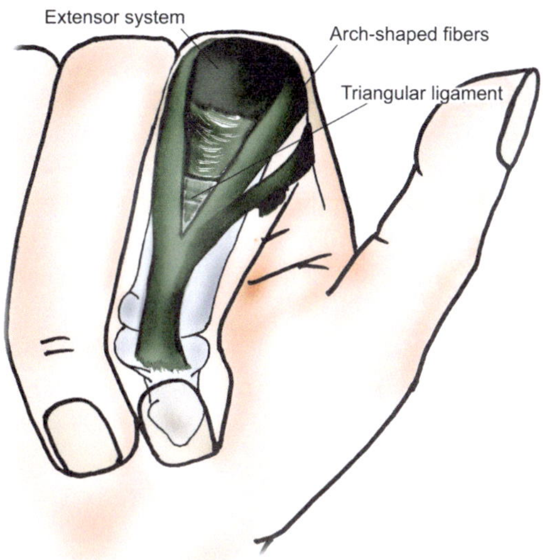

Fig. 1.24 The dorsal retinacular ligament (triangular ligament + arch-shaped fibers) opposes the ventralization of the lateral strips

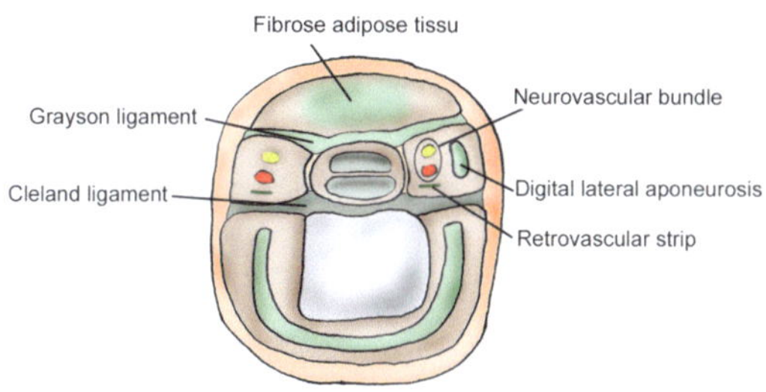

Fig. 1.25 Retinacular partitioning of the neurovascular pedicles

The most radial fibers of the palmar aponeurosis run towards the thumb to divide into two planes (instead of three for the fingers), one superficial on the dermis and the other deeper on the sheath of the flexor pollicis longus.

The natatory ligament extends radially to form the distal commissural ligament, which attaches to either side of the flexor pollicis longus sheath.

The superficial transverse ligament extends radially to form the proximal commissural ligament which ends on the sheath of the flexor pollicis longus, forming with the termination of the distal commissural ligament a major fibrous knot at the base of the thumb.

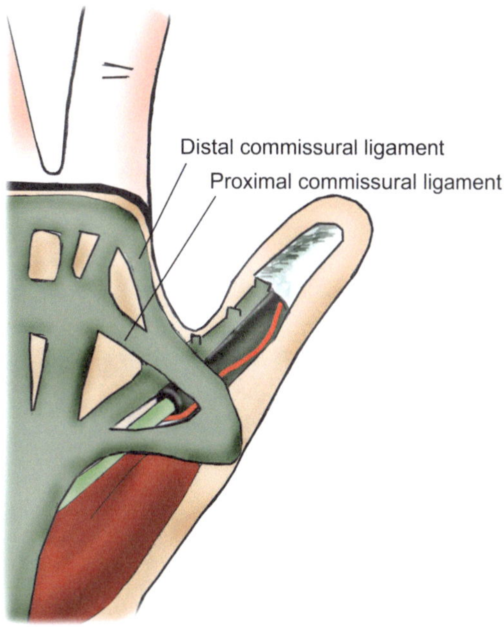

Fig. 1.26 Aponeurosis system of the first finger (according to M. Merle)

Anatomy and Physiology of Extensor Tendons

The extensor system is composed of an extrinsic system and an intrinsic system that work in synergy during the digital extension.

It is extra-synovial, except at the level of the extensor retinaculum where it is surrounded by a synovial sheath allowing its lubrication and nutrition [18] (Fig. 1.27).

In the hand and the forearm, the tendons are flat, composed of longitudinal fibers and located directly under the skin. In the fingers, the extensor system looks more like aponeuroses than like tendons.

Topographic Anatomy

The International Federation of Societies for Surgery of the Hand made a classification allowing us to study their physiology depending on their topography (Fig. 1.28).

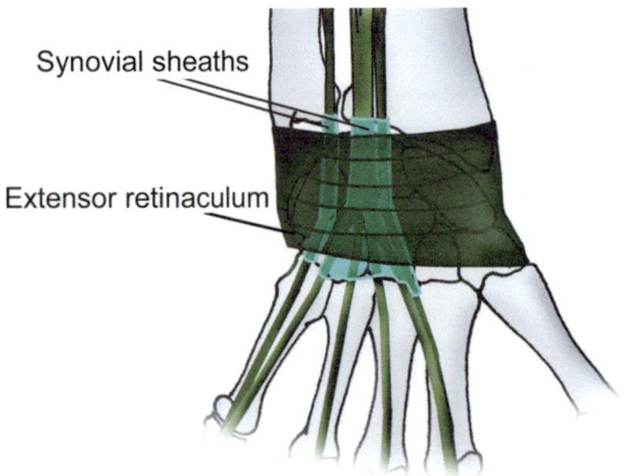

Fig. 1.27 The extensor digitorum and the extensor indicis pass through the fourth synovial sheath of the extensor system. The extensor has its own sheath in the ulnar side (fifth synovial sheath)

Fingers

➔ Zone 1

It is the area where the lateral strips end; they come together and insert on the base of the dorsal side of the third phalanx. The tendon is not vascularized much at this level.

The injuries lead to a mallet finger, characterized by a drop in flexion of the distal phalanx (Fig. 1.29).

These deformities can evolve into a swan-neck deformity, especially when the volar plate of the proximal interphalangeal joint is slack [19] (Fig. 1.30).

➔ Zone 2

In this zone we find the lateral strips, next to the diaphysis of the second phalanx. The deformity is the same as in zone 1, but there can be an associated injury of the oblique retinacular ligament, leading to a faster swan-neck deformity, especially if the volar plate of the proximal interphalangeal joint is slack.

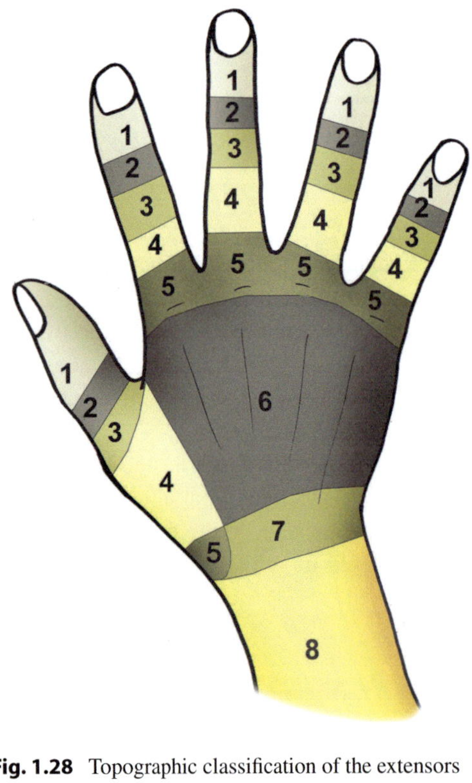

Fig. 1.28 Topographic classification of the extensors

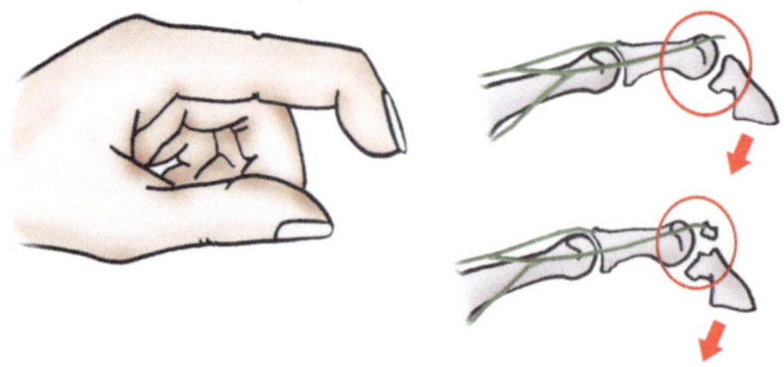

Fig. 1.29 Mallet finger

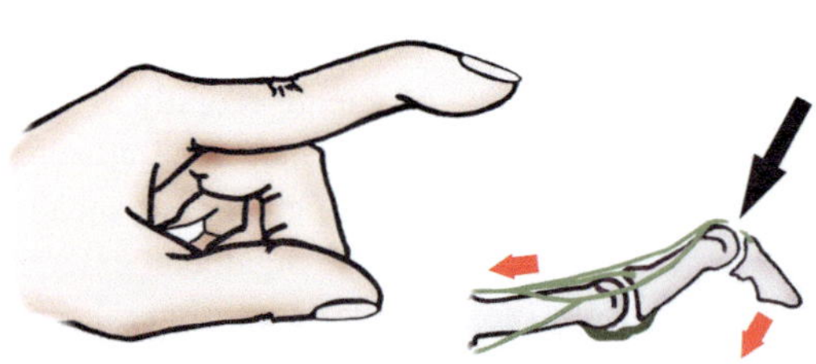

Fig. 1.30 Swan-neck deformity after a mallet finger badly treated. The tension normally applied on the second and third phalanges is now only applied on the second phalanx. In case of slackness of the proximal interphalangeal joint, this excess of tension leads to a joint in hyper-extension

➔ Zone 3

Next to the proximal interphalangeal joint, it is the area of trifurcation of the extensor system, forming the two lateral strips and the median strip ending on the base of the second phalanx.

An isolated injury of the median strip leads to a boutonnière deformity (Fig. 1.31). The lateral strips go to palmar, putting the proximal interphalangeal joint in flexion and the distal interphalangeal joint in extension.

➔ Zone 4

It is the zone next to the diaphysis of the first phalanx, at the level of the dorsal expansion of the interossei.

➔ Zone 5

It is the zone next to the metacarpophalangeal joint. At this level, the extensor tendons are stabilized on the metacarpals by the sagittal strips that insert on both sides of the tendon, on the interglenoidal ligaments (Fig. 1.32).

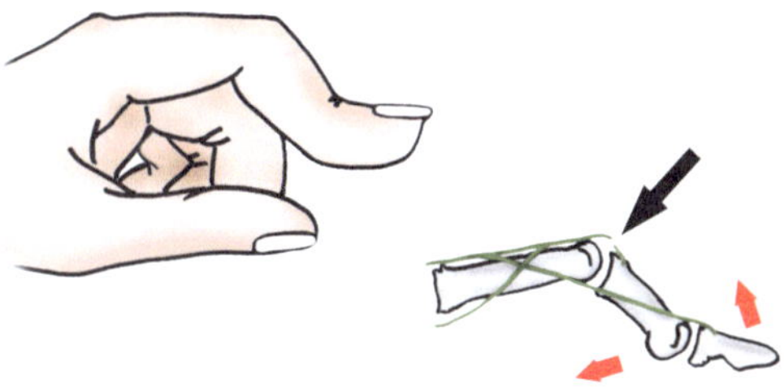

Fig. 1.31 Boutonnière deformity

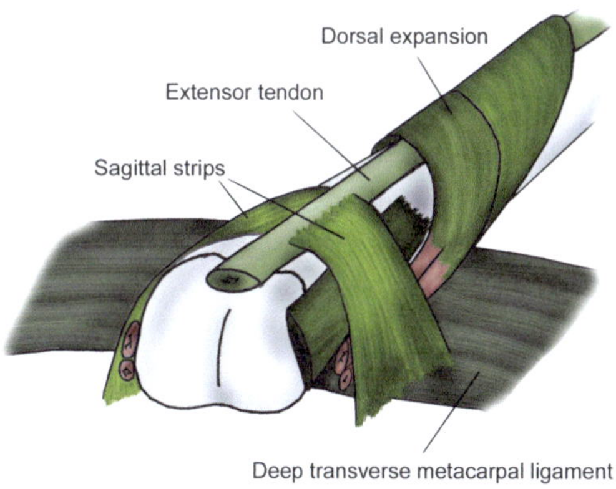

Fig. 1.32 At the level of the metacarpophalangeal joints, the sagittal strips stabilize the extensor tendons in the frontal plane

These stabilizing elements are tensed when the metacarpophalangeal is flexed and relaxed when it is extended.

An injury in the radial sagittal strip leads to a dislocation of the extensor tendon in the ulnar intermetacarpal area, as the extensor system is decentered relative to the axis of the metacarpophalangeal joints. Therefore, the injuries of the ulnar sagittal strip do not lead to a dislocation of the extensor tendon in the radial intermetacarpal area (Fig. 1.33).

➔ Zone 6

The extensor tendons pass along the dorsal side of the metacarpals. At this level, there are some inter-tendinous junctions that connect the extensor tendons.

If there is an injury above the inter-tendinous junctions, the extension deficit will be small, because it is partly compensated by the adjacent tendons (Fig. 1.34).

➔ Zone 7

The tendons slide in the synovial sheath next to the extensor retinaculum. Unlike the extensor indicis, the extensor digiti minimi has its own sheath.

➔ Zone 8

It is the zone above the extensor retinaculum, until the myotendinous junction.

Thumb

The extensor system of the thumb also depends on an extrinsic system made by the extensor pollicis brevis and the extensor pollicis longus, and an intrinsic system made by the sesamoid muscles. The abductor pollicis brevis and the flexor pollicis brevis form the radial part of the dorsal expansion, and the adductor pollicis forms the ulnar part.

The extensor tendons of the thumb pass through six zones, four of which are specific to the thumb and are preceded by the letter T (thumb): TI, TII, TIII, TIV. Two zones are shared with the extensors of the fingers: zones VII (wrist) and VIII (forearm).

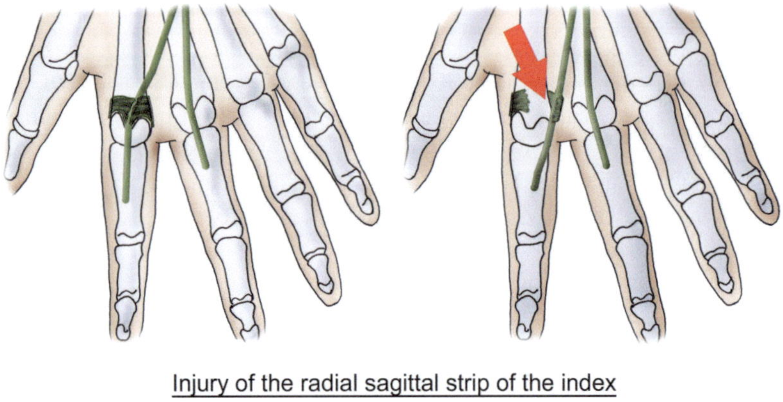

Fig. 1.33 The sagittal strips avoid the dislocation of the extensor tendons in the ulnar inter-metacarpal area

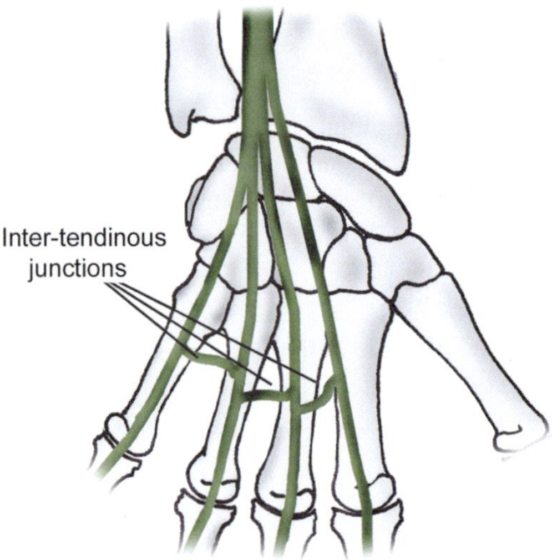

Fig. 1.34 Inter-tendinous junctions in the back of the hand

Physiology

Nutrition of the Extensor Tendons

As in flexor tendons, the nutrition of the extensor tendons depends on an intrinsic system and an extrinsic system. Unlike the flexor tendons, the extrinsic system is the main actor during tendon healing.

The extensor system is, in fact, mostly extra-synovial, which limits the synovial imbibition role it has at the level of the extensor retinaculum (intrinsic healing by a "synovial pump" effect) and favors vascular healing "storms" with fibroblast invasion (extrinsic healing).

This type of healing leads to important adherences.

Biomechanics

The finger extension depends on two synergic systems (Fig. 1.35):

➔ Extrinsic System

This system is made of the extensor digitorum, the extensor indicis, and the extensor digiti minimi.

Its isolated contraction brings the metacarpophalangeal joint in extension but does not lead to an extension of the interphalangeal joints. The extensor digitorum exhausts its action on its proximal insertions, leading to a "claw" deformity.

➔ Intrinsic System

It is composed of the interossei and the lumbrical muscles that join the extrinsic system at the level of the dorsal expansion of the interossei to form a complex group that ensures the harmony of the digital extension.

The interossei have various endings along the digital chain, which allows them to have various actions, depending on the situation:

- On a deep plane, the endings on the lateral tubercles of the first phalanx allow them to separate the fingers and bring them closer to each other and to participate in the lateral stability of the metacarpophalangeal joint.

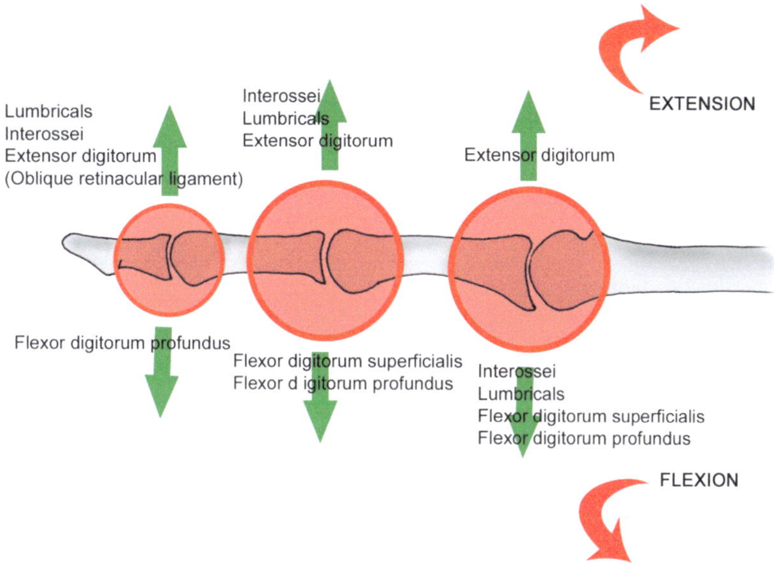

Fig. 1.35 Motor muscles for the extension and flexion of the fingers. The importance of each muscle decreases from top to bottom

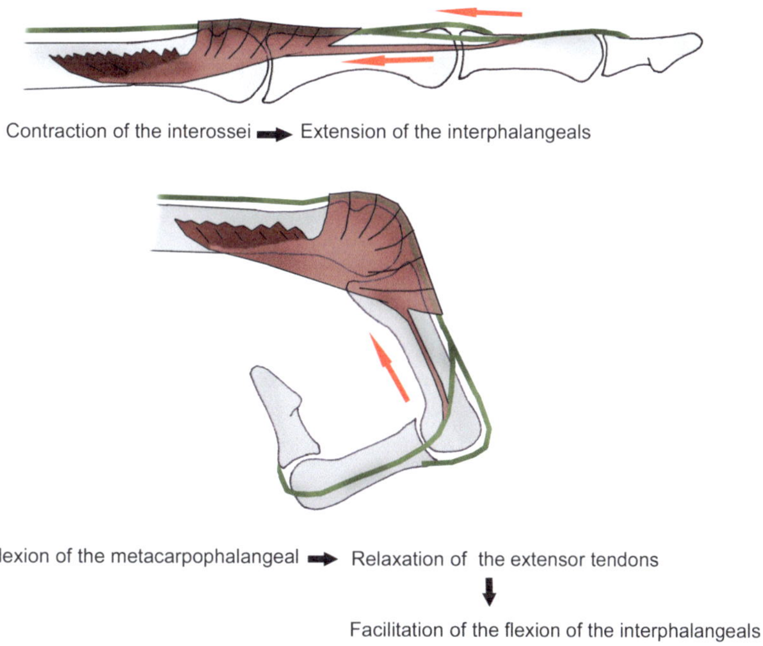

Fig. 1.36 Relaxation of the extensor system at the digital level in flexion of the metacarpophalangeal joint

- On a superficial plane, they form the dorsal expansion of the interossei next to the metacarpophalangeal joint and give off more distal fibers that reinforce the median strip of the extensor tendon, and others associated to the corresponding lumbrical to join the lateral strips. If the metacarpophalangeal joint is extended, the contraction of the interossei brings the interphalangeal joints in extension. If the metacarpophalangeal is flexed, it favors the interphalangeal flexion by relaxing the extensor system (Fig. 1.36).

The lumbrical muscles insert on the flexor digitorum profundus at the level of the palm, pass in front of the inter-glenoidal ligament on the radial side, and end on the corresponding lateral strip. They play a proprioceptive role, dividing

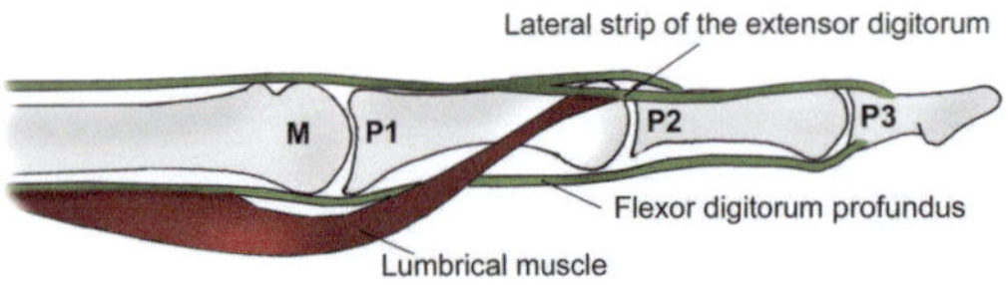

Fig. 1.37 The lumbrical muscles distribute the tension between the flexor and extensor systems

the tension between the two systems, which explains the incredible number of mechanoreceptors they contain (Fig. 1.37).

They also have an extension action in the distal phalanx, regardless of the position of the metacarpophalangeal joint.

Extension Dynamic and Tendon Race

The extension of the fingers starts with the metacarpophalangeal joint, through the action of the extensor digitorum.

The contraction of the lumbrical muscles opposes the tension of the flexor digitorum profundus and therefore the formation of a "claw."

The contraction of the interossei also participates, through the dorsal expansion, in this fight against the "claw." Combined with the contraction of the extensor digitorum, it brings the proximal interphalangeal joint in extension. The extension of the distal interphalangeal joint happens, thanks to the tension in the oblique retinacular ligament and the action of the lateral strips.

The tendinous race of the extensor system during the complete extension of the fingers is around 35 mm in the wrist, 10 to 15 mm in the metacarpophalangeal joints, 2 to 3 mm in the proximal interphalangeal joint, and lower than 1 mm in the distal interphalangeal joint [20].

Anatomy and Physiology of Flexor Tendons

The flexor tendons are part of the extrinsic system (from the forearm) and are responsible for the flexion of the proximal interphalangeal joint for the flexor digitorum superficialis and the distal interphalangeal joint for the flexor digitorum profundus.

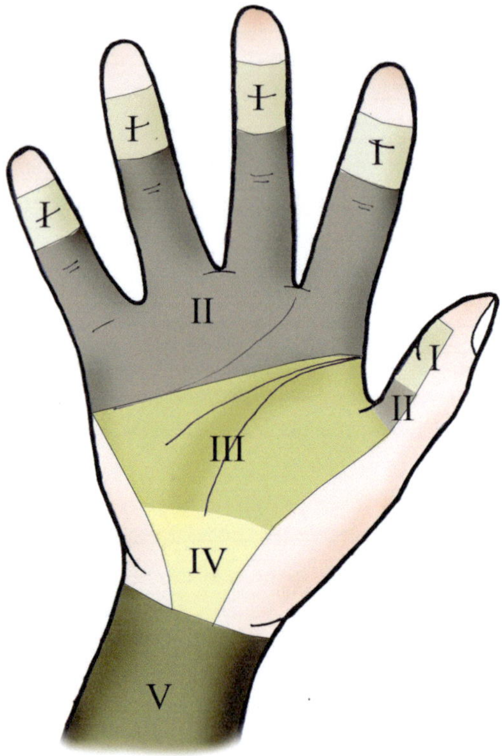

Fig. 1.38 Topographic classification of the flexor tendons according to Verdan and Michon

Their helix structure gives them an important resistance to the constraints imposed on them.

Topographic Anatomy

The Verdan and Michon classification allows us to approach their physiology according to five topographic zones (Fig. 1.38):

Fingers

➔ **Zone 1**

Located below the distal insertion of the flexor digitorum superficialis, it is the area of the distal insertion of the flexor digitorum profundus. It is one of the areas where the tendon is poorly vascularized, which makes its healing longer and random in the case of injury.

➔ Zone 2

It starts at the entrance of the digital sheath and ends at the medium part of the second phalanx (lower than the two tendon strips of the flexor digitorum superficialis).

This zone is used to be called the "no man's land" by Bunnell, because it seemed impossible to repair the injuries that occurred there. The injuries in that zone are still the most complex to treat.

The two flexors share the digital canal, made up of the periosteum and the palmar ligaments of the metacarpophalangeal and proximal interphalangeal joint from behind, and the annular ligaments and cruciate pulleys in the front (Fig. 1.39).

The aim of these pulleys and annular ligaments is to maintain the flexors against the bone levers, thus permitting the complete finger winding and avoiding the "bowstring" effect.

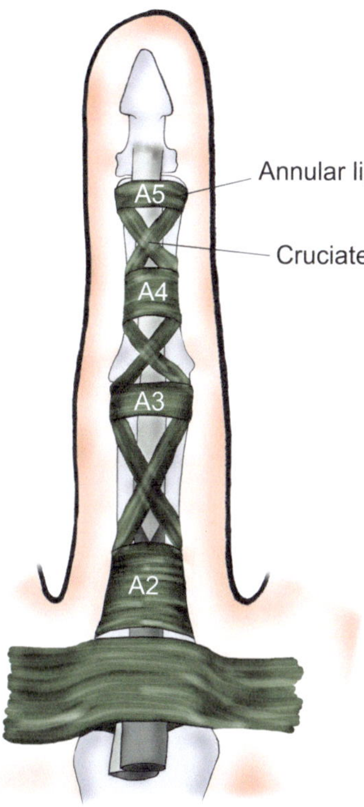

Fig. 1.39 Location of the annular ligaments and cruciate pulleys

Lastly, the flexor digitorum superficialis splits into two strips near the base of the first phalanx to let the flexor digitorum profundus pass. Below this chiasma, the flexor digitorum profundus becomes superficial and the flexor digitorum superficialis becomes deep [3] (Fig. 1.40).

➔ Zone 3

Located between the distal part of the flexor retinaculum (or transverse carpal ligament) and the entrance of the digital sheath.

➔ Zone 4

It corresponds to the carpal tunnel where the flexor retinaculum acts as the first pulley for the flexor system.

➔ Zone 5

Located between the musculotendinous junction proximally (inferior third of the forearm) and the proximal part of the flexor retinaculum.

Thumb

The only extrinsic muscle that makes the flexion of the thumb is the flexor pollicis longus.

The T1 zone corresponds to the ending of the flexor pollicis longus, and the T2 zone is between the A1 pulley and the proximal part of the A2 pulley. The T3 zone is located at the level of the thenar eminence (possible area of adherences with the two heads of the flexor pollicis brevis) (Fig. 1.41). Zones 4 and 5 are the same than for the fingers.

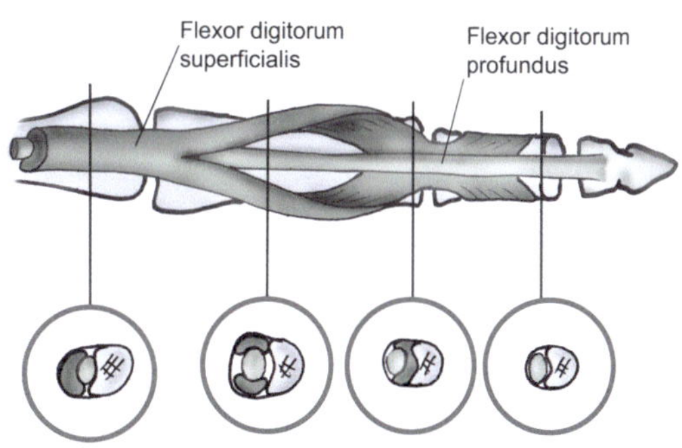

Fig. 1.40 Flexor digitorum superficialis' chiasma (area of frequent adherences)—according to Kapandji

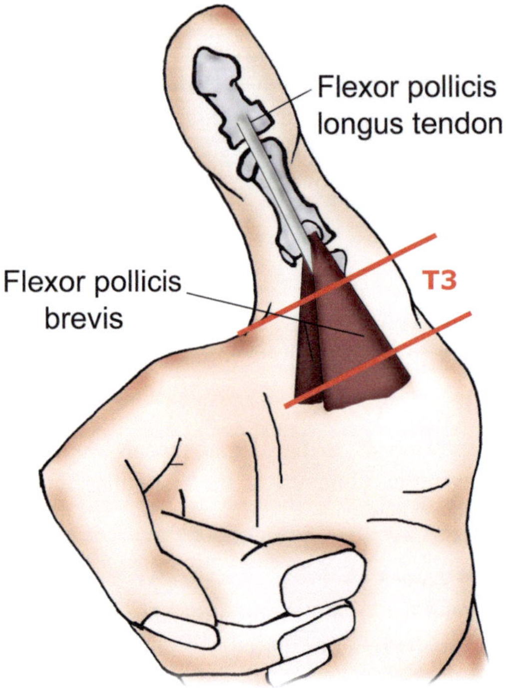

Fig. 1.41 Trajectory of the flexor pollicis longus between the two heads of the flexor pollicis brevis

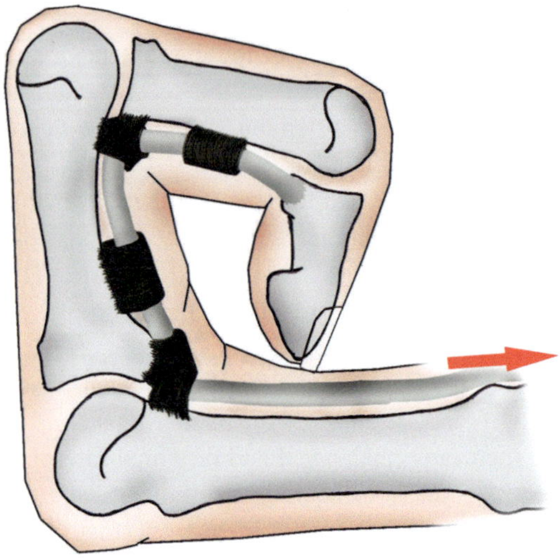

Fig. 1.42 The pulleys keep the flexor tendons against the skeleton to avoid the "bowstring" effect

Pulleys

They are fibrous bands maintaining the flexor system in contact with the skeleton and therefore avoiding the "bowstring" effect [21, 22] (Fig. 1.42).

There are five annular ligaments and three cruciate pulleys at the digital level, to which must be added the flexor retinaculum at the level of the carpal tunnel (Fig. 1.43).

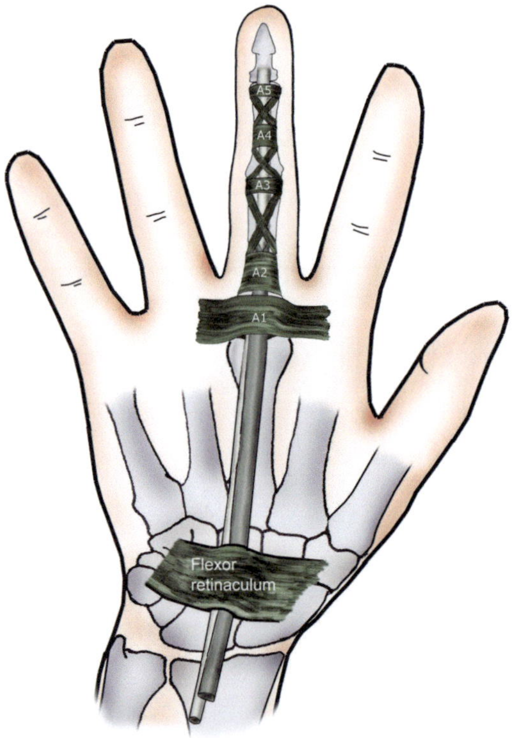

Fig. 1.43 The flexor retinaculum participates in the action of the digital pulleys

Nutrition

It depends on two complementary systems:

The Vascular System

Outside the digital sheath: the flexor tendons are vascularized from their two endings (periosteum and musculotendinous junction) and by the intratendinous vascular system for the areas far from the extremities of the tendon.

The paratendon, surrounding the tendon, sends a structure to carry the vessels (the mesotendon) which enters the tendon, allowing its vascularization.

Inside the digital sheath, the mesotendon condenses to form vincula, supplied by anastomoses with the collateral arteries.

The two flexors each have two vincula, a short one near their ending and a long one higher, which infuse their dorsal part.

There still are three areas that are badly vascularized, in front of the A2 and A4 pulleys. The first one is proximal to the flexor digitorum superficialis' chiasma, and the two others are above and below the vinculum longus that approaches the flexor digitorum profundus at the level of the proximal interphalangeal joint (Fig. 1.44).

The Synovial Pump

The synovial sheaths have different organizations, depending on the finger (Fig. 1.45). The flexor pollicis longus has its own sheath, from zone 4 to the T1 zone.

The index, middle, and ring fingers share a sheath with the little finger in zone 4. They each have their individual sheath in the digital canal. The little finger's sheath, shared with the other fingers, continues until the digital canal.

The synovial fluid in the sheaths plays an important role of lubrication and nutrition, by soaking the tendons in the digital canal [24].

It is important to note that, in the digital canal, the nutrition of the flexor digitorum superficialis is twice as important through this method as through the vascular system, and five times more important for the flexor digitorum profundus.

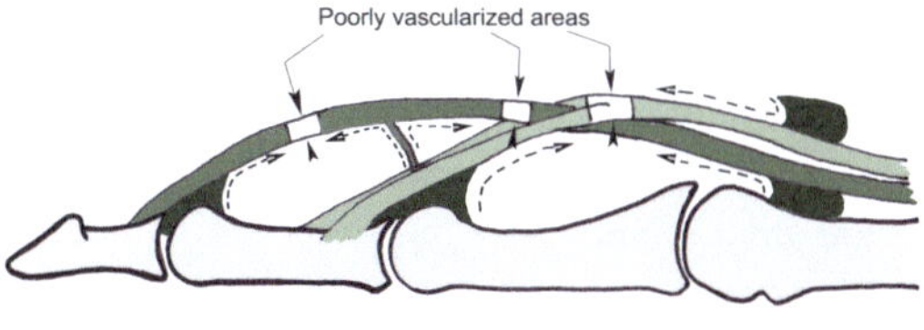

Fig. 1.44 Vincula system, participating in the vascularization of the flexor system but leaving some avascular areas

Thanks to these two systems, we obtain the healing of the tendon by extrinsic healing (vascular mechanism) and intrinsic healing (synovial pump).

The extrinsic healing corresponds to a fibroblastic invasion, which causes adherences. On the other hand, the intrinsic healing is related to a phenomenon of synovial imbibition that does not create adherences.

A surgery as atraumatic as possible and an immediate active rehabilitation favor the intrinsic healing, providing a better functional recovery.

The Quadriga Effect

Blocking the flexor digitorum profundus of a finger by forcibly extending the distal interphalangeal joint with the wrist in extension prevents the flexion of the distal interphalangeal joint of the other fingers but allows the flexion of the proximal interphalangeal joint (Fig. 1.46).

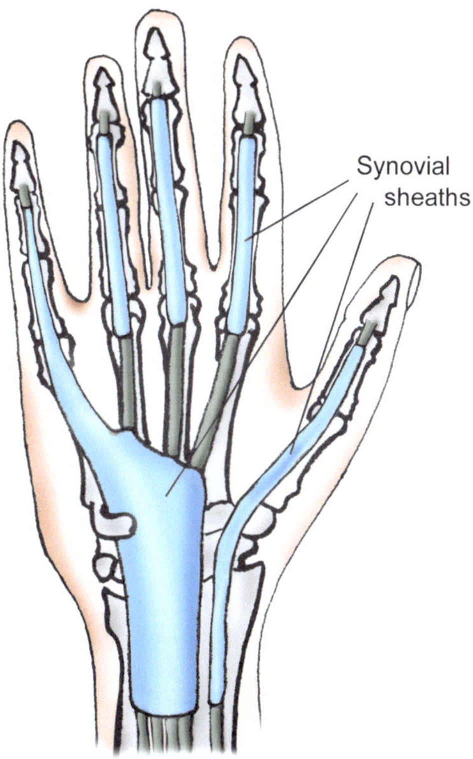

Fig. 1.45 Usual topography of the synovial sheaths

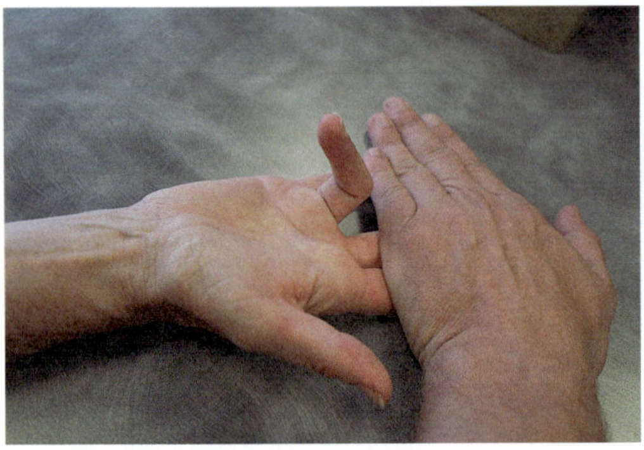

Fig. 1.46 The quadriga effect; it is impossible to flex the distal interphalangeal joint in one finger if the others are maintained in extension, because the flexor digitorum profundus is the same for all the fingers and the proper tendons of each finger become individual very distally

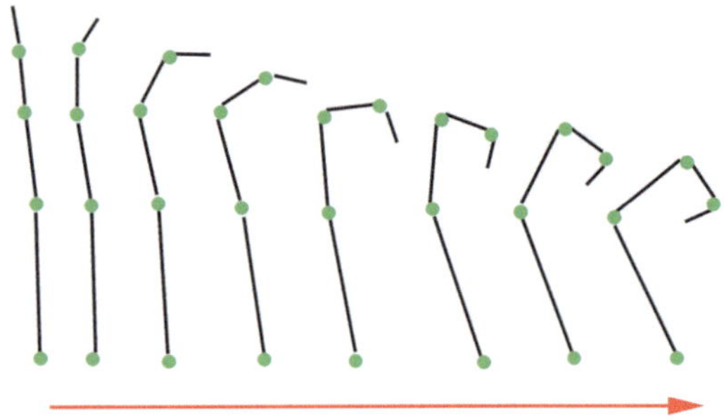

Fig. 1.47 The dynamics of finger winding

This phenomenon can be explained by the fact that the flexor digitorum superficialis tendons are very well individualized in the forearm, whereas the flexor digitorum profundus tendons are individualized only in the hand, thus preventing (or limiting) their isolated contraction.

Winding Dynamics and Tendon Gliding

From an analytic point of view, the role of each tendon during the finger flexion is well known and defined:

- Flexion of the distal interphalangeal joint produced by the flexor digitorum profundus.
- Flexion of the proximal interphalangeal joint produced by the flexor digitorum superficialis.
- Flexion of the metacarpophalangeal joint produced by the interossei through the dorsal expansion.

Finger winding starts with the proximal interphalangeal joint up to 10°, then it is limited by the oblique retinacular ligament that brings the proximal interphalangeal joint in flexion. The flexion of the interphalangeal joints is then proportional up to 80°, where the expansion of the interossei has glided distally enough along the first phalanx to favor the action of the interossei in the flexion of the metacarpophalangeal joint (Fig. 1.47).

The race of the flexor tendons in full flexion is 85 mm anterior to the wrist, of which 25 mm is related to the digital winding (outside the wrist) [23].

The metacarpophalangeal joint provides 77% of the range of motion, the proximal interphalangeal joint 20%, and the distal interphalangeal joint 3%.

Nerve Anatomy

Median Nerve (Fig. 1.48)

It is a mixed nerve (motor, sensorial, and neurovegetative role).

It comes from roots C6 to T1 and passes through the posterior cord (C6–C7) and medial cord (C8–T1), then through the brachial canal until the Struthers ligament (inconstant) above the medial epicondyle, to reach the bicipital groove.

It then passes between the two heads of the pronator teres where it gives off the anterior interosseous branch. This nerve innervates the flexor indicis profundus, the flexor pollicis longus, and the pronator quadratus, as well as a part of the wrist joints.

The median nerve then passes under the flexor digitorum superficialis.

The palmar cutaneous branch of the median nerve arises from its lateral side 6 cm above the

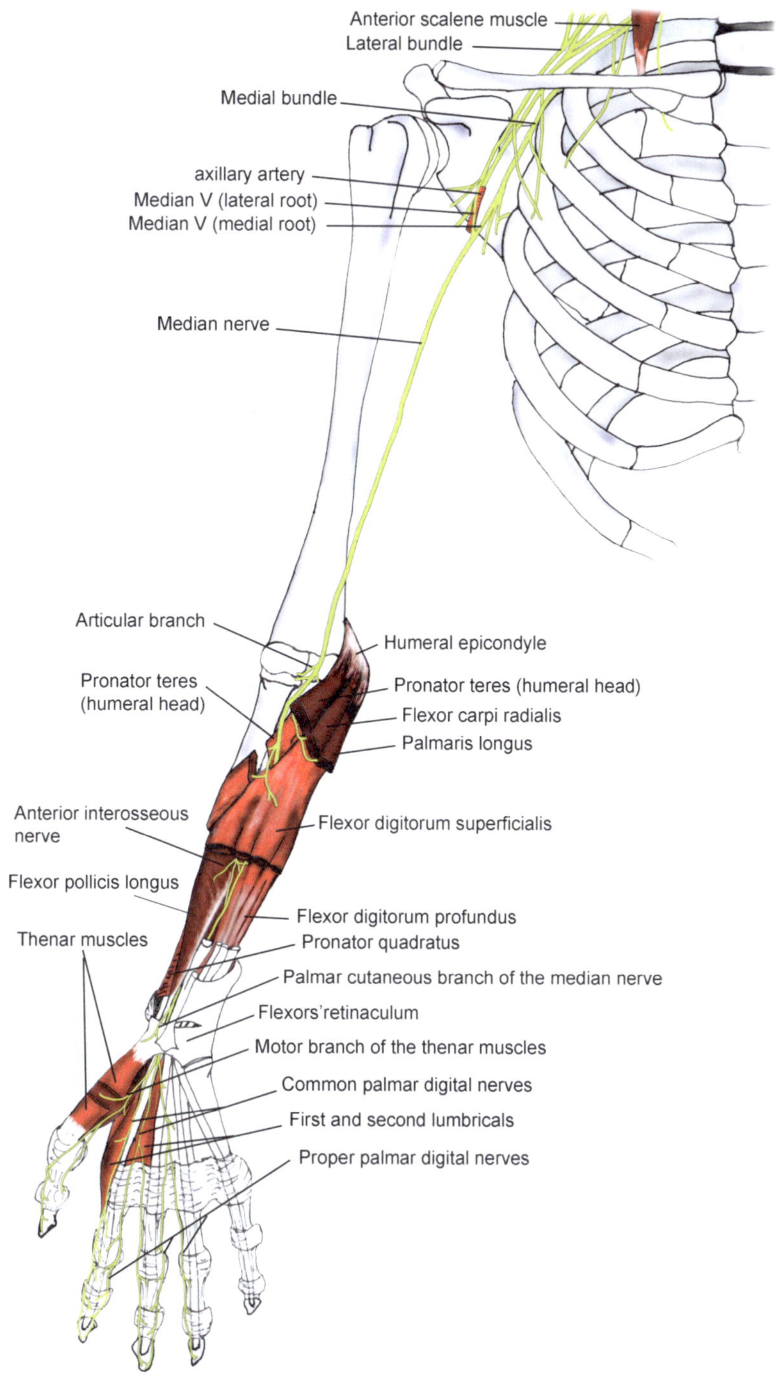

Fig. 1.48 Anatomical situation of the median nerve

palmar flexion crease of the wrist, passes between the flexor carpi radialis and the palmaris longus, then passes through the ante-brachial aponeurosis above the wrist to give off its terminal branches (sensitivity of the thenar compartment).

It enters the hand at the level of the carpal tunnel, which is an hourglass-shaped inextensible osteo-fibrous tunnel. Its narrow part is the hamulus.

It is formed dorsally by the palmar concave osteo-ligamentous groove and closed in the front by the flexors' retinaculum composed of two layers:

- The superficial layer and the antebrachial fascia prolonged distally by the palmar aponeurosis.
- The deep layer with the carpi volare proximally, then from the distal palmar crease of the wrist: the flexor retinaculum that spreads from the pisiform to the apophysis of the sesamoid inward, and from the scaphoid's tubercle to the trapezium outward. Its distal part is covered by fat tissues that form the fat pad of Kaplan and Milford, which contains the superficial palmar arch.

Between these two layers and the two compartments, there is the fascia of Mirza.

Its most internal part forms the floor of the Guyon's canal, limited inward by the insertion of the flexor carpi ulnaris on the pisiform and in the front by the antebrachial fascia.

The carpal tunnel contains the nine flexor tendons with their synovial sheath and the median nerve, organized in three planes [25]:

- Deep plane with the four deep flexor tendons.
- Medium plane with the superficial flexors (the tendons of the flexor indicis and flexor digiti minimi are deeper and more lateral than the flexor tendons of the third and fourth fingers).
- Superficial plane with the median nerve, located in front of the flexor indicis and outside the axis of the fourth finger.

The flexor carpi radialis passes through its own canal, separated from the carpal tunnel by a sagittal connective partition.

Mechanically, the flexors' retinaculum is the first reflection pulley of the flexor system and therefore optimizes the tendons' action, making them more efficient and avoiding the "bowstring" effect. It plays an important role in the strength of the grips.

Distally to the carpal tunnel, the median nerve gives off its terminal branches (Fig. 1.49):

- The thenar branch usually comes from the radial side of the nerve, half the time beyond the inferior side of the ligament, in 30% of the cases behind the ligament bypassing its inferior part, and in 20% of the cases behind the ligament, passing through it. It rarely comes from the anterior side or the medial part of the nerve.
- The proper palmar digital nerve of the thumb.
- The interdigital nerve: in 90% of the cases, there is an anastomosis between the nerve of the third space and the one of the fourth space (terminal branch of the ulnar nerve from the Guyon's canal). It is called the anastomosis of Berrettini, located in the fat pad

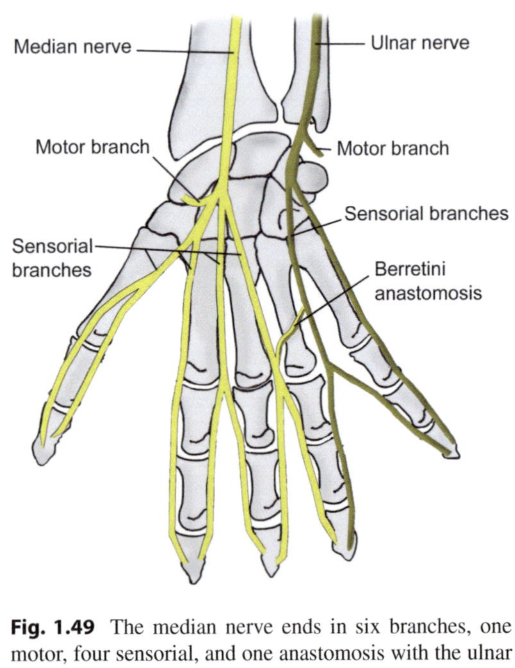

Fig. 1.49 The median nerve ends in six branches, one motor, four sensorial, and one anastomosis with the ulnar nerve (Berretini)

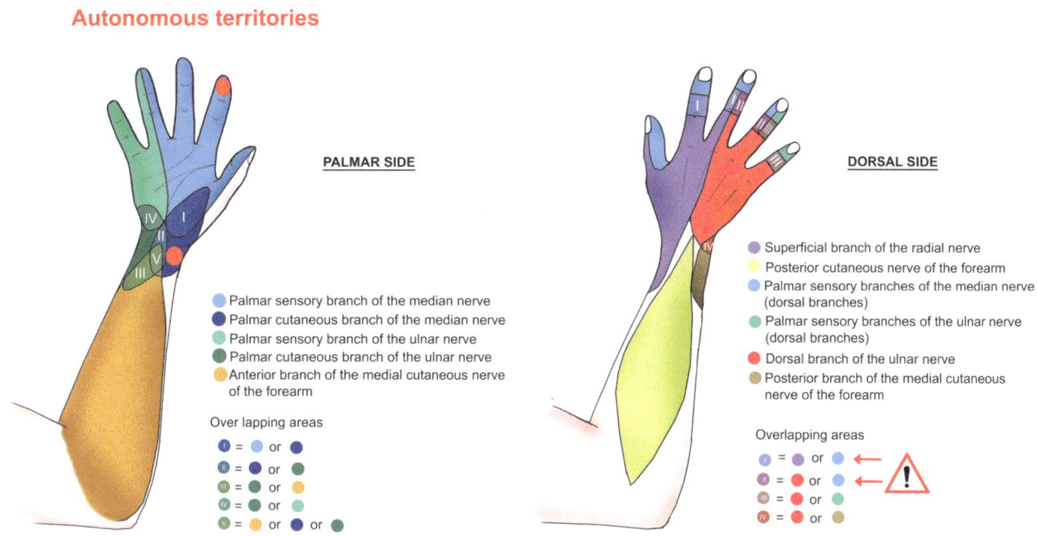

Fig. 1.50 Sensory innervation of the median nerve (the red dots are autonomous territories)

with the superficial palmar aponeurosis and therefore exposed during surgery (especially endoscopy).

Therefore, at the motor level, it innervates:

- The anterior compartment of the forearm, except the flexor carpi ulnaris and the two medial heads of the flexor digitorum profundus (innervated by the ulnar nerve).
- The two radial lumbrical muscles (branches from the first and second spaces) and the external thenar muscles (abductor pollicis and superficial fascicle of the flexor pollicis brevis, as the deep fascicle of the flexor pollicis brevis and the adductor pollicis are the medial thenar muscles innervated by the ulnar nerve) innervated by the thenar branch.

At the sensorial level, it innervates:

- The palmar side of the three first fingers and the radial half of the fourth finger.
- The dorsal side of the two distal phalanges of the index and the third finger, and the radial side of the two distal phalanges of the fourth finger.

In more detail, the sensory innervation associated with the median nerve is divided between its palmar sensory branch and its palmar cutaneous branch. There are individual variations, and the territories described may be dependent on the other nerves of the hand, except for autonomous territories [26] (Fig. 1.50).

Radial Nerve (Fig. 1.51)

The radial nerve is a mixed nerve from the posterior branches of the spinal nerves C5, C6, C7, C8, and sometimes T1. After passing in the lower triangular space of the axilla, it enters the humeral groove. Then at about 10 cm above the epicondyle, it pierces the external intermuscular septum to enter the anterior compartment of the arm, coursing in the external bicipital compartment considered to be the "top floor" of the radial tunnel.

The "medium floor" goes from the humeral condyle to the inferior part of the radial head; in this part the nerve splits into the posterior interosseous nerve (motor innervation) and the superficial branch of the radial nerve (sensorial innervation).

The anterior branch is antero-internal and courses on the brachialis muscle. The posterior branch courses laterally between the brachialis and the brachioradialis.

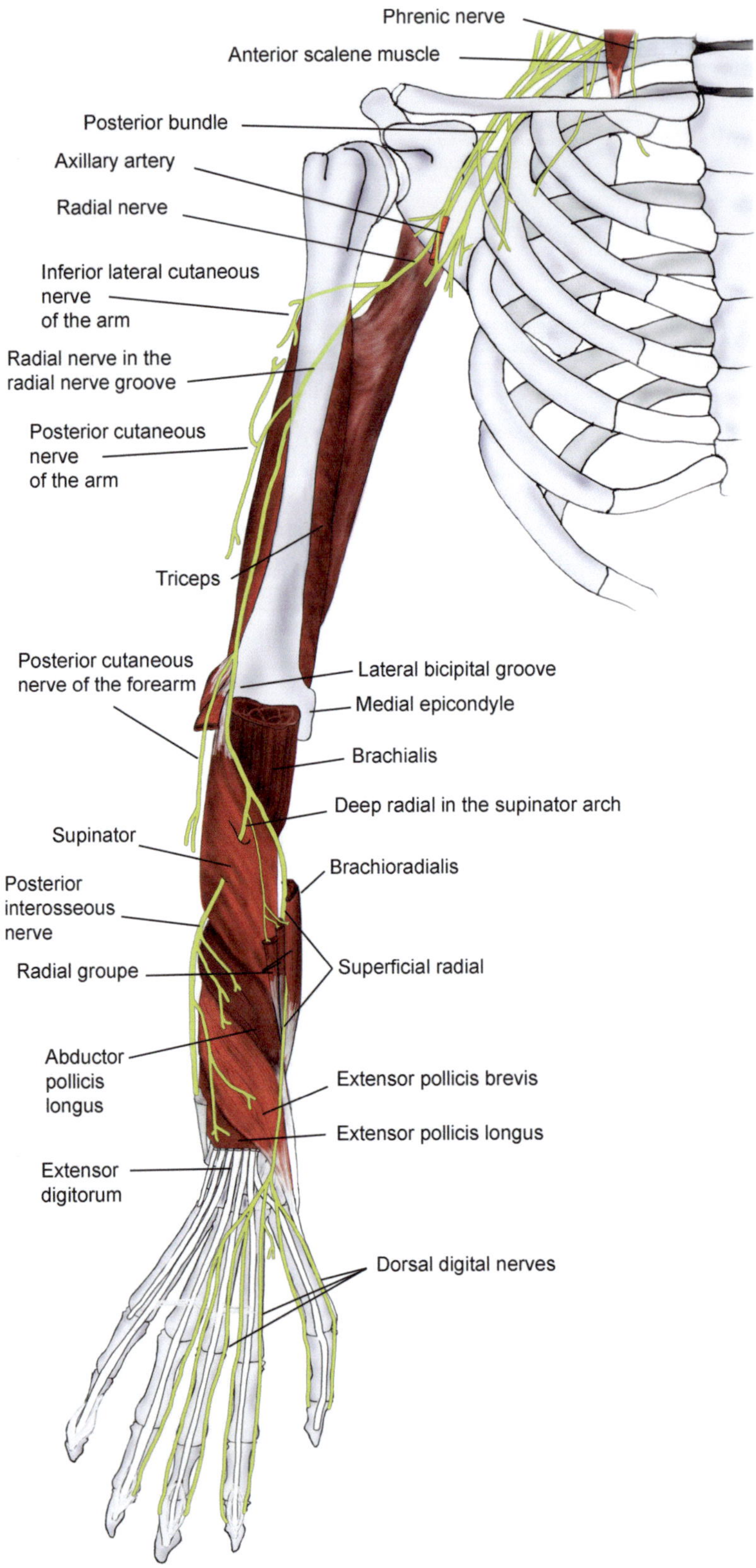

Fig. 1.51 Anatomical situation of the radial nerve

The "lower floor" corresponds to the posterior interosseous nerve passing between the superficial and deep bundles of the supinator, through a muscular or fibrous arcade called the arcade of Fröhse (30% of the cases).

The radial nerve gives off a posterior branch that innervates the extensor carpi ulnaris, the extensor digitorum, and the extensor digiti minimi with its posterior branch, and the abductor pollicis longus, the extensor pollicis brevis, the extensor pollicis longus, and the extensor indicis with its anterior branch.

The anterior sensorial branch passes along the posterior side of the brachioradialis, then gets closer to the radial artery and avoids the lateral side of the radius to cross the abductor pollicis longus, extensor pollicis brevis, and extensor carpi radialis tendons.

The nerve reaches the dorsal side of the wrist then splits into four dorsal digital branches.

From a sensory point of view, it mainly innervates the dorso-radial part of the hand, but, like the median nerve, there are individual variations, and the territories described may be dependent on the other nerves of the hand, except for autonomic territories [26] (Fig. 1.52).

Ulnar Nerve (Fig. 1.53)

The ulnar nerve is a mixed nerve and therefore has a motor, sensory, and neuro-vegetative function.

It originates from the C8 and T1 nerve roots and goes along the internal side of the arm, along the internal head of the triceps and crosses the arcade of Struthers towards the ulnar canal of the elbow. This canal is made of a ligamentous floor (medial collateral ligament), bony walls (epitrochlear-olecranon groove), and a fibrous roof (retinaculum of the ulnar canal).

The ulnar nerve then goes between the two heads of the flexor carpi ulnaris under Osborne's fascia.

It continues its path under the flexor carpi ulnaris and above the flexor digitorum superficialis, behind the arcade of Amadio and Beckenbaugh.

In the middle of the forearm, it gets ventral and goes along the flexor digitorum superficialis towards the Guyon's canal in the wrist.

In the inferior third of the forearm, it splits in two to give off the dorsal part of the ulnar nerve and continues towards the Guyon's canal (Fig. 1.54).

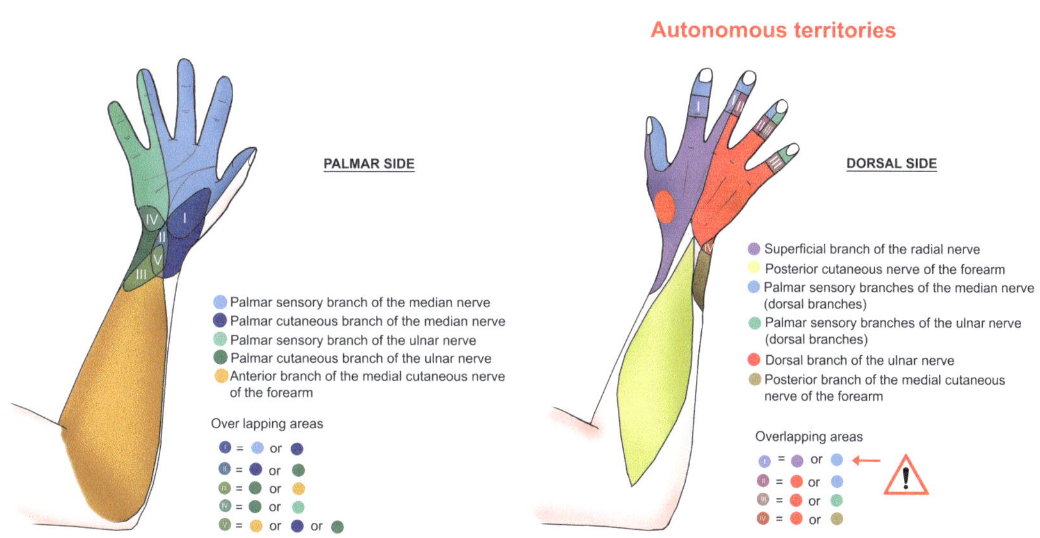

Fig. 1.52 Sensory innervation of the radial nerve by its superficial branch (the red dots are autonomous territories)

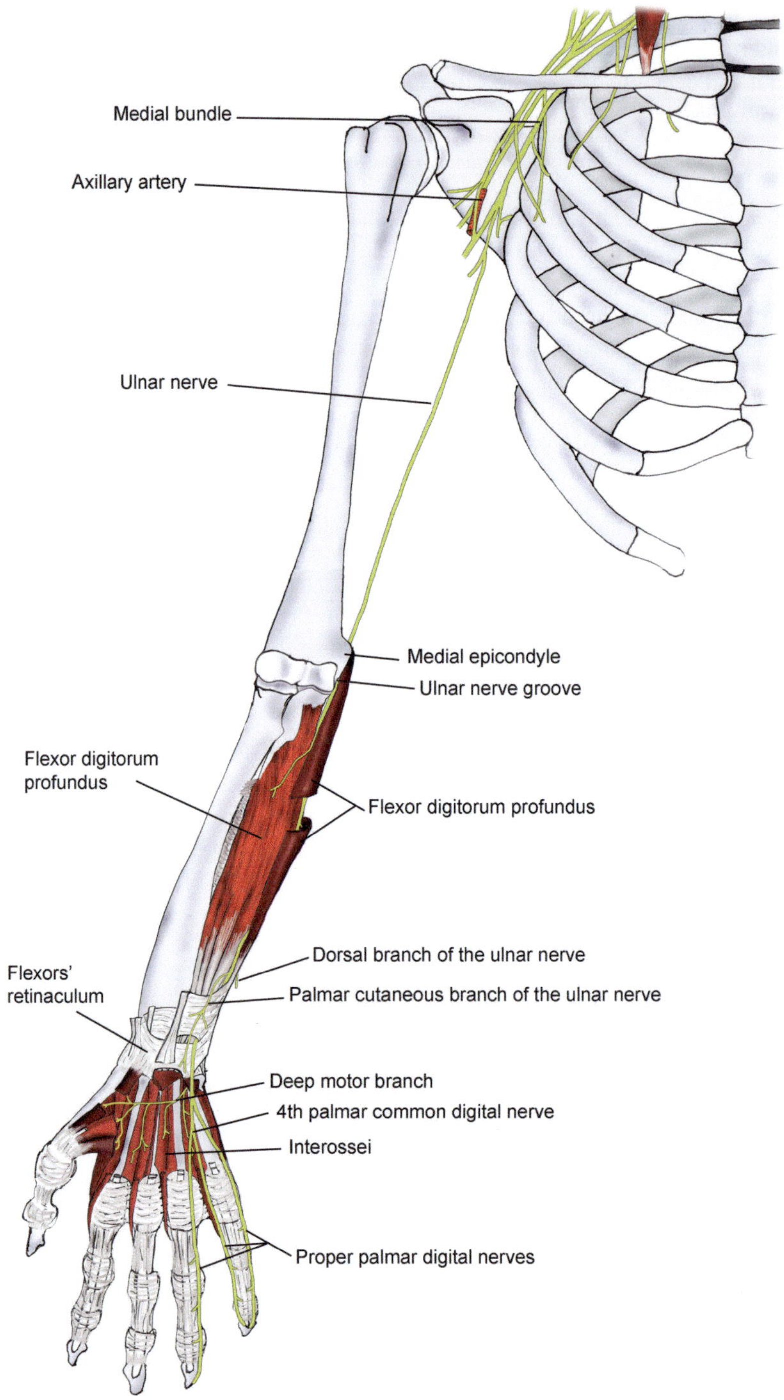

Fig. 1.53 Anatomical situation of the ulnar nerve

It then splits in four branches, the most ulnar being motor (hypothenar eminence, interossei, third and fourth lumbricals, adductor pollicis, deep bundle of the flexor pollicis brevis).

The two medium branches are the sensory nerves of the fifth and half of the fourth finger. The most radial branch forms the Berrettini anastomosis with the median nerve.

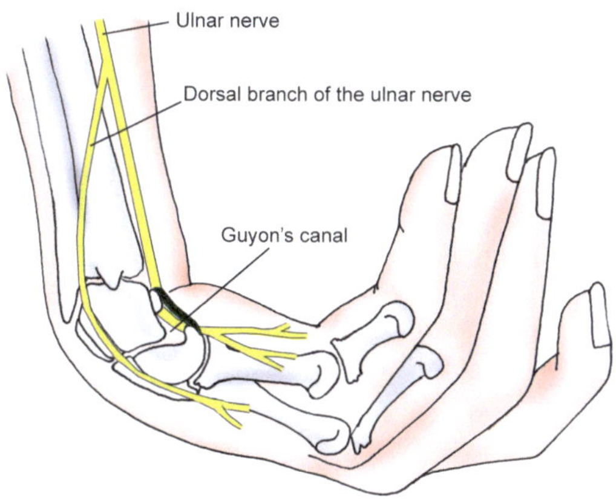

Fig. 1.54 Path of the ulnar nerve in the Guyon's canal

At the motor level, it innervates the flexor carpi ulnaris and the two medial heads of the flexor digitorum profundus in the forearm.

In the hand, it innervates all the intrinsic muscles except for the two radial lumbricals, the opponens pollicis, the abductor pollicis brevis, and the superficial bundle of the flexor pollicis brevis.

From a sensory point of view, it innervates the little finger and the ulnar half of the ring finger, but, like the median and ulnar nerves, there are individual variations, and the territories described may be dependent on the other nerves of the hand, except for autonomous territories [26] (Fig. 1.55).

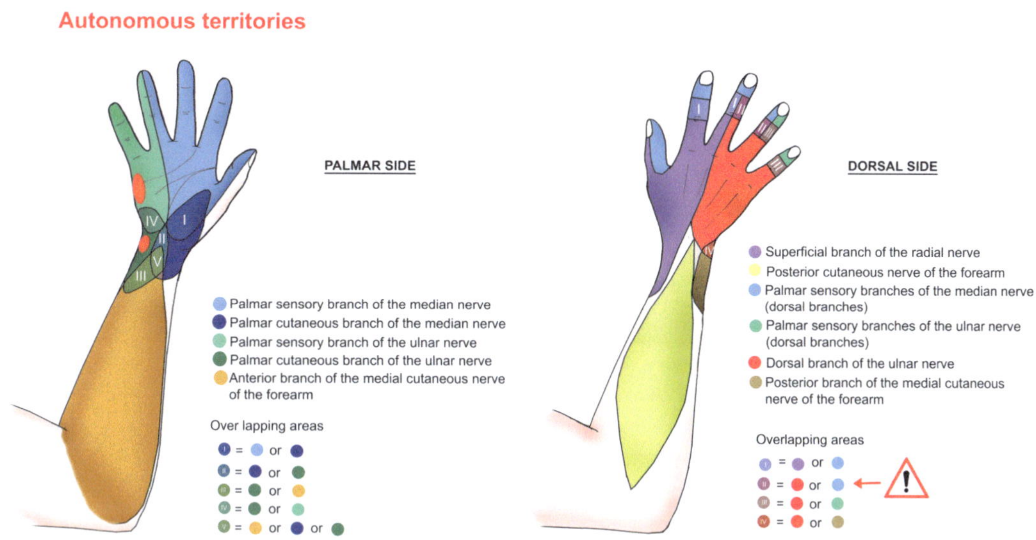

Fig. 1.55 Sensory innervation of the ulnar nerve (the red dots are autonomous territories)

Hand Vascularization

The cutaneous circulation of the hand presents anatomical and physiological variations that are related to the distal location and the special exposure to thermal and postural variations. There are an arterio-venous circulation and a capillary circulation, which is very dense and can vary significantly under the influence of several factors such as the temperature or the position of the hand.

The arterio-capillary system has an autonomic regulation to maintain its tone in an adapted manner but can be influenced by various factors such as pain, emotions, forced inspiration, and tobacco inhalation. During sleep, this tone decreases, which may explain the vasodilatation of the extremities (hand and foot).

The hand is vascularized mainly by the radial and ulnar arteries, which form arterial arches through their anastomoses. The main arteries are the superficial and deep palmar arches and secondarily the carpal, dorsal, and palmar arches.

The superficial palmar arch results from the anastomosis between the ulnar artery and the palmar branch of the radial artery.

The ulnar artery splits into two branches at Guyon's canal: a deep branch that helps to form the deep palmar arch, and a superficial branch that descends vertically and radially from the unciform process of the hamate, crossing the origin of the hypothenar muscles and entering the middle palmar compartment.

The anterior branch of the radial artery runs inferiorly and medially, crossing the upper end of the thenar eminence and joining the ulnar artery to form the superficial palmar arch. In practice, this arch is essentially formed by the ulnar artery, as the anterior branch of the radial artery is often small. It gives off the four palmar digital arteries.

The deep palmar arch results from the anastomosis between the radial artery and the deep branch of the ulnar artery.

The radial artery bypasses the radiocarpal joint at the level of the wrist, enters the anatomical snuffbox, then enters the first interosseous muscle, and reaches the palm of the hand. It runs transversely and medially to join the deep branch of the ulnar artery and form the deep palmar arch.

The deep branch of the ulnar artery arises at the level of the pisiform, then enters the hypothenar eminence, and runs laterally towards the radial artery.

The deep palmar arch gives off the palmar metacarpal arteries (Fig. 1.56).

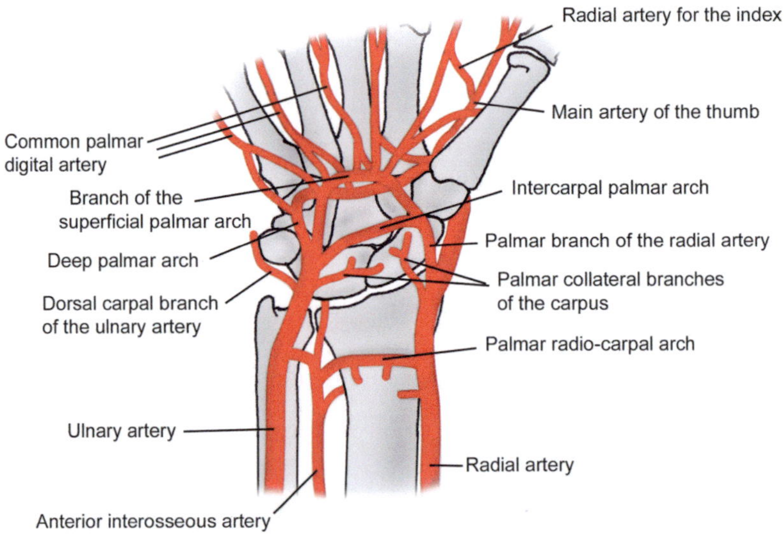

Fig. 1.56 Hand vascularization (anterior part)

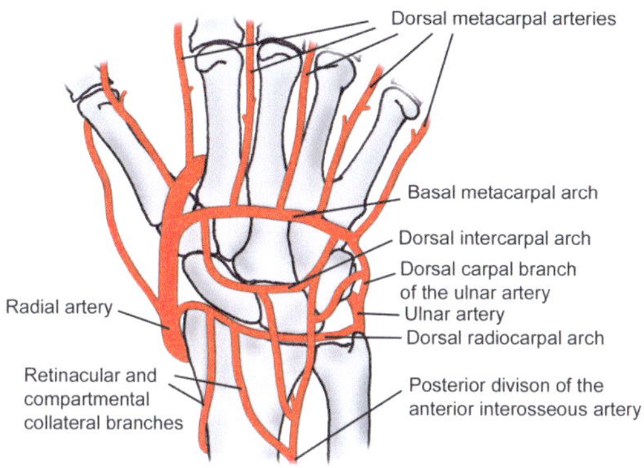

Fig. 1.57 Hand vascularization (posterior part)

Dorsally, vascularization is provided by the dorsal radiocarpal arch, the dorsal intercarpal arch, and the basal metacarpal arch (Fig. 1.57).

The fingers are vascularized by the interosseous arteries and the palmar digital arteries, which anastomose to form the palmar collaterals of the fingers via proximal and distal perforators. These arteries are superficial from the commissure of the fingers. For each finger, there are two palmar collateral arteries, one internal (ulnar) and one external (radial), which have palmar transverse anastomoses between them and end at the level of the pulp by anastomosing again.

Skin Covering

Palmar Skin

The palmar skin is the functional surface of the hand.

Its integumentary physiology is similar to that of other parts of the skin, but it has several unique characteristics.

It is made up of a thick corneous layer (up to 1 to 2 mm) that is resistant because it is well hydrated by the sweat glands.

It is relatively supple but not very extensible, as it is anchored to the deep plane, which helps to ensure a firm grip.

This palmar skin is rich in mechanoreceptors, due to its organization into papillary ridges. The junction between the dermis and the epidermis is marked by alternating dermal and epidermal projections: the epidermal ridges. This organization and the presence of tact receptors in the dermal papillae provide exceptional sensitivity. Pressure exerted perpendicular to the skin is transmitted by the epidermis and stimulates the papilla and the receptor it contains, as well as receptors in adjacent papillae (Fig. 1.58).

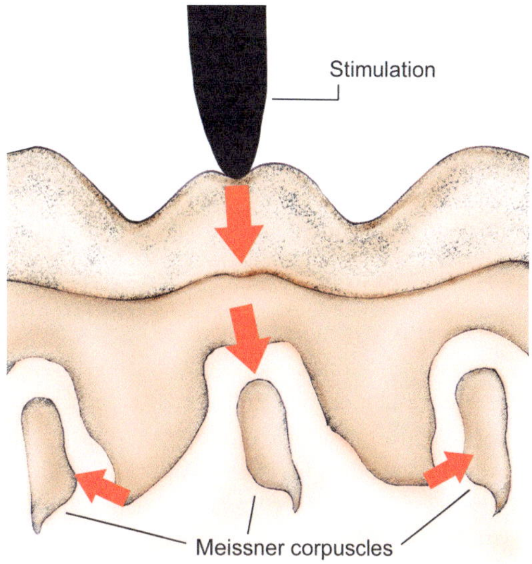

Fig. 1.58 Papillary structure of the palmar skin allowing the presence of more skin receptors (increased surface area) and the recruitment of several receptors for a localized stimulation

The papillary ridges are macroscopically the fingerprints, and their role is to ensure a better grip.

The palmar surface of the hand is made up of numerous fat pads. They improve the congruence between the hand and the object. They are delimited by a system of fibrous tracts that fix the skin to the various aponeurotic planes.

There are three of them:

- The thenar pad, which covers the inner part of the thenar eminence muscles.
- The hypothenar pad, which covers the hypothenar muscles and the inner edge of the hand.
- The metacarpophalangeal pad, which extends transversely from the ulnar edge to the radial edge of the hand in front of the base of the fingers. It is thicker in the interdigital spaces.

The fingers also have a pad on each phalanx. On the third phalanx, the pulp plays a full part in the quality of the grip, not only because of its structure but also because of its wealth of different types of receptors.

Dorsal Skin

The dorsal skin is the social side of the hand.

Unlike the palmar skin, this part is highly extensible and loose in relation to the underlying tissue to allow the flexion of the fingers and wrist. Its surface area then increases by 20%. This flexibility, especially in the metacarpals, is fundamental to the flexion of the metacarpophalangeal joints [27]. The flexion of the proximal and distal interphalangeal joints is made possible by the dorsal skin reserves located at the back of these joints (Fig. 1.59).

The dorsal skin, on the other hand, is very fragile. Its layers are similar to those of the palmar skin, but the corneous layer is thin (0.02 mm). This fragility increases with age.

The ungual part should also be noted, where the nail serves as a support for the palmar pulp when gripping. It also helps to improve sensitivity by reflecting the waves emitted by touch.

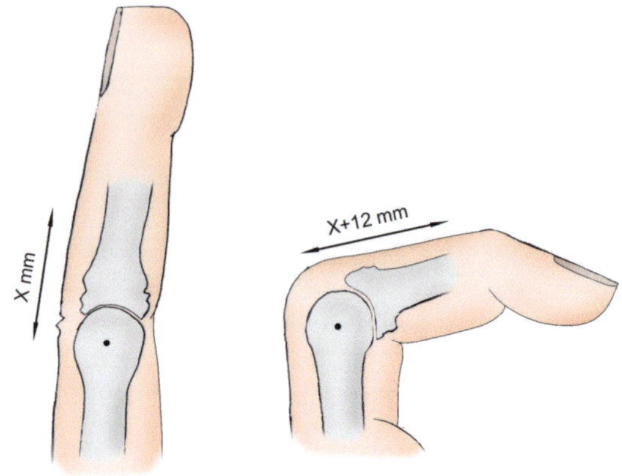

Fig. 1.59 "Excess" cutaneous tissue at the level of the back of the interphalangeal joints allows flexion in these joints

Functional Units

The functional units are the most mobile areas of skin tissue on the palmar and dorsal surfaces. The surgeon's approach must avoid passing through these areas but follow the limits of these functional units to avoid adherent or hypertrophic scars. If this is not possible, a "Z" incision will be made around the unit (Fig. 1.60).

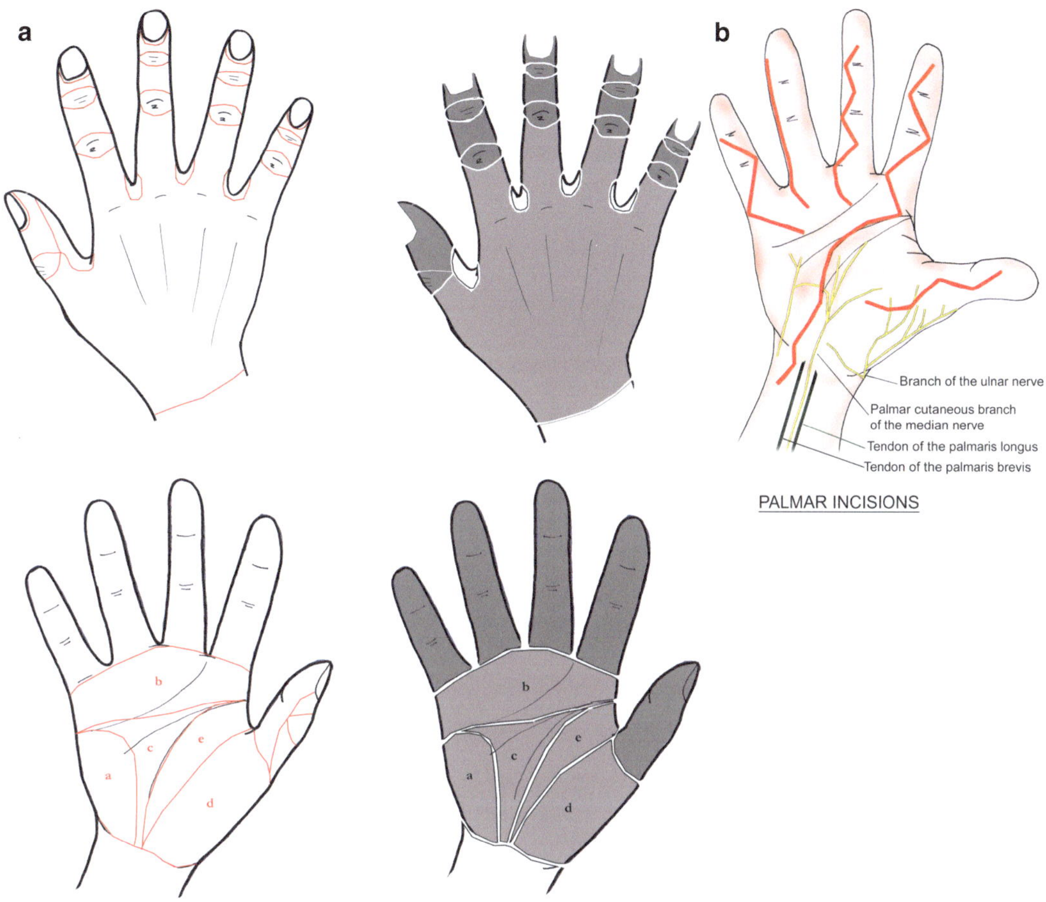

Fig. 1.60 Ideal surgical approach (**a**) avoiding flexion folds (Langer lines) or (**b**) not crossing them transversely

Bibliography

1. Wills BP, et al. The effect of metacarpal shortening on digital flexion force. J Hand Surg Eur. 2013;38(6):667–72.
2. Park AE, et al. The Fibonacci sequence: relationship to the human hand. J Hand Surg Am. 2003;28(1):157–60.
3. Kapandji, I.A., Physiologie articulaire tome 1 – Membre supérieur. 2005: Maloine.
4. Sun Y, et al. In vivo metacarpophalangeal joint collateral ligament length changes during flexion. J Hand Surg Eur Vol. 2017;42E(6):610–5.
5. Bain GI, et al. The functional range of motion of the finger joints. J Hand Surg Eur. 2015;40(4):406–11.
6. Allison DM. Anatomy of the collateral ligaments of the proximal interphalangeal joint. J Hand Surg Am. 2005;30(5):1026–31.
7. Sandhu SS, Dreckmann S, Binhammer PA. Change in the collateral and accessory collateral ligament lengths of the proximal interphalangeal joint using cadaveric model three-dimensional laser scanning. J Hand Surg Eur. 2016;41(4):380–5.
8. Pang EQ, Yao J. Anatomy and biomechanics of the finger proximal interphalangeal joint. Hand Clin. 2018;34(2):121–6.
9. Bowers WH, et al. The proximal interphalangeal joint volar plate. I. An anatomical and biomechanical study. J Hand Surg Am. 1980;5(1):79–88.
10. Bowers WH. The proximal interphalangeal joint volar plate. II: a clinical study of hyperextension injury. J Hand Surg Am. 1981;6(1):77–81.
11. Saito S, Suzuki Y. Biomechanics of the volar plate of the proximal interphalangeal joint: a dynamic ultrasonographic study. J Hand Surg Am. 2011;36(2):265–71.
12. Ladd AL, et al. The 2014 ABJS Nicolas Andry award: the puzzle of the thumb: mobility, stability, and demands in opposition. Clin Orthop Relat Res. 2014;472(12):3605–22.
13. Garcia-Elias M, et al. Trapeziometacarpal ligaments biomechanical study: implications in arthroscopy. J Wrist Surg. 2016;5(4):277–83.

14. Mobargha N, et al. The effect of individual isometric muscle loading on the alignment of the base of the thumb metacarpal: a cadaveric study. J Hand Surg Eur. 2015;41:374.
15. Thompson JS, Littler JW, Upton J. The spiral oblique retinacular ligament (SORL). J Hand Surg Am. 1978;3(5):482–7.
16. Ueba H, et al. An anatomic and biomechanical study of the oblique Retinacular ligament and its role in finger extension. J Hand Surg Am. 2011;36(12):1959–64.
17. Zwanenburg RL, Werker PM, McGrouther DA. The anatomy and function of Cleland's ligaments. J Hand Surg Eur. 2014;39(5):482–90.
18. Iwamoto A, et al. An anatomic and biomechanic study of the wrist extensor retinaculum septa and tendon compartments. J Hand Surg Am. 2006;31(6):896–903.
19. Chinchalkar SJ, Lanting BA, Ross D. Swan neck deformity after distal interphalangeal joint flexion contractures: a biomechanical analysis. J Hand Ther. 2010;23(4):420–5.
20. Boyes W. Bunnell's surgery of the hand. JB Lippincott Philadelphia; 1970.
21. Mallo GC, et al. A2 and A4 flexor pulley biomechanical analysis: comparison among gender and digit. Hand (N Y). 2008;3(1):13–6.
22. Doyle JR. Anatomy of the finger flexor tendon sheath and pulley system. J Hand Surg Am. 1988;13(4):473–84.
23. Strickland JW. The scientific basis for advances in flexor tendon surgery. J Hand Ther. 2005;18(2): 94–110.
24. Gonzalez MH, et al. Biomechanics of the digit. J Am Soc Surg Hand. 2005;5(1):48–60.
25. Rotman M, Donovan J. Practical anatomy of the carpal tunnel. Hand Clin. 2002;2002(18):219–30.
26. Spicher C, Desfoux N, Sprumont P. Atlas des territoires cutanés du corps humain: esthésiologie de 240 branches. Sauramps Medical; 2010.
27. Girbon JP, Oddou L. La mobilité cutanée du dos de la main lors de la flexion. Enroulement des doigts longs. Annales de kinésithérapie. 2000;27:348–52.

Further Reading

Kamata Y, et al. How the lumbrical muscle contributes to placing the fingertip in space: a three dimensional cadaveric study to assess fingertip trajectory and metacarpophalangeal joint balancing. J Hand Surg Eur. 2016;41(4):386–91.
Crowley JS, et al. The Lumbricals are not the workhorse of digital extension and do not relax their own antagonist. J Hand Surg Am. 2021;46(3):232–5.
Tang JB. Clinical outcomes associated with flexor tendon repair. Hand Clin. 2005;21(2):199–210.

Part II

Osseous and Capsulo-Ligamentous Injuries in the Hand and Thumb

Fractures of Metacarpals and Phalanges

2

Grégory Mesplié and Nicolas Christiaens

Physiopathology and Types of Fractures

Fractures of the Metacarpals

Fractures of the Base

The stable and extra-articular fractures do not present an important risk of secondary displacement, if the treatment is correctly done.

On the contrary, the joint fractures are potentially unstable and source of secondary arthrosis.

- The fracture of the base of the fifth metacarpal: the radial fragment stays in contact with the base of the fourth metacarpal and the hamate, while the extensor carpi ulnaris tends to move the rest of the metacarpal dorsally, proximally and medially (Fig. 2.1).
- The joint fractures in the base of the second and third metacarpals present the same risk of instability, because of the action of the radial extensors of the carpus [1].

The joint fractures in the base of the first metacarpal can be of two types:

- The Bennett fracture, with an anterior fragment (the "beak" of the first metacarpal) that remains blocked in the trapezium recess [2] and the rest of the base of the metacarpal moving radially because of the abductor pollicis longus. The thenar muscles (mainly the adductor pollicis) tend to move the metacarpal towards adduction (Fig. 2.2).
- The Rolando fracture, which is a fracture with one metaphyseal fracture line and two epiphyseal fracture lines (T-shaped or V-shaped) (Fig. 2.3).

Fractures of the Diaphysis

As in base fractures, the therapist must consider the exact site of the injury, to anticipate the contractions that may cause deformity (Fig. 2.4).

➔ Fingers

They can be transverse, in spiral, or comminuted (Fig. 2.5).

The transverse fractures can lead to an anterior tilt of the part distal to the fracture, because of the action of the interossei and flexor muscles (Fig. 2.6).

In the case of spiral fractures, we must check if there are any rotatory disorders, sometimes increased by the contraction of the interosseous muscles. This tendency can be demonstrated by

G. Mesplié (✉) · N. Christiaens
Institut Sud Aquitain de la Main et du Membre Supérieur (ISAMMS), Biarritz, France

G. Mesplié (ed.), *Hand Functional Anatomy and Therapy*,
https://doi.org/10.1007/978-3-031-92505-4_2

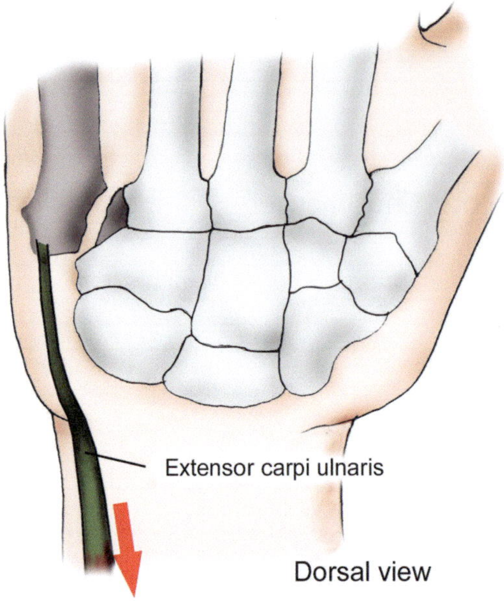

Fig. 2.1 In the fractures of the base of the fifth metacarpal, the extensor carpi ulnaris can cause instability of the fracture (left hand on the picture)

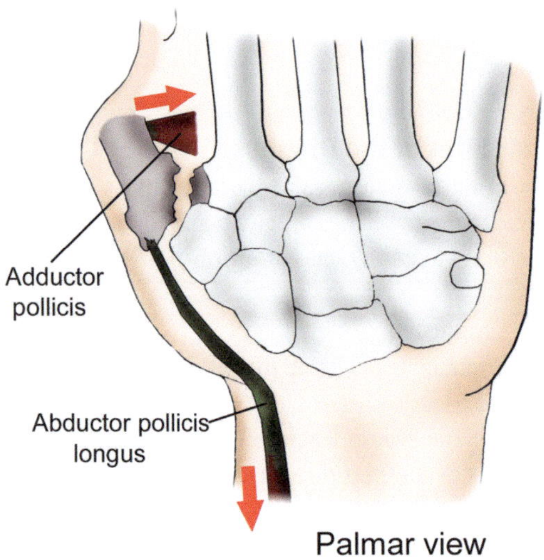

Fig. 2.2 Bennet fractures, possibly unstable because of the effect of the abductor pollicis longus and the thenar muscles

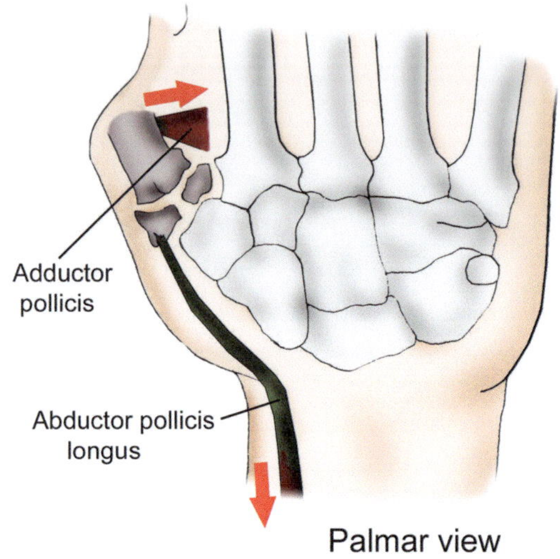

Fig. 2.3 Rolando fractures, possibly unstable because of the effect of the abductor pollicis longus and the thenar muscles

asking the patient to perform a global flexion of the fingers. A misalignment of the metacarpal in relation to the adjacent fingers is then observed.

In this type of deformity, the two radial metacarpals most often pronate excessively, whereas the two ulnar metacarpals tend to supinate excessively when the fingers are flexed [3] (Fig. 2.7). Comminuted fractures are the most complex and cause secondary stiffening more often.

➔ **Thumb** We can observe a palmar tilt of the distal part, because of the effect of the expansion made by the flexor pollicis brevis, the abductor pollicis brevis, and the adductor pollicis (Fig. 2.8).

Fracture of the Neck of the Metacarpals

The fractures of the neck are the most frequently observed, mainly in the fourth and fifth metacarpals. This "bad boxer's fracture" is often due to a punch with an impact on the ulnar side (the "good

Bone	Zone	Regional deformation forces	Type of fracture
Metacarpal		**Intrinsic muscles** ⟶ distal flexion	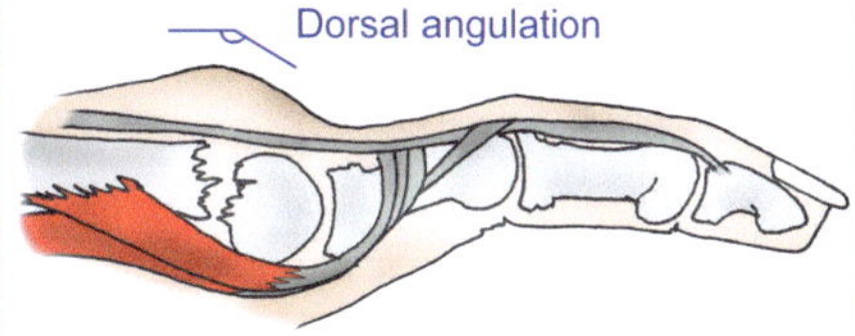
Proximal phalanx		**Intrinsic muscles** ⟶ proximal flexion **Extensor system** ⟶ distal extension	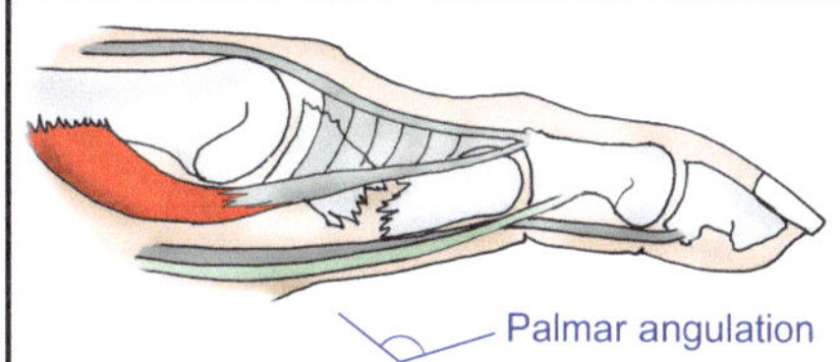
Medial phalanx	Proximal 1/3	**Central tendon of the extensor** ⟶ proximal extension **Flexor digitorum superficialis** ⟶ distal flexion	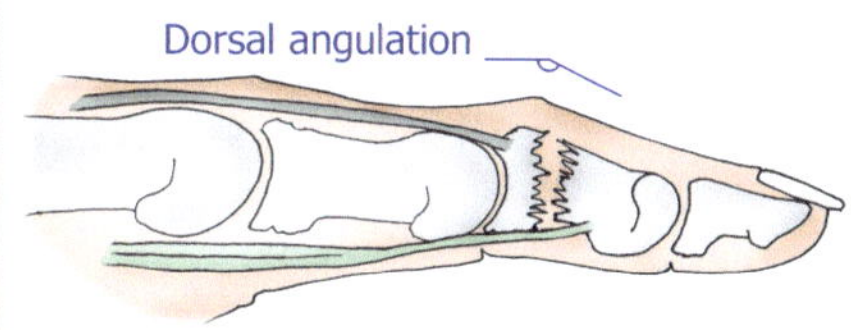
	Distal 1/3	**Extensor tendon** ⟶ distal extension **Flexor digitorum superficialis** ⟶ proximal flexion	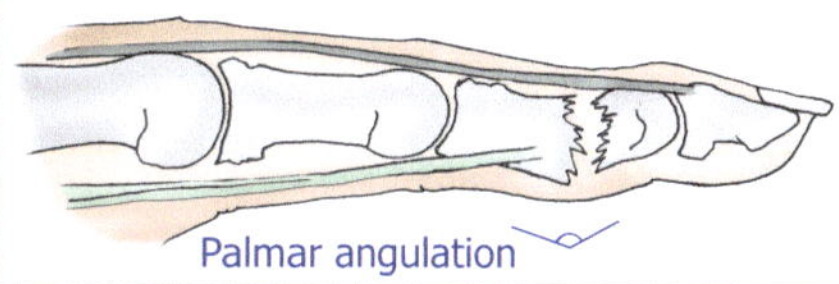
Distal phalanx	Diaphysis	**Extensor tendon** : all clear (but injury of the nail matrix) **Flexor digitorum profondus** ⟶ distal flexion	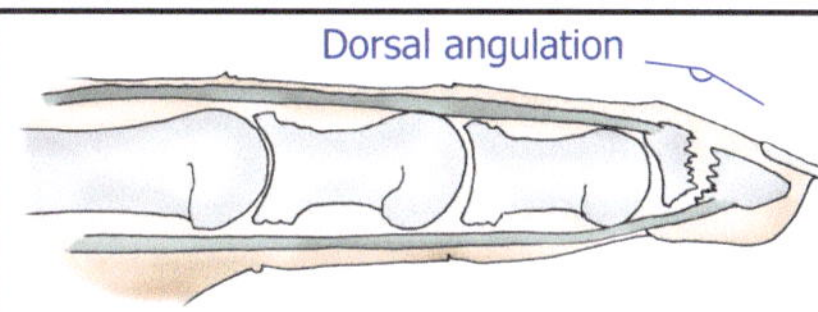
	Head	No tendinous insertion	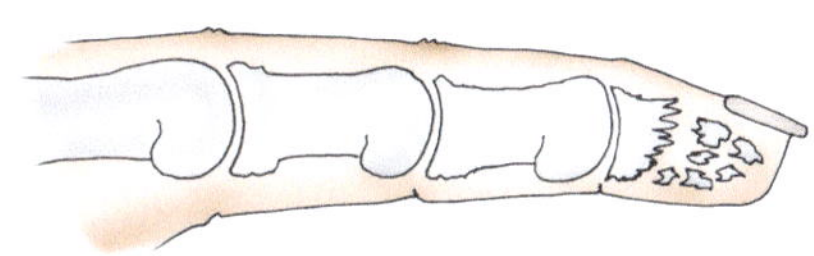

Fig. 2.4 Tendinous insertions that can cause a vicious callus if the fracture is not stabilized

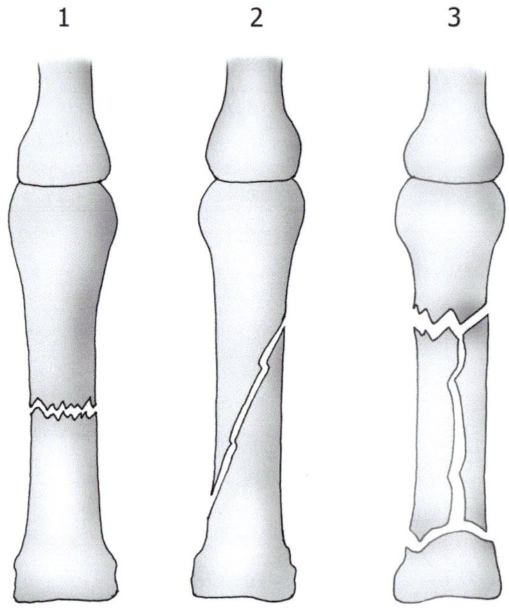

Fig. 2.5 The three main types of fractures of the diaphysis

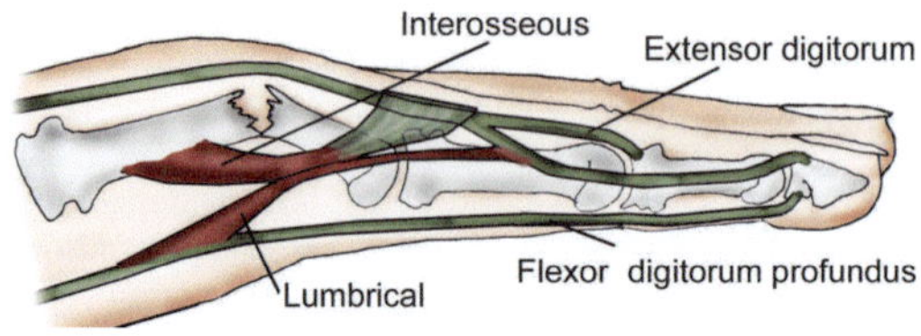

Fig. 2.6 Anterior tilt of the distal part of the fracture because of the action of the interossei and flexors

Fig. 2.7 In fractures of the metacarpal with vicious rotation, the radial metacarpals tend to have an excessive pronation, unlike the ulnar metacarpals

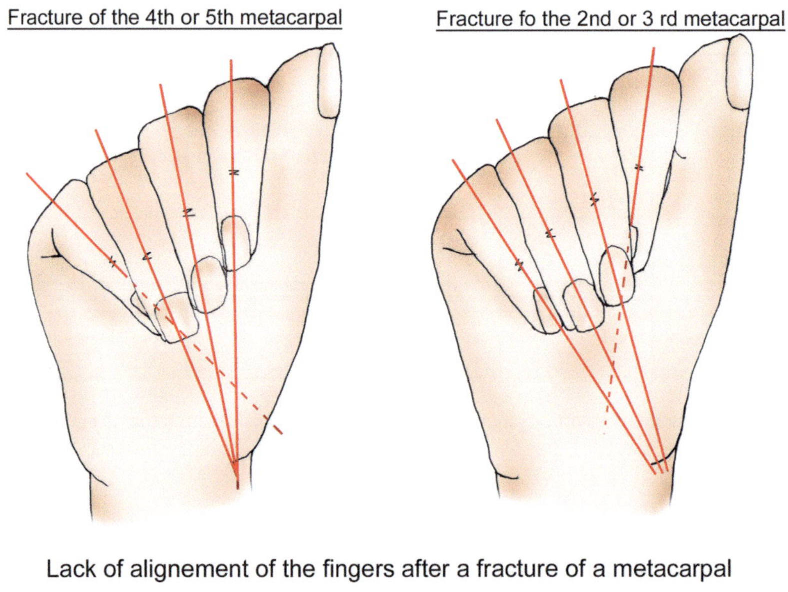

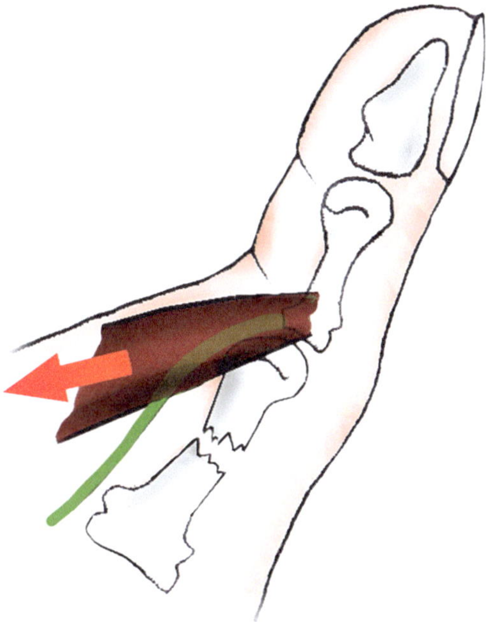

Fig. 2.8 Anterior tilt of the distal fragment in the thumb

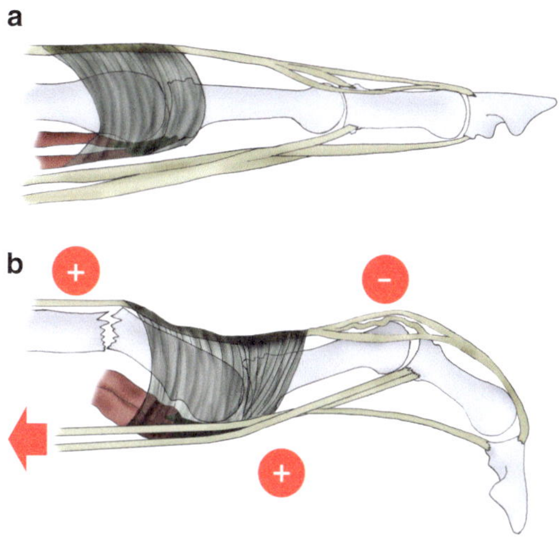

Fig. 2.9 Pseudo-claw after a metacarpal neck fracture with anterior tilt of the distal fragment: this tilt puts tension on the extensor system proximally to the metacarpophalangeal joint but relaxes it distally

boxers" usually use the two radial metacarpals that are more fixed), leading to an anterior tilt of the head of the metacarpal.

In that case, like in the fractures of the diaphysis, the dorsal expansion of the interossei (or the thenar muscles—except the opponent—for the thumb) increases the palmar displacement of the metacarpal head. This tilt may cause a "pseudo" claw, due to the concomitant effect of relaxing the extensor system at the digital level and tensioning the flexor system (Fig. 2.9).

Joint Fractures of the Metacarpal Head

These fractures are a source of stiffness in the case of prolonged immobilization [4] and of arthrosis in the case of badly reduced displacement, at the level of the thumb or the fingers.

Fractures of the Phalanges

Joint Fractures

The joint fractures, like in every other joint, present a risk of stiffness and secondary arthrosis in the case of prolonged immobilization and/or bad restoration of the joint surfaces.

We must be very vigilant because some of these fractures are in fact ligamentous or tendinous injuries, which must be imperatively identified quickly (Fig. 2.10).

Fractures of the Diaphysis

➔ First Phalanx

As in the metacarpals, these fractures can be transverse, spiral, or comminuted. In the case of a transverse fracture, the proximal fragment tends to glide towards the palmar side (because of the dorsal expansion of the interossei), and the distal fragment tends to glide towards the dorsal side (because of the extensor system).

➔ Second Phalanx

In transverse fractures, when the fracture line is proximal to the end of the flexor digitorum superficialis, the proximal fragment is pulled backwards by the median strip of the extensor system, and the distal fragment is pulled frontwards by the flexor digitorum superficialis.

When the fracture line is distal to the end of the flexor digitorum superficialis, the proximal fragment moves frontwards, and the distal fragment moves backwards.

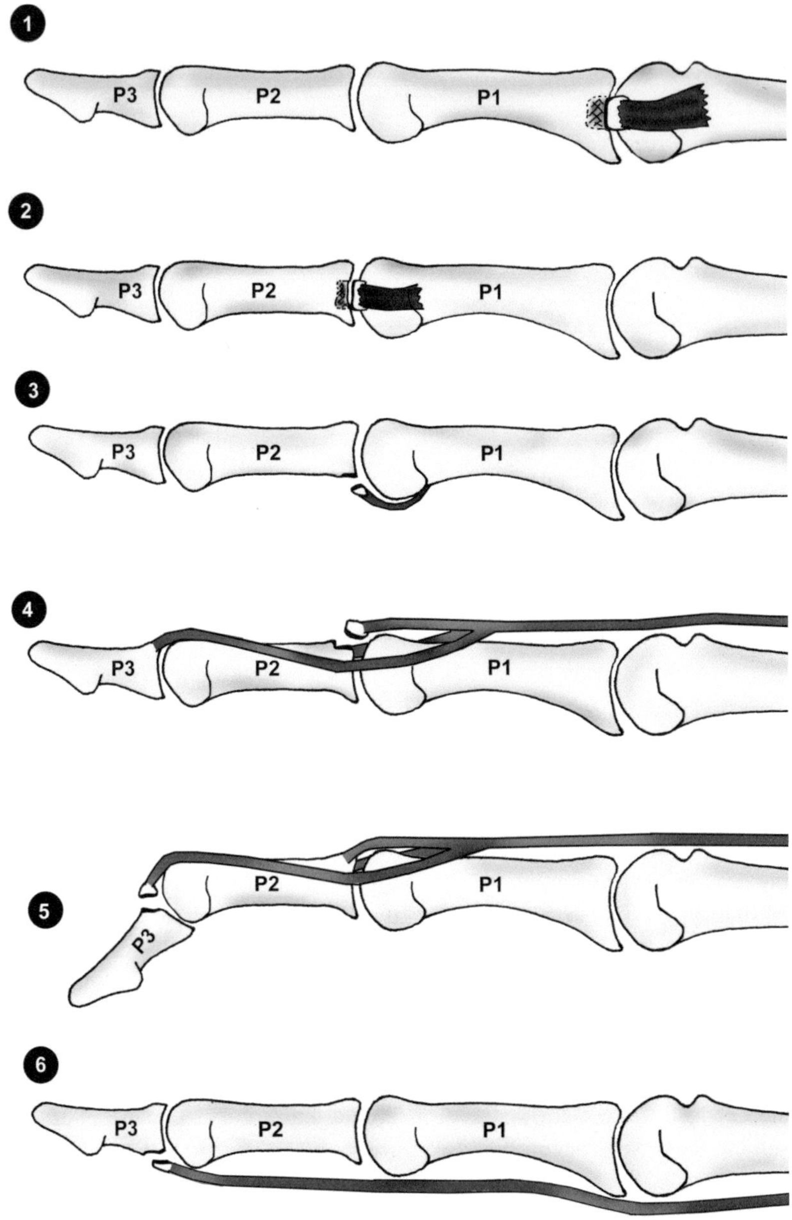

Fig. 2.10 Joint fractures

➔ Third Phalanx

The fractures of the diaphysis of the third phalanx are often the consequence of a crushing trauma, leading to trophic disorders and a prolonged pain. They usually do not cause residual stiffness.

Therapeutic Process

Our therapeutic process depends on the type of injury. The priority would be allowing the early mobilization of the damaged finger without disturbing the osseous healing. In fact, any fracture in

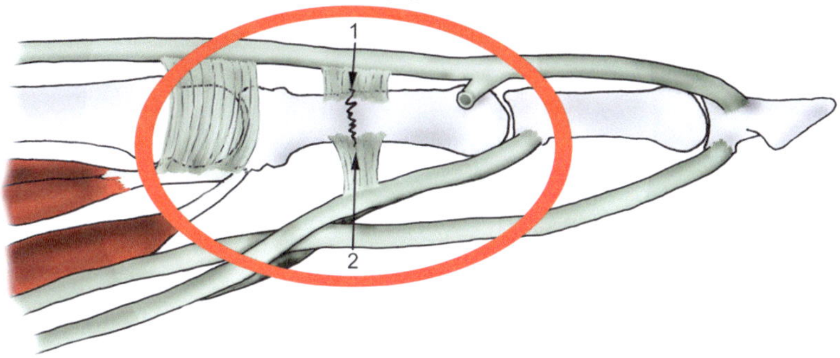

Fig. 2.11 Any fracture in the hand creates a "zone of injury", a source of adherences between all the elements next to the fracture site

the hand creates a "zone of injury" that is a source of adherences between all the elements in the immediate vicinity of the fracture site (Fig. 2.11).

Orthopedic Treatment

This treatment is based on the use of thermoformable orthoses, which ideally adapt to the patient's morphology and leave the unaffected joints free.

Allowing Early Mobilization

It is the treatment that obtains the best results [5, 6], but it can be used only in stable fractures. The orthosis must allow the osseous healing and at the same time maintain the movements that do not put excessive constraints on the callus.

The evolution is regularly controlled (by clinical and radiological assessments) to limit the risk of secondary displacements.

Immobilization

This is the default choice, when there is a counterindication for surgery and the fracture is displaced or unstable. The orthosis is more constraining and immobilizing to improve osseous healing, but it must allow a soft mobilization of the joints that are not concerned by the fracture. The orthosis is also worn longer, which can lead to secondary stiffness in the immobilized joints.

Surgical Treatment (Fig. 2.12)

The surgical treatment is used in the case of displaced fractures with a functional tolerance of 30° of tilt for the fractures of the diaphysis of the fourth or fifth metacarpals [7], and 5° of tilt for the fractures of the diaphysis of the second or third metacarpals.

Every other displacement (phalanges tilt, rotatory disorders, etc.) and unstable fractures need a surgical intervention. The goal of this surgery is to stabilize the fracture site, being as minimally invasive as possible [4], to allow early mobilization of the injured hand, thus reducing edema, stiffness, and tendon adherences.

Percutaneous Techniques

They are used in case of reducible closed injuries.

Their interest is to limit the risk of secondary displacements and to allow an early mobilization, with an adapted orthosis.

Open Osteosynthesis

These techniques concern the open and unstable fractures, or the non-reducible ones, and the joint fractures. Screwed plates, screws, Bilboquets, or external fixators can be used, among others (Fig. 2.12).

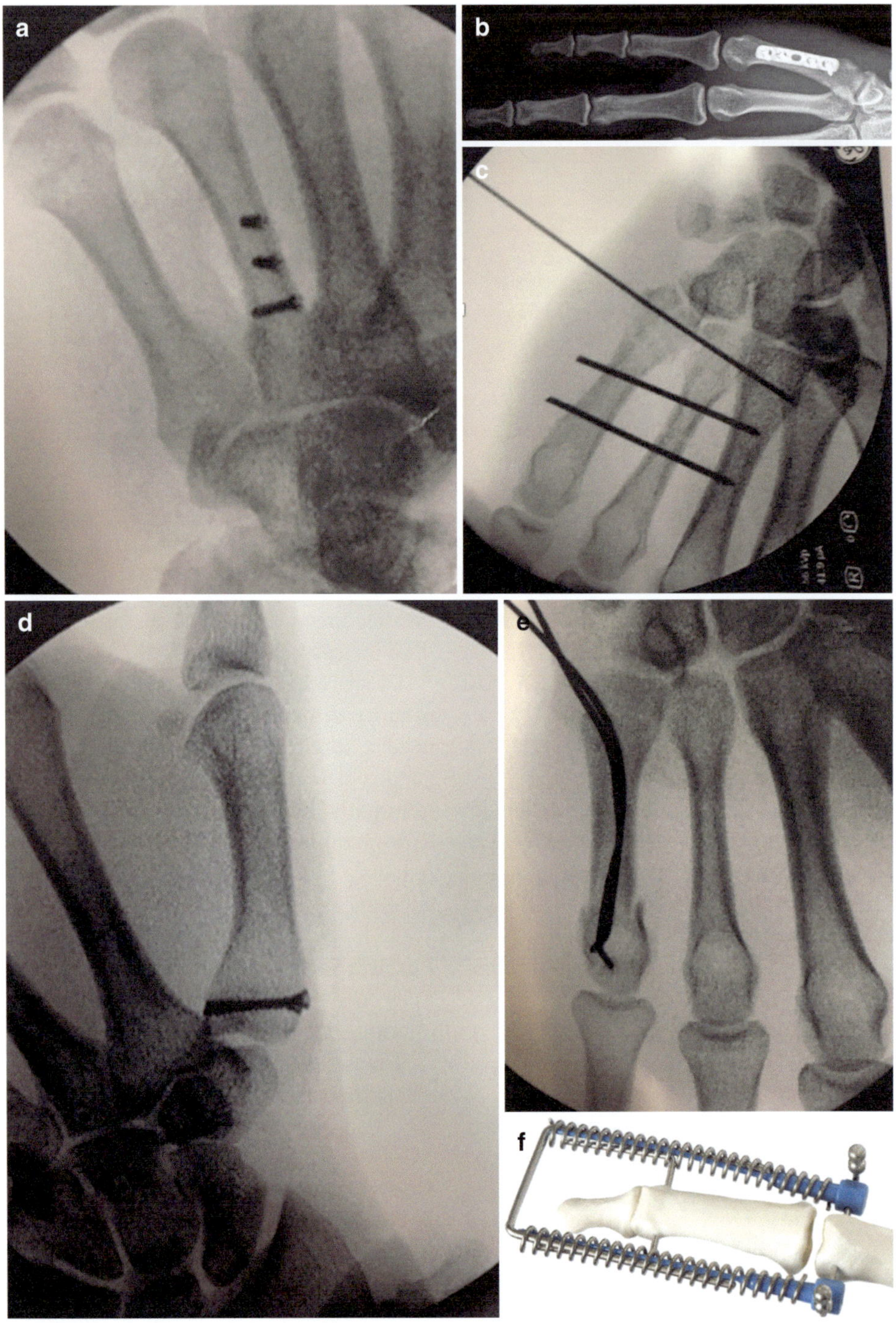

Fig. 2.12 Examples of surgical techniques. (**a**) Osteosynthesis with screws of a spiral fracture of the third metacarpal diaphysis. (**b**) Osteosynthesis with plate fixation of a fracture of the fifth metacarpal diaphysis. (**c**) Osteosynthesis with intermetacarpal pin of a fracture of the base of the fifth metacarpal. (**d**) Screw fixation of the anterior beak of the first metacarpal in a Bennet fracture with a large fragment. (**e**) Osteosynthesis of a neck fracture of the fifth metacarpal using a centro-medullar pin. The entry point of the pin is at the dorso-ulnar part of the base of the fifth metacarpal. (**f**) Ligamentotaxor® that can be used for early mobilization under traction of the proximal interphalangeal joint after a joint fracture. (Pictures by Grégory Mesplié)

Rehabilitation and Orthoses

Orthotic Immobilization Treatment

The type of orthosis depends on the location of the fracture, its displacement, and its stability. The described orthoses are the same with or without surgery.

Fingers

➔ Stable Fracture of the Metacarpal Base

We realize the orthosis putting the wrist in 20° of extension [1], combined with a syndactyly with the adjacent finger opposed to the tendency of bad rotation. If there is no such tendency assessed, the syndactyly is preferably realized between the fourth and fifth fingers or the second and third fingers (Fig. 2.13).

➔ Stable Fracture of the Metacarpal Diaphysis

A metacarpal gauntlet maintains the metacarpal architecture (transversal and longitudinal metacarpal arches), combined with a syndactyly, following the same principles as before (Fig. 2.14).

In the case of a slight rotatory disorder (spiral fracture), a derotation wedge can be used to correct the fingers winding, while allowing the fingers to be mobilized quickly [8].

➔ Unstable Fracture of the Metacarpals

We realize a "Thomine" orthosis, placing the wrist in 20° of extension and the metacarpophalangeal joints in 70° of flexion. The interphalangeal joints stay free (Fig. 2.15).

In the case of a neck fracture with anterior tilting of the distal fragment, with a pseudo ulnar claw attitude, we use an orthosis with a dorsal shell. This shell allows the patient to be main-

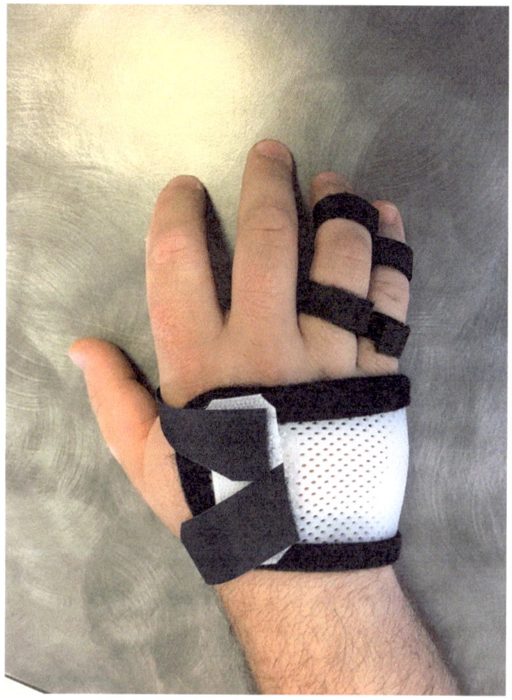

Fig. 2.14 Metacarpal gauntlet and syndactyly between the fourth and fifth fingers after a stable fracture of the diaphysis of the fifth metacarpal. (Pictures by Grégory Mesplié)

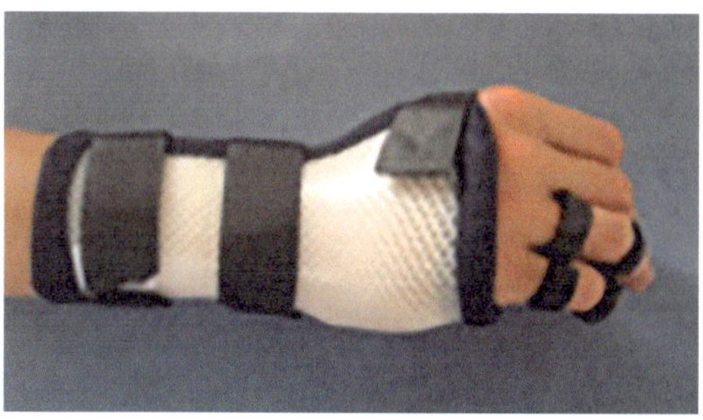

Fig. 2.13 Orthosis placing the wrist in 30° of extension and syndactyly between the fourth and fifth fingers after a stable fracture of the base of the fifth metacarpal. (Pictures by Grégory Mesplié)

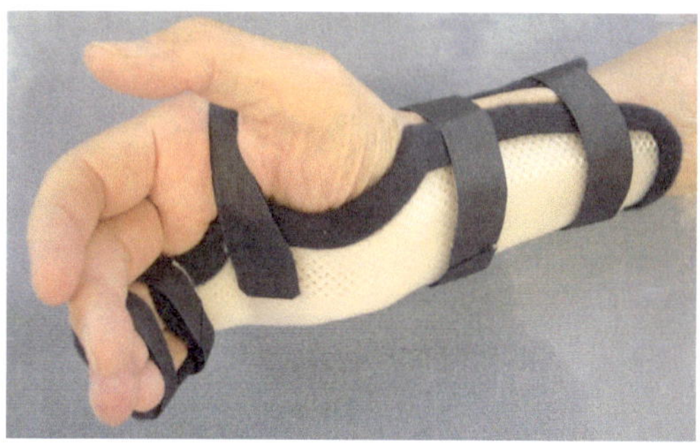

Fig. 2.15 Orthosis placing the wrist in 30° of extension, the metacarpophalangeal joints in 70° of flexion and the interphalangeal joints free in flexion/extension after an unstable fracture of the metacarpals. (Pictures by Grégory Mesplié)

tained in interphalangeal extension during the day, which prevents a possible flessum of the proximal interphalangeal joint. It also allows the patient to perform regular self-rehabilitation exercises in flexion (series of 10 repetitions every hour).

This orthotic treatment of unstable fractures is only used in cases where surgery is not possible, as it requires a greater immobilization to maintain the reduction, and during a longer time, which is a significant source of complications (complex regional pain syndrome, stiffness, etc.).

➔ Stable Fracture of the First and Second Phalanges

A syndactyly is enough, associating the second and third fingers or the fourth and fifth fingers (Fig. 2.16). The syndactyly can be made of thermoformable plastic to protect the injury site from impact.

➔ Unstable Fracture of the Base or Diaphysis of the First Phalanx

We realize a metacarpal gauntlet that maintains the metacarpal arches and places the metacarpophalangeal joints in 70° of flexion (Fig. 2.17). As in fractures of the necks of the metacarpals, in the case of a pseudo-ulnar claw attitude, due to an anterior tilt of the proximal fragment of the first phalanx, we use an orthosis with a dorsal shell.

➔ Unstable Fracture of the Head of the First or Second Phalanx

The orthosis realized is a digital tube. An early liberation of the distal interphalangeal joint is made in case of a fracture of the head of the first phalanx or the base of the second phalanx if the osseous callus evolves well (after a radiographic control).

It is also possible to use an orthosis creating a joint distraction, allowing early mobilization of the injured joint under traction [9].

➔ Stable or Instable Fracture of the Third Phalanx

A thermoformed "thimble" is made, leaving the proximal interphalangeal joint free (Fig. 2.18). Letting the distal interphalangeal joint free in the distal injuries of the third phalanx is technically very difficult and the patients tend to lose their orthosis, especially during the night.

Thumb

➔ Stable Fracture of the Base of the First Metacarpal

We realize an orthosis placing the wrist in a neutral position and the metacarpophalangeal joint in a functional position (Fig. 2.19). We do not let the

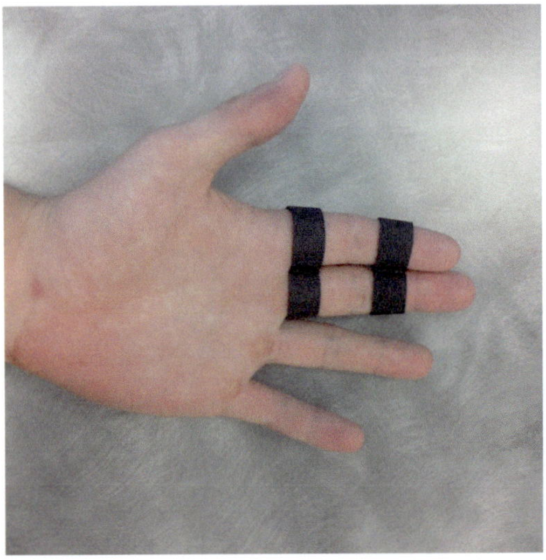

Fig. 2.16 Simple syndactyly after stable fractures of the first or second phalanx. (Pictures by Grégory Mesplié)

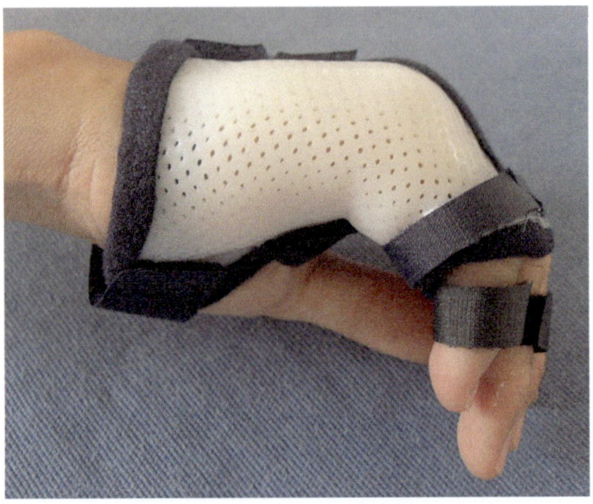

Fig. 2.17 Orthosis placing the metacarpophalangeal joints in 70° of flexion and conserving the metacarpal arches in unstable fractures of the base or the diaphysis of the first phalanx. (Pictures by Grégory Mesplié)

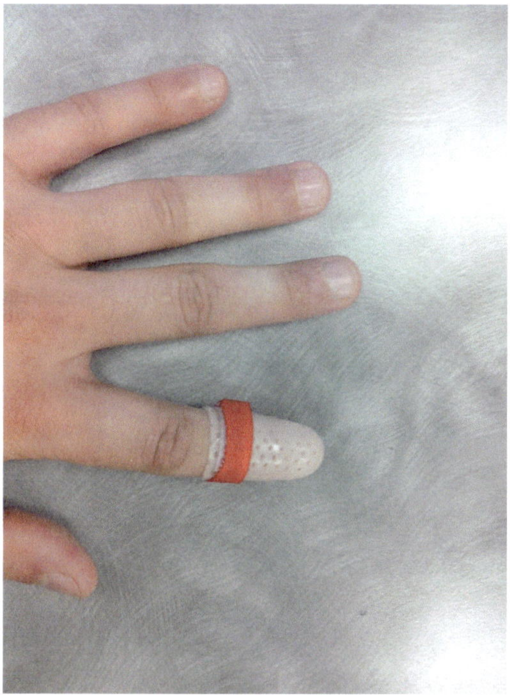

Fig. 2.18 Orthosis after a fracture of the third phalanx letting the proximal interphalangeal joint free. (Pictures by Grégory Mesplié)

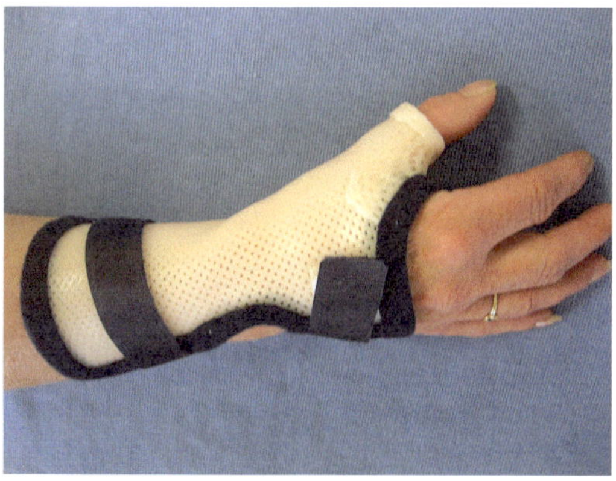

Fig. 2.19 Orthosis immobilizing the wrist and the metacarpophalangeal joint in a neutral position after a stable fracture of the base of the first metacarpal. (Pictures by Grégory Mesplié)

metacarpophalangeal joint free in this case, as the patient can be tempted to grab things between the thumb and the fingers, which can lead to excessive constraints on the base of the first metacarpal.

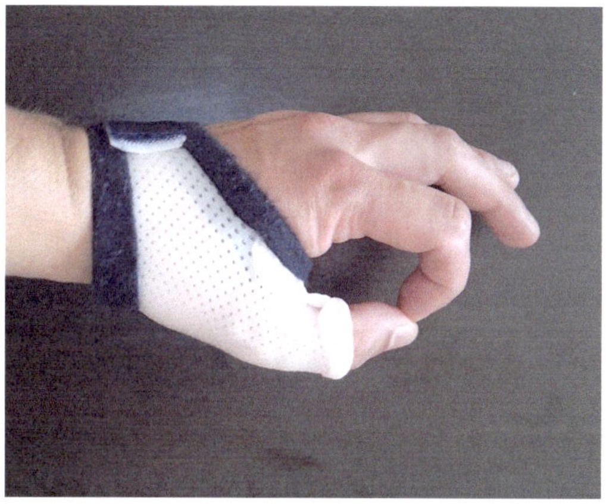

Fig. 2.20 Orthosis after a stable fracture of the diaphysis of the first metacarpal. (Pictures by Grégory Mesplié)

➔ Stable Fracture of the Diaphysis of the First Metacarpal

The orthosis lets the wrist free but maintains the thumb in a functional position, with a good commissural opening (Fig. 2.20).

➔ Unstable Fracture of the First Metacarpal

We realize the same orthosis than for the fracture of the base of the first metacarpal.

➔ Stable Fracture of the Base of the First Phalanx

The orthosis places the metacarpophalangeal joint in a functional position, with the interphalangeal joint free.

Careful: some patients have a very wide first phalanx head, in comparison to the diaphysis. This particularity makes it impossible to mold the orthosis as close as possible to the first phalanx, as the orthosis could be impossible to take off. In these cases, we immobilize the interphalangeal straight, at least until the first radiologic control (D15).

➔ Stable Fracture of the Diaphysis of the First Phalanx

We place the metacarpophalangeal joint in a functional position and the interphalangeal joint straight (Fig. 2.21).

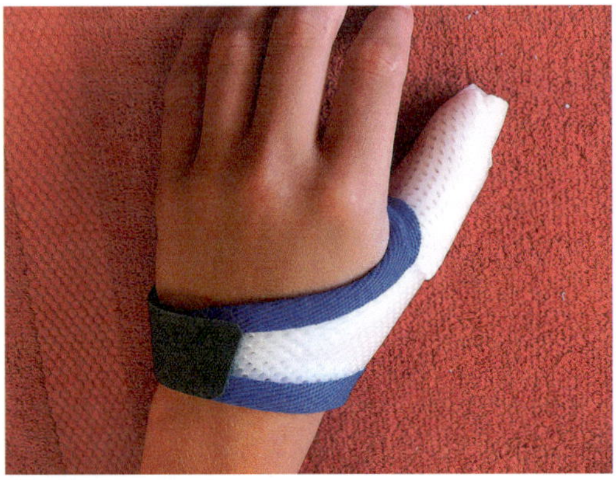

Fig. 2.21 Orthosis after a stable fracture of the diaphysis of the first phalanx, metacarpophalangeal joint in a functional position and interphalangeal joint straight. (Pictures by Grégory Mesplié)

➔ Stable Fracture of the Head of the First Phalanx
The orthosis is a tube placing the interphalangeal joint straight (Fig. 2.22).

➔ Unstable Fracture of the First Phalanx
We immobilize the metacarpophalangeal joint in a functional position and the interphalangeal joint straight.

➔ Stable or Unstable Fracture of the Second Phalanx
A "thimble" places the interphalangeal joint straight.

Rehabilitation

Describing a specific protocol for each type of fracture does not have any practical interest. In this type of pathologies, the surgeon faces six different situations:

- Immediate mobilization for partial and/or stable fractures.
- Orthotic immobilization for unstable fractures when it is impossible to realize an osteosynthesis (deteriorated general condition of the patient, refusal to undergo surgery, etc.)
- Orthopedic reduction with a good stability allowing early mobilization.
- Orthopedic reduction, with instability requiring percutaneous techniques for an early mobilization.
- Bloody reduction and "unstable" osteosynthesis, leading to immobilization (3 to 6 weeks).
- Strong osteosynthesis and early mobilization.

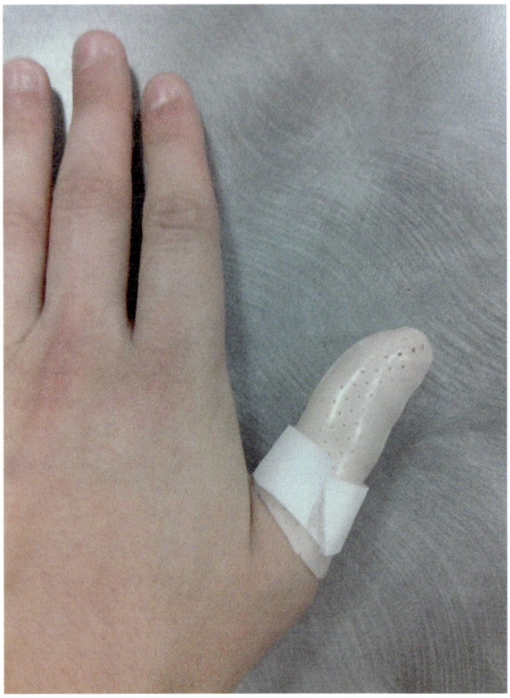

Fig. 2.22 Orthosis placing the interphalangeal joint straight after a stable fracture of the head of the first phalanx. (Pictures by Grégory Mesplié)

The therapist is then left with two situations:

- Immediate mobilization, in the case of stable fracture or after a strong osteosynthesis. This is the ideal option because it allows early mobilization, which is essential for good functional results and limited complications such as stiffness or the development of complex regional pain syndrome (CRPS) [10–12].
- Immobilization after unstable fracture (with or without osteosynthesis).

Rehabilitation Protocol (Fig. 2.23)

The described protocol concerns the fractures that need immobilization. When the immediate

a Fractures of the metacarpals and phalanges

	Post-operative (A)	Relative fragility (B)	Consolidation phase (C)
REHABILITATION	<u>Therapeutic goals</u> : 1- Fight against trophic disorders 2- Fight against pain 3- Prevent stiffness 4- Prevent fonctional exclusion <u>Techniques:</u> 1- Draining massages and compressive bandage, vacuotherapy, electrotherapy (tonolysis) 2- Cryotherapy, TENS, TVS (100Hz) 3- Passive then active mobilizations of the free joints (until tension) 4- TVS (70-80Hz) and varied sensitive stimulation (without constraint) <u>Risks:</u> Stiffness and/or trophic disorders if inadequate mobilizations, type 1 CRPS, vicious callus/pseudarthrosis (especially if there is an orthopaedic treatment)	<u>Therapeutic goals :</u> 1- Same as in phase A, intensify si necessary 2- Total recovery of joint amplitudes (pain free) 3- Muscular awakening <u>Techniques:</u> 1- Pressotherapy (drainage), vacuotherapy (scar) and defibrosing massage if the scar is closed and non-inflammatory (A1), manipulations of light objects (A4) 2- Electrostimulation, fluidotherapy, passive then active mobilizations (except in joint fractures) soft postures and intrinsic stretching (except if they put contraints on the callus) 3- After D45, static then dynamic contractions of the muscle opposed to the potential deformation, with moderate resistance <u>Risks:</u> Same as phase A , functional exclusion (especially index)	<u>Therapeutic goals :</u> 1- Save as in previous phases, intensify si necessary 2- Complete fonctional recovery <u>Techniques:</u> 1- Intensify the specific joint mobilizations, stretching of the intrinsic musculature, postures and electrostimulation (B2) 2- Functional activities adapted to the patient's professional and sporting needs, recovery of normal muscular ratios <u>Risks:</u> Same as in phases A and B
ORTHOSIS	Immobilization orthosis adapted to the type of fracture - worn constantly except during rehabilitation	1- Progressively taking the immobilization orthosis off (night, light activities → more intense activities) 2- Postural orthosis after D45 (soft tension but worn during large periods)	1- Progressively taking the immobilization orthosis off (more intensive activity → high-risk activities) 2- Postural orthosis, adapting the modalities of the results are not satisfactory
	D3 to D21/45	D21/45 to D90	After D90

b

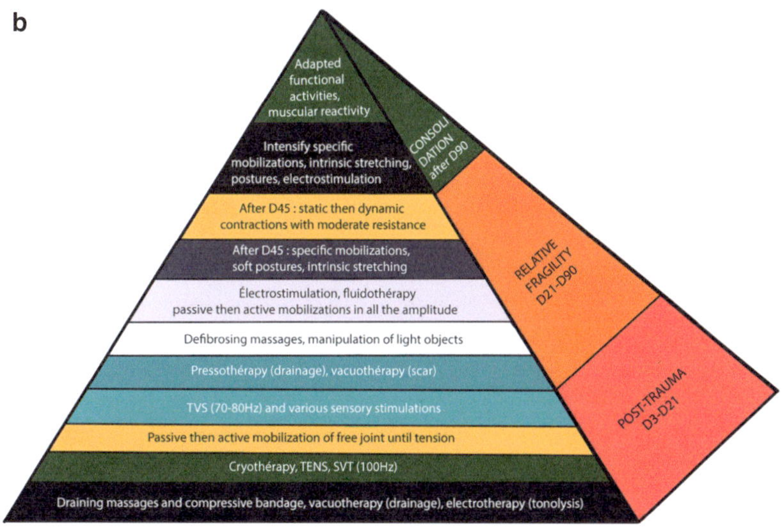

Fig. 2.23 Rehabilitation protocol (**a**) and progression pyramid (**b**)

mobilization is possible, the protocol starts in phase (B), or fragility phase, using techniques with an increasing intensity for trophic disorders and pain.

➔ Immobilization Phase—D3 to D21 (Orthopedic Treatment) or D21/45 (Osteosynthesis)

In this phase rehabilitation is often limited to self-rehabilitation exercises and control of the orthosis. However, some other things can be done if there is a bad evolution or if the initial trophic disorders are important. The period from D0 to D3 is a period of strict immobilization with a compression dressing, allowing the hand to rest and limiting the risk of edema and/or pain developing (Fig. 2.24).

- *Fight Against Trophic Disorders and Pain*

The treatment is based on the PRICE protocol:

- P for protection of the fracture site throughout this whole phase, achieved by immobilization and making the patient aware of the fragility of the tissue.
- R for rest of the traumatized area, which should not be used during the entire immobilization period, apart from self-rehabilitation exercises provided by the rehabilitator.
- I for "ice" with icing of the fractured area several times a day. This technique is sometimes poorly tolerated digitally and in this case should be applied proximally to the traumatized area.
- C for compression, with a compression bandage worn at night if the edema is under control, but which may be worn permanently in the opposite case. The use of a wide, stretchable, and elastic bandage in the width and length directions makes it possible to limit the thickness of the system so as not to prevent daytime mobilization (Fig. 2.25).
- E for elevation of the hand for the same anti-edematous purpose.

- *Active Self-Mobilizations of the Free Joints*

This essential work to prevent the onset of stiffness [13] allows maintaining joint amplitude, mobilizing tendinous and retinacular elements in relation to the fracture site, and improving the overall trophicity of the hand by stimulating the "vis a latere" (muscular venous pump).

The exercises include analytical and then global mobilizations, as well as tendon gliding exercises [14]. They are performed every hour in sets of 10 repetitions, except in the case of pain or increased edema, when they are temporarily stopped.

- *Maintaining the Motor Pattern*

The use of Transcutaneous Vibratory Stimulation (TVS) at a frequency of 70–80 Hz at the myotendinous junctions stimulates the motor

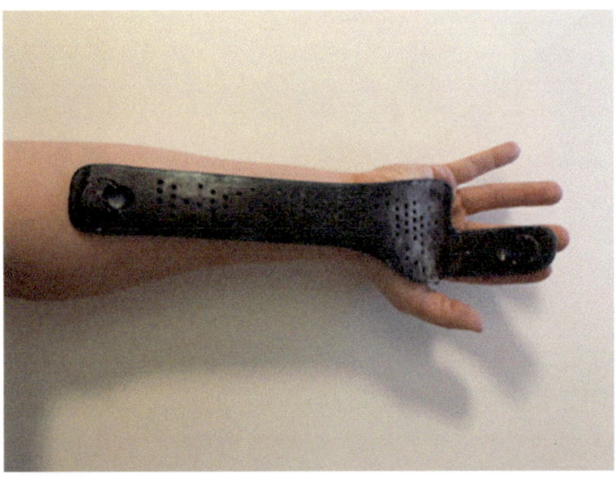

Fig. 2.24 Orthosis printed with a 3D printer (Xkelet©) to immobilize the hand in a suitable position, combined with a compressive bandage for the first 3 days post-trauma/surgery. (Pictures by Grégory Mesplié)

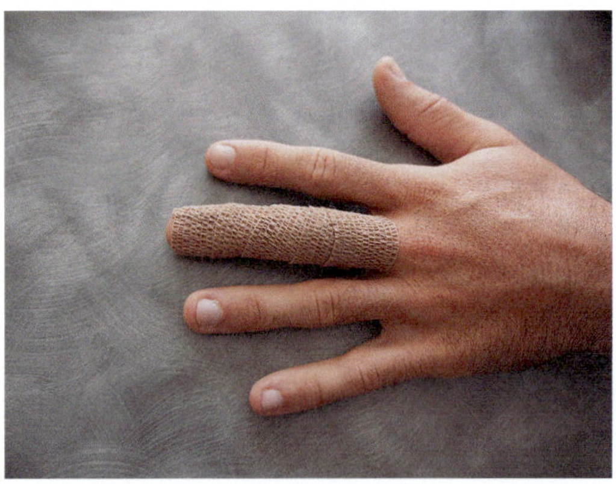

Fig. 2.25 Compressive bandage to fight against trophic disorders. (Pictures by Grégory Mesplié)

and pre-motor areas, limiting disturbances to the motor pattern and proprioception [15].

- *Orthosis Control and Fight against a Possible Angulation/Bad Rotation*

A regular control of the orthosis is realized to check if there aren't any problems of fulcrum, bad rotation, or bad angulation.

When these troubles are moderate, the orthosis can be adapted to limit their evolution (foam spacers opposed to the angulation, syndactyly with the finger opposed to the rotatory trouble, etc.). But above all, it is important to inform the surgeon about this type of evolution, in order not to lose time if another surgery is necessary.

➔ Relative Fragility Phase—D21 (Orthopedic Treatment) or D21/45 (Surgery) to D90

- *Fight Against Trophic Disorders and Pain*

This is an essential element, as it determines our possibilities for the other goals. Therefore, it is the essential and priority element in this phase and can use:

- In the event of surgery, massages around the scar may be done if the recoloration time in the vitro-pressure test is greater than 2 s. Relaxing massages of the forearm can also be performed if hypertonia of the extrinsic musculature is observed, which is often the case.
- Analgesic or tenolysis electrotherapy can be used, using the methods described in the chapter "Physical Agents" in Volume 1 [16, 17].
- Pressotherapy with stepped compression at the proximal and distal ends, which helps to drain the hand (see chapter "Physical Agents—Pressotherapy" in Volume 1). At this stage, the technique may not be well tolerated by the patient, in which case we will use it later.

Transcutaneous vibratory stimulation and infrasound are used for their analgesic and vasomotor effects, as described in chapter "Physical Agents—Mechanical Waves" in Volume 1 [17]. Out of caution, vibrations with an amplitude greater than 1 mm are performed far from the fracture site to avoid the risk of disrupting the healing process.

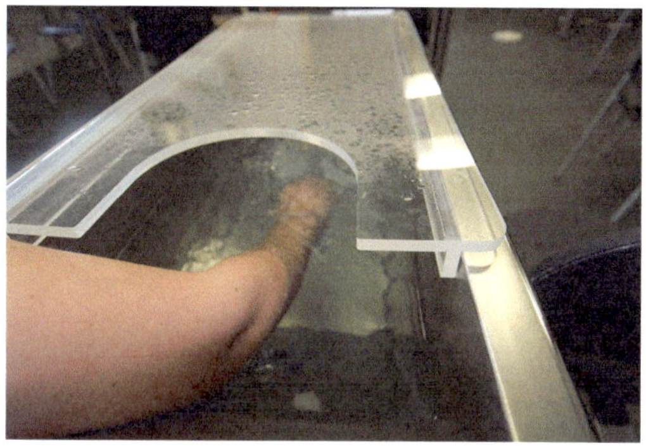

Fig. 2.26 Soft active mobilization in hot baths, improving viscoelasticity of the connective tissue. (Pictures by Grégory Mesplié)

- *Soft Recovery of the Amplitudes in the Immobilized Joints*
- *Fluidotherapy* (Fig. 2.26)

These techniques (hot water, corn dust, hot air, etc.) increase the viscoelasticity of the tissues and therefore improve mobility. We ask the patient to realize slow active mobilizations until he feels a sensation of tension during the whole treatment (approximately 20′).

- *Depressotherapy*

It is mainly used after a surgery around the scar but can also be interesting if there are adherences in the extensor system (frequent after this kind of injuries).

- *Massages Against Adherences*

Like depressotherapy, these massages are important mainly after a surgery around the scar. They also help fighting against fibrosis, which is present as well when there is no surgery.

- *Active Electrotherapy*

It is usually used after relaxing the retracted tissues, to limit the resistances when mobilizing, which can lead to tendinopathies of the "motor" muscles.

We ask the patient to actively mobilize his fingers during the electrostimulation, to maintain his motor pattern and optimize the recuperation of the joint amplitudes. This exercise is realized in all the areas with a deficit of mobility.

- *Active and Passive Manual Mobilizations*

Like electrotherapy, we use these techniques after relaxing the fingers using massages and fluidotherapy to limit the resistances when mobilizing, which can lead to tendinopathies in the working muscles.

During this relative fragility phase, we first use active exercises, which are more reassuring for the patient as he can control the tension in his retracted or adherent tissues. This active mobilization also allows tendon gliding, especially in relation to the fracture site [18].

Passive mobilizations are also used with grips close to the stiff joint, to avoid imposing shear force on it. The mobilization force used may create a feeling of tension or discomfort but must never be painful.

In the case of a joint fracture, there can exist a "came effect" (see chapter "Hand and Wrist Mobilizations" in Volume 1) that limits the mobilization. In this case, strength techniques must not be used, as it could accelerate the degenerative processes occurring in the joint. A radiologic exam is therefore essential before starting to recuperate the amplitudes.

From D45, if the radiological assessment shows that the fracture site is stable, specific gentle and painless mobilization maneuvers can be initiated. These are described in detail in the techniques used in the solidity phase.

- *Stretching of the Intrinsic Muscles*

These stretchings are realized if the Finochietto test is positive, which means there is a retraction of the intrinsic muscles, quite frequent in these traumas (Fig. 2.27).

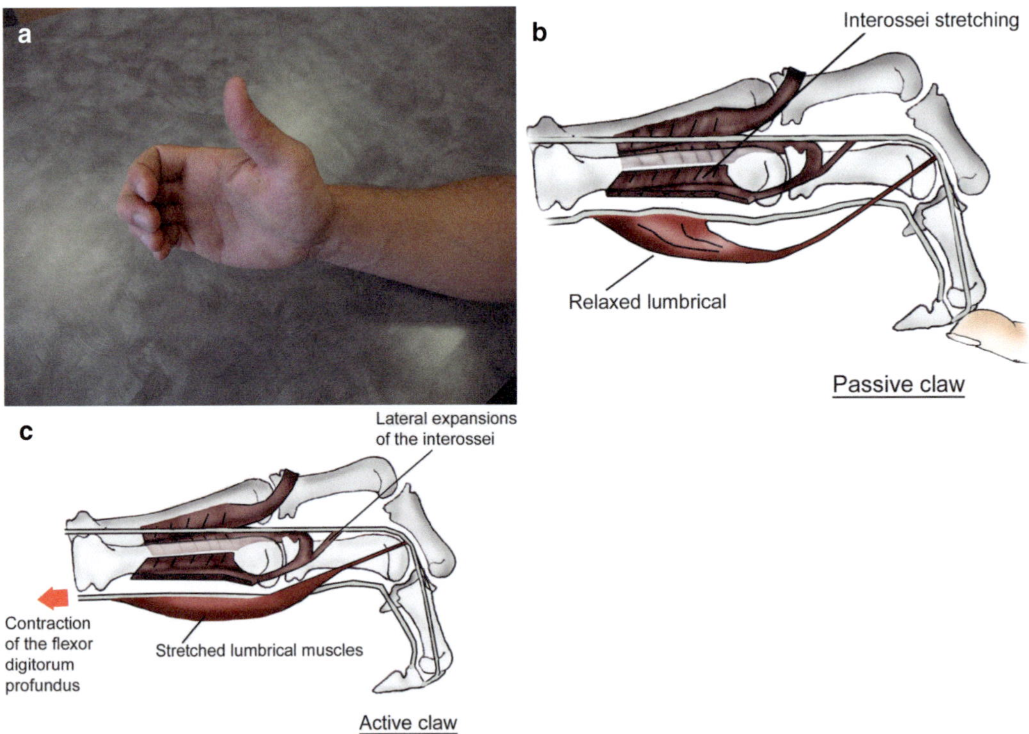

Fig. 2.27 (**a**) Positive Finochietto test; the retraction of the intrinsic muscles makes it impossible to realize active mobilizations in the extrinsic + position. (**b**) The passive placement in the extrinsic + position stretches the interossei but not the lumbrical muscles. (**c**) The extrinsic + position combined with a wrist extension stretches the lumbrical muscles by creating a disto-proximal displacement of the flexor tendons

We stretch these muscles passively putting the hand in an "extrinsic +" position. To stretch the lumbrical muscles, we add a wrist extension to this position to put tension on the proximal part of the lumbrical muscles.

These stretchings must be soft and well tolerated by the patient. If they are not tolerated in this phase, we postpone the application of this technique.

- *Computerized Imitation Exercises*

The patient must imitate exercises displayed on a screen. The models are defined depending on the patient's joint limitations.

- *Proprioceptive Abilities*

It is important to propose a coherent evolution for the exercises depending on the healing phase, in order not to disturb the consolidation process. The recovery stage of the proprioceptive abilities must also be considered so that the patient does not develop compensative pathologies such as tendinopathies or reflex contractures.

- *Perception of Joint Position (Hagert's Stage 3)*

It is defined as the ability to precisely reproduce a given joint angulation [19].

The rehabilitation of this perception is done in three steps. In the first step, the therapist places the patient's wrist in a defined joint position and controls the joint amplitude with a goniometer.

In the second step, the wrist is placed in another position, indifferently. In the third step, the patient must place his forearm in the first position [19, 20].

The exercise is realized with the patient's eyes closed to avoid any visual afference.

This test is highly correlated with the hand's sensorimotor abilities [20] and must therefore be done before any evolution of the rehabilitation protocol—especially before Hagert's stage 5.

- *Kinesthesia (Hagert's Stage 4)*

It is defined as the ability to detect a passive movement. The therapist realizes the movement while the patient keeps his eyes closed and tells him when he perceives the movement.

This exercise is easy to realize at the physiotherapy office or at home but does not allow a precise analysis regarding the patient's perception threshold.

Using an arthromotor device allows analyzing more precisely the movement speed and the studied angular sector.

A laser can also be a very helpful tool to improve conscious proprioceptive abilities. The patient must follow trajectories becoming increasingly complex, going faster and faster.

- *Conscious Neuromuscular Rehabilitation (Hagert's Stage 5)*

Several strengthening modes have been described to improve neuromuscular abilities. They help increase the basic muscle tone and therefore the joint's dynamic stability [21].

We ask the patient to realize isometric contractions with a low intensity during 6 s. Thirty repetitions or less are done, considering that it must not create any pain or secondary trophic disorder.

The contractions must under no circumstances put torsion or distraction constraints on the callus, as it is not strong in this phase.

The exercises depend on where the fracture is:

- Fracture of the base of the fifth metacarpal: exercise for the intrinsic muscles in the axis of the fingers, sustain of the palmar side of the metacarpals (Fig. 2.28). No solicitation of the extensor carpi ulnaris that tends to displace the osseous fragment.
- Fracture of the base of the second and third metacarpals: exercise for the intrinsic muscles in the axis of the fingers, with a palmar sustain. No work with the radial extensors of the carpus that end on the base of the second and third metacarpals.
- Fracture of the base of the first metacarpal: exercise for the opponent pollicis sustaining the palmar side of the first metacarpal. No work with the abductor pollicis longus that ends on the radial side of the base of the first metacarpal. Working with the abductor pollicis brevis and the flexor pollicis brevis

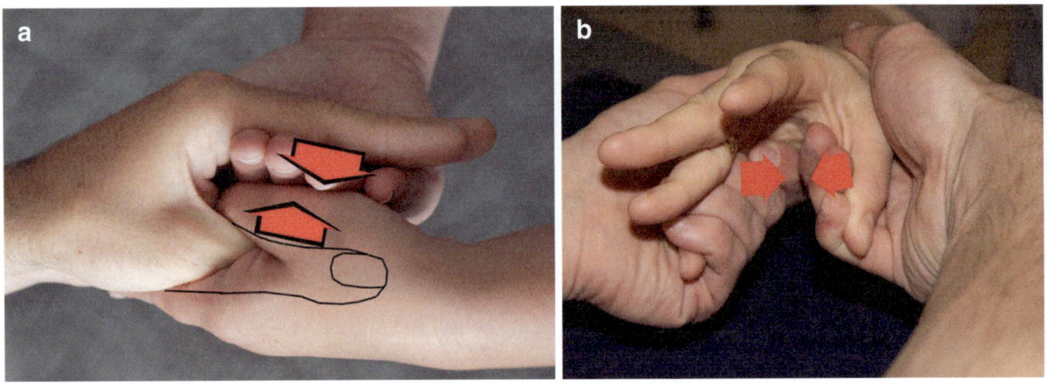

Fig. 2.28 Exercise for the intrinsic muscles after a fracture of the base of the metacarpals. This exercise is not realized at this stage in the fractures of the diaphysis of the metacarpals, as it can favor the anterior tilt of the distal fragment

tends to displace the first metacarpal in a palmar direction and therefore is not recommended.

- Fracture of the diaphysis of the metacarpals: muscular awakening of the thenar and hypothenar muscles. No work with the interossei, because their role of flexion of the metacarpophalangeal joints tends to displace the distal fragment in a palmar direction. To limit this tendency for the head of the metacarpal to tilt anteriorly, it is better to ask for a contraction of the interosseous muscles when the metacarpophalangeal joint is extended. In this position, the dorsal expansion slides from distal to proximal without applying anterior force to the head of the metacarpal.
- Fracture of the diaphysis of the first phalanx: same as before, because the interossei tend to displace the proximal fragment in a palmar direction. We do not work with the extensor system that tends to displace the distal fragment dorsally.
- Fracture of the diaphysis of the second phalanx: no work with the flexor digitorum superficialis and the extensor system that tend to displace the fragments in one direction or another depending on the localization of the fracture line.

Active electrostimulation of the abovementioned muscles can also be done according to the methods described in the chapter "Electrotherapy" of Volume 1 [17].

- *Proprioceptive and Functional Exercises*

This is achieved by realizing prehension, dexterity, and intermuscular coordination exercises.

➔ Consolidation Phase (After D90)

- *Full Recovery of the Joint Amplitudes*

We intensify the techniques used in the previous phase and add some specific mobilization techniques, realized in a decoaptation position, especially in joint fractures.

- *Fingers*
  - The metacarpophalangeal joint (Fig. 2.29): in the sagittal plane, the kinematics of the metacarpophalangeal joint allow a flexion/extension movement completed by a sliding movement, depending on the concavity rule (Fig. 2.30).

  In the frontal plane, the joint also allows an abduction/adduction movement in the extension position only, because in this position the collateral ligaments are relaxed [22] (Fig. 2.31). In the transversal plane, there are automatic axial rotation movements accompanying the sagittal movements (Fig. 2.32).
- Rotation during flexion is slightly pronator for the index finger and supinator for the other three fingers, with an increasing amplitude towards the ulnar fingers [23].
  - The proximal interphalangeal joint: in the sagittal plane, there are two simultaneous

Fig. 2.29 Summary table of the movement combinations when mobilizing the metacarpophalangeal joints

	Mobilization in flexion	Mobilization in extension
Frontal plane	-	Abduction/adduction
Transversal plane	Index : slight pronation Other fingers : supination	Index : slight supination Other fingers : pronation
Gliding	Anterior	Posterior

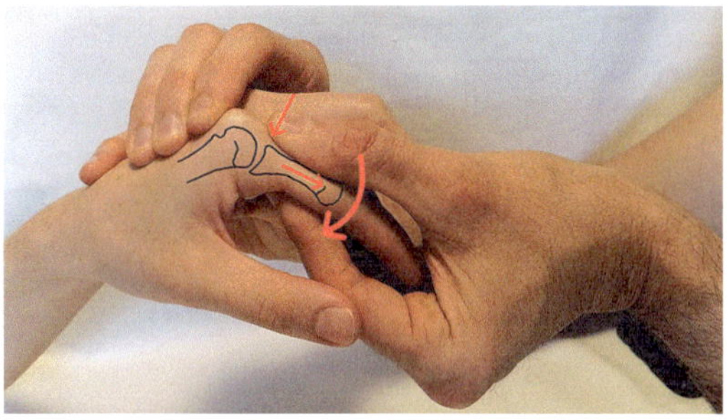

Fig. 2.30 Mobilization / gliding of the metacarpophalangeal joint in flexion

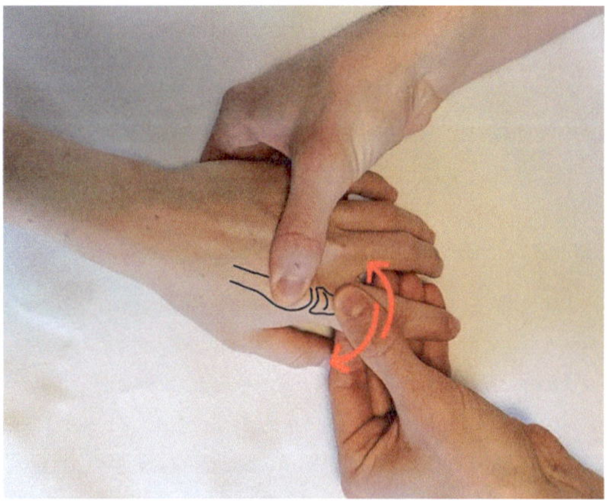

Fig. 2.31 Mobilization / gliding of the metacarpophalangeal joint in abduction/adduction

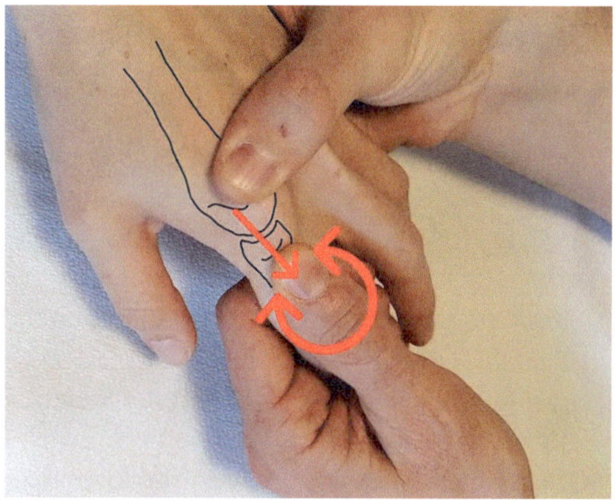

Fig. 2.32 Mobilization / gliding of the metacarpophalangeal joint in rotations

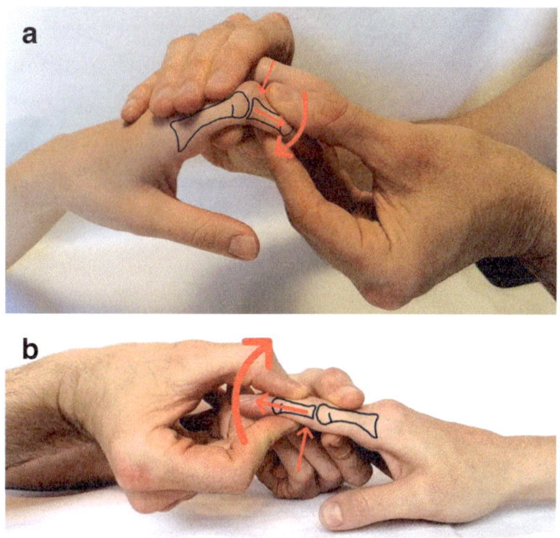

Fig. 2.33 Mobilization / gliding of the proximal interphalangeal joint in flexion/extension

rotational movements around two different centers. One of the centers corresponds to the center of the bending radius of the condyles of the head of the first phalanx, while the second center of rotation corresponds to the center of the bending radius of the cheeks of the base of the second phalanx. In practice, in the sagittal plane, the proximal interphalangeal joint performs a flexion/extension movement, whose instantaneous center of rotation moves with the movement, associated with a translational movement that complies with the concavity rule (Fig. 2.33).

In the frontal plane, the degree of freedom concerns the lateral movements in abduction and adduction. However, these movements are

Fig. 2.34 Summary table of the movement combinations when mobilizing the proximal interphalangeal joints

	Mobilization in flexion	Mobilization in extension
Transversal plane	Index : slight pronation Other fingers : supination	Index : slight supination Other fingers : pronation
Gliding	Anterior	Posterior

stabilized by the collateral ligaments throughout the flexion/extension range, with a position of maximum stability in extension [24].

- In the transversal plane, as with the metacarpophalangeal joints, there is an automatic axial rotation which makes it possible to oppose the pulp of the finger with the pulp of the thumb. This rotation follows the same pattern as for the metacarpophalangeal joints, with a tendency towards pronation for the index finger and towards supination for the other fingers [23]. The kinematics of the proximal interphalangeal joint therefore includes a flexion/extension movement coupled with a sliding movement and an axial rotation movement (Fig. 2.34).
  - The distal interphalangeal joints have been very little studied in the scientific literature. In the sagittal plane, the kinematics of the distal interphalangeal joint combines a flexion/extension movement with a sliding movement in accordance with the concavity rule (Fig. 2.35).
- *Thumb*
  - The trapezo-metacarpal joint: the mobilization techniques should focus on both angular and accessory movements. The therapist's proximal hand immobilizes the base scaphoid/trapezium/trapezoid between its thumb and index. The distal hand grasps the base of the first metacarpal. The therapist then mobilizes the joint along the different axes of angular movement (Fig. 2.28). For an easier joint mobilization, it may be useful to apply a slight decoaptation force through the thumb. Moreover, this axial traction allows mobilizing the joint glidings from distal to proximal.
- For the other accessory movements, dorsopalmar and radioulnar analytical glides are performed. A sliding movement in circumduction can be used to work on accessory movements in a global way (Fig. 2.36).
  - The metacarpophalangeal joint: with one hand, the therapist immobilizes the metacarpal between his thumb and index. With the other, he grasps the first phalanx and creates flexion and extension movements, combining them with accessory movements. For an easier manipulation, the distal hand also applies a decoaptor traction (Fig. 2.37).
  - The interphalangeal joint: the therapist immobilizes the head of the first phalanx and grasps the last phalanx between his index and thumb. With a gentle traction, the therapist mobilizes the joint in flexion and extension with a slight glide in accordance with the rule of concavity (Fig. 2.38).

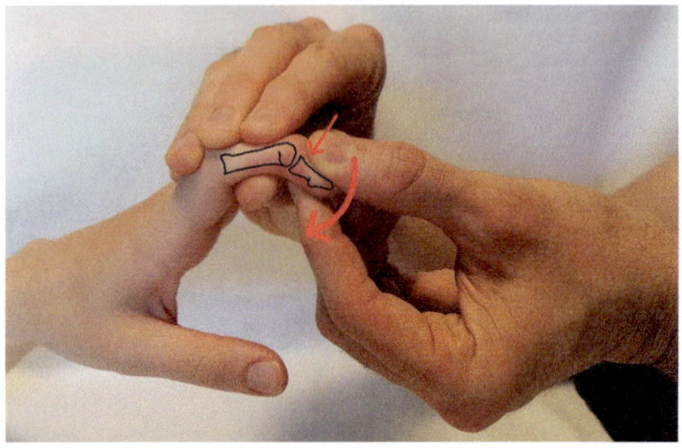

Fig. 2.35 Mobilization / gliding of the distal interphalangeal joint in flexion/extension

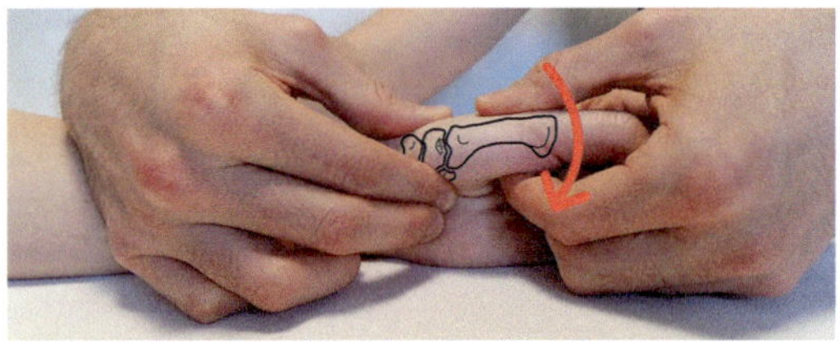

Fig. 2.36 Circumduction of the trapezio-metacarpal joint

- *Full Recovery of Proprioceptive Abilities*

An auxotonic contraction is realized in the forearm and hand muscles to regain the initial strength and the muscular balance between the intrinsic and extrinsic muscles, often impaired in these traumas (Fig. 2.39).

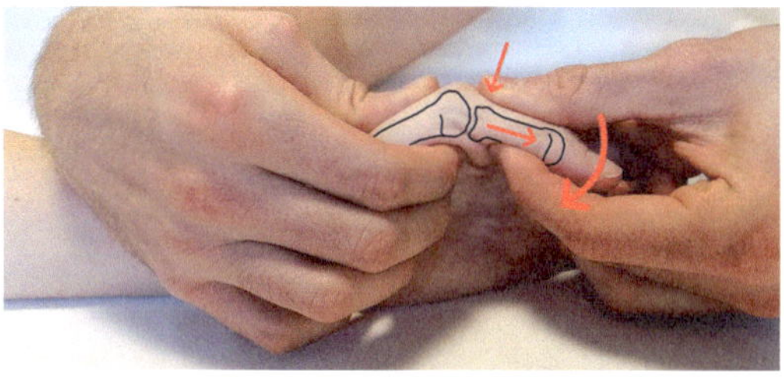

Fig. 2.37 Mobilization / gliding of the thumb's metacarpophalangeal joint in flexion

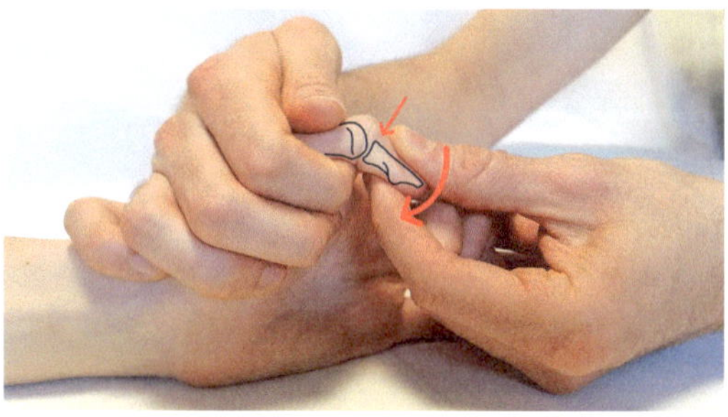

Fig. 2.38 Mobilization / gliding of the thumb's interphalangeal joint in flexion

- *Functional Recovery*

A specific treatment adapted to the patient's needs is made, allowing him to regain an optimal function (proprioception, dexterity, coordination).

Orthotic Treatment to Gain Amplitude

Since the second phase of rehabilitation and in the absence of counter indication related to the evolution of the osseous callus, it is sometimes necessary to realize an orthosis to gain amplitude to optimize the rehabilitation (see chapter "Common Hand and Wrist Orthoses" in Volume 1).

In case of passive and active stiffness, their goal is to increase mobility through an external force. The effectiveness of these orthoses depends on the intensity and duration of the force applied [25]. The best efficiency, which results in tissue growth (rather than elongation of existing fibers), is obtained by applying a low-intensity force (between 100 and 250 g) for a long period (at least 6 hours a day) [26, 27].

In addition, the results obtained are optimized if this protocol is put in place no later than 2 to 3 months after the trauma [27].

In some chronic stiffnesses, especially for the flessum of the proximal interphalangeal joint, they can be worn for several days with satisfactory results [28].

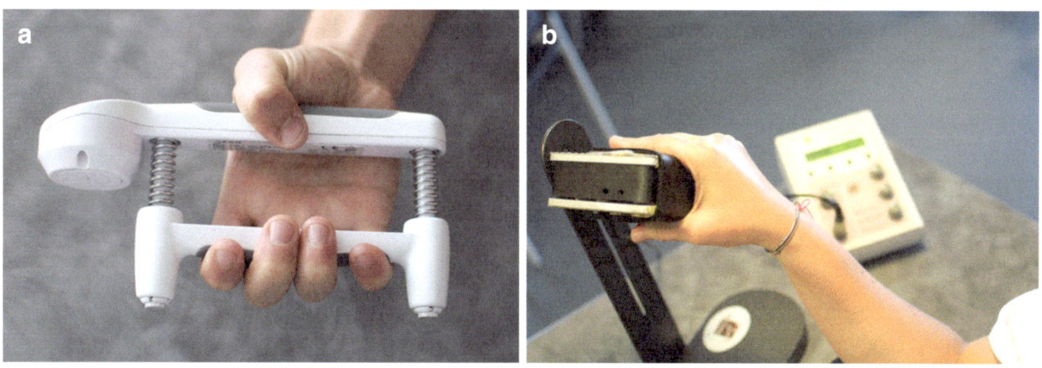

Fig. 2.39 Dynamometer allowing the assessment and the strengthening of the extrinsic (**a**) or intrinsic (**b**) muscles. The goal in this phase is to recover muscular ratios comparable with the healthy side. (Pictures by Grégory Mesplié)

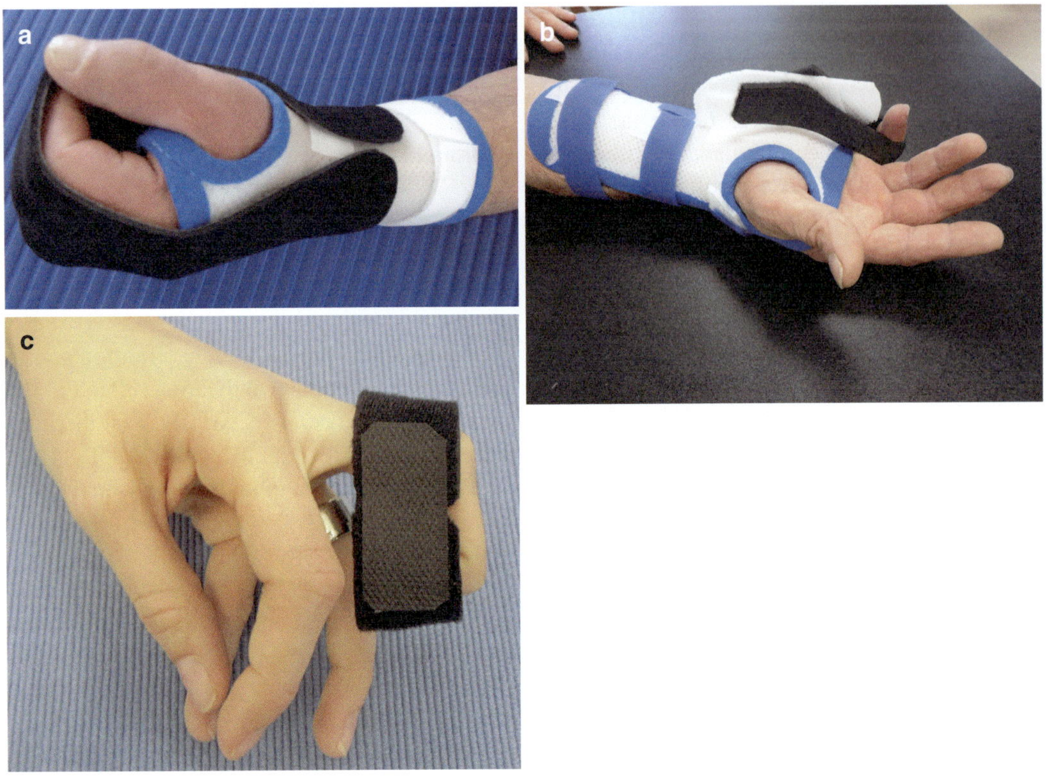

Fig. 2.40 Global winding orthosis (**a**), selective on the metacarpophalangeal joint (**b**) or on the interphalangeal joints (**c**). They are worn several times during the day, 15 minutes each time. (Pictures by Grégory Mesplié)

As the flexion position is very restrictive at the vascular level, winding orthoses are worn for several relatively short diurnal postures (around 20′) (Fig. 2.40), while extension orthoses are more easily supported for a continuous night wear.

Extension orthoses are worn at night and can be global or selective (Fig. 2.41).

In the case of a more marked deficit in active mobility or a disturbance in the motor pattern, the use of torque transmission orthoses is a very good option. The goal of these orthoses is to redirect the internal forces of one or more joints, favoring the action of one muscular system over another. Most often, the effect is obtained by blocking "normal" joints to redirect the muscle power towards the stiff joint [29] (see chapter "Common Orthoses of the Hand and Wrist" in Volume 1).

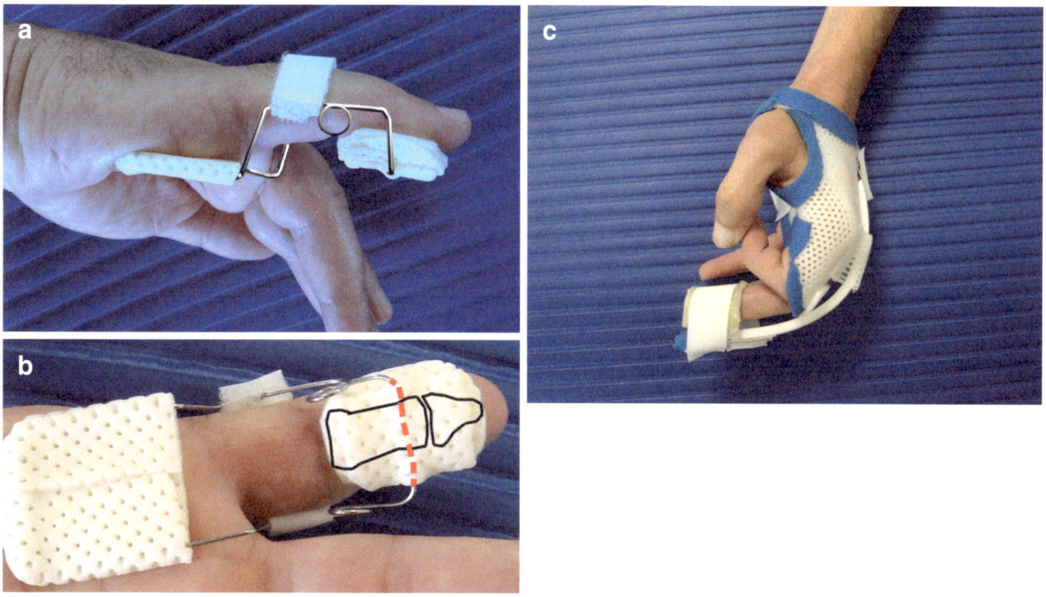

Fig. 2.41 Extension orthosis for the proximal interphalangeal joint (Capener) (**a** and **b**), or global extension orthosis (Levame) (**c**). They are worn during the night. (Pictures by Grégory Mesplié)

Bibliography

1. Toemen A, Midgley R. Hand therapy management of metacarpal fractures: an evidence-based patient pathway. Hand Therapy. 2010;15(4):87–93.
2. Edmunds JO. Traumatic dislocations and instability of the trapeziometacarpal joint of the thumb. Hand Clin. 2006;22(3):365–92.
3. Le Nen D. Extra-articular fractures of the digital metacarpals and phalanges of the long fingers. Chir Main. 2014;33(1):1–12.
4. Liodaki E, et al. Management of difficult intra-articular fractures or fracture dislocations of the proximal interphalangeal joint. J Hand Surg Eur Vol. 2015;40(1):16–23.
5. Peyronson F, et al. Nonoperative versus operative treatment for displaced finger metacarpal shaft fractures: a prospective, noninferiority, randomized controlled trial. J Bone Joint Surg Am. 2023;105(2):98–106.
6. Baratz ME, Divelbiss B. Fixation of phalangeal fractures. Hand Clin. 1997;13(4):541.
7. Beredjiklian PK. Small finger metacarpal neck fractures. J Hand Surg Am. 2009;34(8):1524–6.
8. Khan A, Giddins G. The outcome of conservative treatment of spiral metacarpal fractures and the role of the deep transverse metacarpal ligaments in stabilizing these injuries. J Hand Surg Eur Vol. 2015;40(1):59–62.
9. O'Brien L, Presnell S. Patient experience of distraction splinting for complex finger fracture dislocations. J Hand Ther. 2010;23(3):249. quiz 260
10. Diaz-Garcia R, Waljee JF. Current management of metacarpal fractures. Hand Clin. 2013;29(4):507–18.
11. Markiewitz AD. Complications of hand fractures and their prevention. Hand Clin. 2013;29(4):601–20.
12. Balaram AK, Bednar MS. Complications after the fractures of metacarpal and phalanges. Hand Clin. 2010;26(2):169–77.
13. Meals C, Meals R. Hand fractures: a review of current treatment strategies. J Hand Surg Am. 2013;38(5):1021–31. quiz 1031
14. Ataker Y, et al. Early active motion after rigid internal fixation of unstable extra-articular fractures of the proximal phalanx. J Hand Surg Eur Vol. 2017;42E(8):803–9.
15. Roll R, et al. Illusory movements prevent cortical disruption caused by immobilization. NeuroImage. 2012;62(1):510–9.
16. Mesplié G. Physical agents. In: Hand and wrist therapy : clinical examination and advanced rehabilitation tools. Springer; 2022.
17. Mesplié G. Thérapie de la main, examen clinique et outils de prise en charge rééducative avancée du poignet et de la main. 2021: Sauramps Médical.
18. Hays PL, Rozental TD. Rehabilitative strategies following hand fractures. Hand Clin. 2013;29(4):585–600.
19. Hagert E. Proprioception of the wrist joint: a review of current concepts and possible implications on the rehabilitation of the wrist. J Hand Ther. 2010;23(1):2–16. quiz 17
20. Karagiannopoulos C, et al. Responsiveness of the active wrist joint position sense test after dis-

tal radius fracture intervention. J Hand Ther. 2016;29(4):474–82.
21. Riemann B, Lephart S. The sensorimotor system, part 1: the physiologic basis of functional joint stability. J Athl Train. 2002;37(1):71–9.
22. Sun Y, et al. In vivo metacarpophalangeal joint collateral ligament length changes during flexion. J Hand Surg Eur Vol. 2017;42E(6):610–5.
23. Degeorges R, et al. Rotations of three-joint fingers: a radiological study. Surg Radiol Anat. 2004;26:392.
24. Pang EQ, Yao J. Anatomy and biomechanics of the finger proximal interphalangeal joint. Hand Clin. 2018;34(2):121–6.
25. Nguyen T, et al. Effects of cell seeding and cyclic stretch on the fiber remodeling in an extracellular matrix–derived Bioscaffold. Tissue Eng Part A, 2008.
26. Krotoski J, Breger Stanton DE. The forces of dynamic orthotic positioning: ten questions to ask before applying a dynamic orthosis to the hand. In: Skirven TM, Osterman AL, Fedorczyk J, Amadio PC, editors. Rehabilitation of the hand and upper extremity, 2-volume set: expert consult. Elsevier Health Sciences; 2011.
27. Valdes K, et al. Efficacy of orthotic devices for increased active proximal interphalangeal extension joint range of motion: a systematic review. J Hand Ther. 2018;32:184.
28. Flowers KR, LaStayo PC. Effect of total end range time on improving passive range of motion. J Hand Ther. 1994;25(1):48–54. quiz 55
29. Midgley R, Pisano K. Therapist's management of the stiff hand, in rehabilitation of the hand and upper extremity. Elsevier, Editor; 2021.

3 Capsulo-ligamentous Injuries of the Proximal Interphalangeal Joint

Grégory Mesplié

Volar Plate Sprains

Physiopathology

The volar plate injuries occur during a trauma in hyperextension (Fig. 3.1).

The clinical signs are an important periarticular edema, associated to an anterior hematoma and pain when palpating the anterior part of the joint.

The X-rays can highlight the presence of a little osseous fragment, corresponding to a tearing of the volar plate, always located at the level of the base of the second phalanx [1, 2].

Therapeutical Process and Rehabilitation

If the observed fragment is voluminous, its surgical reinsertion will be realized. It appears that the presence of an avulsion does not have a significant impact on the result obtained when the treatment is carried out correctly [3].

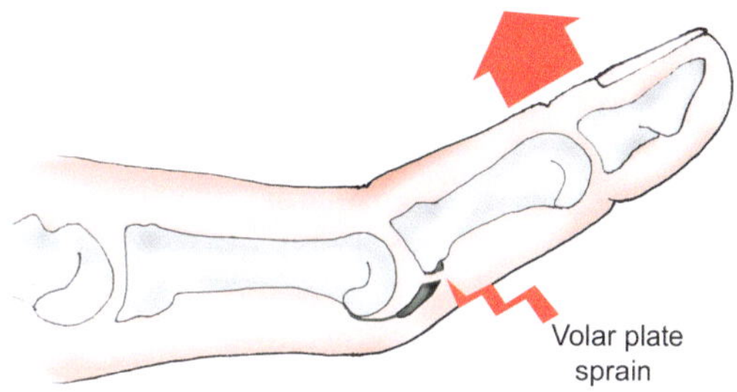

Fig. 3.1 Traumatism in hyper-extension leading to volar plate injuries. (Picture by Josette Mesplié)

In other cases, the treatment is orthotic, combined with an early or immediate mobilization depending on the pain and trophic disorders. The immobilization must not last longer than 3 days to limit the risk of stiffness.

The orthotic treatment consists in realizing a night orthosis placing the interphalangeal joint in extension, and a syndactyly to be worn during the day [4] (Fig. 3.2).

The rehabilitation (Fig. 3.3) must be realized early and with very soft and progressive techniques in order not to "attack" the damaged tis-

G. Mesplié (✉)
Institut Sud Aquitain de la Main et du Membre Supérieur (ISAMMS), Biarritz, France

G. Mesplié (ed.), *Hand Functional Anatomy and Therapy*,
https://doi.org/10.1007/978-3-031-92505-4_3

sues [5–8]. As Madden reminds us: "tissues don't know enthusiasm, but stress."

Acute Phase (D3 to D21)

➔ Fight Against Pain and Trophic Disorders

- Draining massages from distal to proximal, following the neurovascular pedicles.
- Electrotherapy: 1 Hz on the edematous area or 100 Hz for a precise analgesic effect.
- Gaseous cryotherapy allowing a very precise anti-edematous effect on the interphalangeal joint. Cryotherapy also has an interesting analgesic effect (Fig. 3.4).
- Pressotherapy: the device realizes a compression from distal to proximal that drains the hand edema. A soft painless posture in extension can be realized during the treatment. In this phase, this technique can be badly tolerated by the patient, in which case we delay its application.
- Compressive bandage during the night if the edema is important and resistant to treatment [9] (Fig. 3.5).
- Put the hand in an elevated position at home, especially when there is a global edema of the hand (rare case).
- Transcutaneous vibratory stimulations (frequency 50–100 Hz, amplitude >1 mm) are applied on the painful area, moving along the sensitive nerve concerned by the area. If there is pain when contacting with the device, we place it away from the painful area, still on the corresponding nerve. This type of mechanical vibration has a sensorimotor stimulation effect, limiting the risks of functional exclusion.

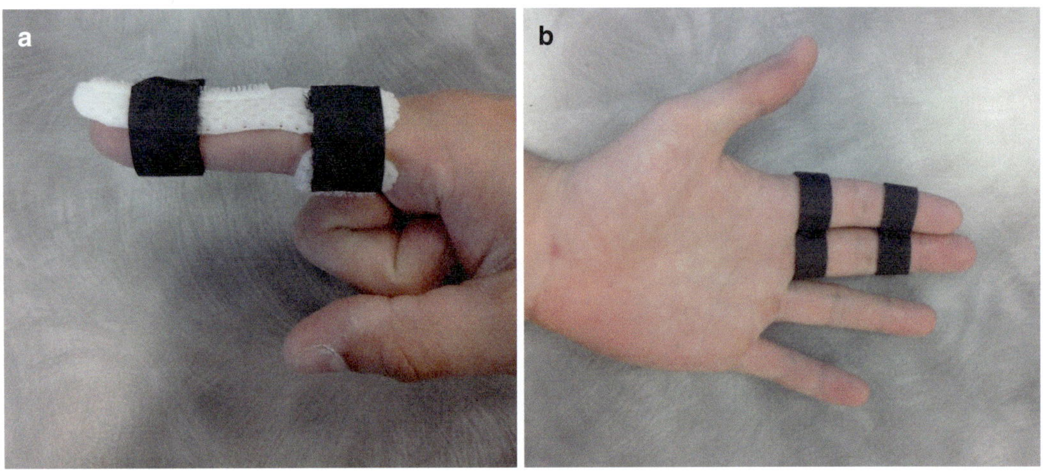

Fig. 3.2 The "proximal interphalangeal stop" in extension is worn during the night (**a**). Diurnal syndactyly liberating the flexion creases of the proximal interphalangeal joint to maintain mobility (**b**). (Picture by Grégory Mesplié)

a

Severe injuries of the volar plate

	Post-trauma (A)	Relative fragility (B)	Consolidation phase (C)
REHABILITATION	**Therapeutic goals** : 1- Decrease trophic disorders 2- Decrease pain 3- Prevent stiffness 4- Prevent fonctional exclusion **Techniques:** 1- Draining massages, vacuotherapy (drainage), electrotherapy (tonolysis) 2- Cryotherapy, TENS, TVS (100Hz) 3- Passive then active mobilizations (until tension) Fluidotherapy (if no inflammation) 4- TVS (70-80Hz) and various sensory stimulations (without constraint) **Risks:** Stiffness and/or trophic disorders if inadequate mobilizations, type 1 CRPS,	**Therapeutic goals :** 1- Same as in phase A, intensify si necessary 2- Total recovery of joint amplitudes **Techniques:** 1- Pressotherapy (drainage) (A1), manipulations of light objects (A4) 2- Electrostimulation, soft joint mobilizations (not antero-posterior), defibrosing, vacuotherapy **Risks:** Same as phase A , functional exclusion (especially index)	**Therapeutic goals :** 1- Save as in previous phases, intensify si necessary 2- Complete fonctional recovery **Techniques:** 1- Postures, intrinsic stretching, electrostimulation (B2) 2- Functional activities adapted to the patient's professional and sporting needs **Risks:** Same as in phases A and B
ORTHOSIS	1- «Proximal interphalangeal stop» (0°) or digital tube in extension during the night + compressive bandage 2- Syndactyly with the adjacent finger during the day +/- compressive bandage	Orthosis to gain amplitude after D45 (soft tension but worn during long periods of time)	Orthosis to gain amplitude, adapting the modalities if the results are not satisfactory
	D3-D21	D21-D60	After D60

b

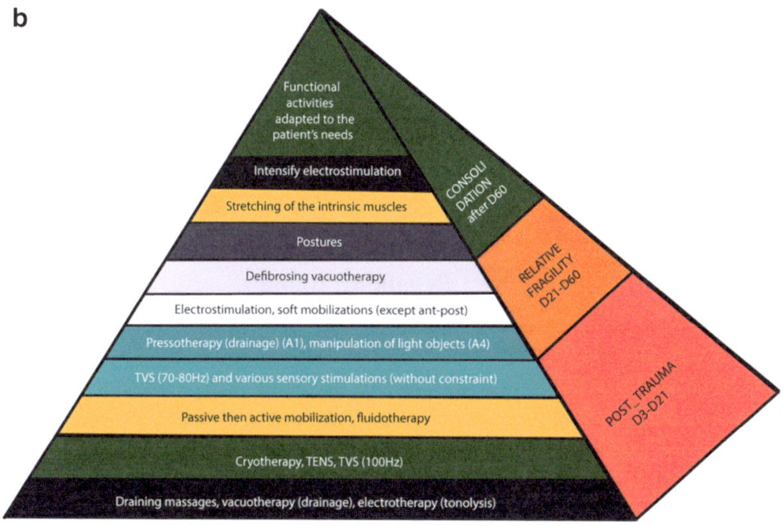

Fig. 3.3 Rehabilitation protocol (**a**) and progression pyramid (**b**) for volar plate sprains. (Picture by Grégory Mesplié)

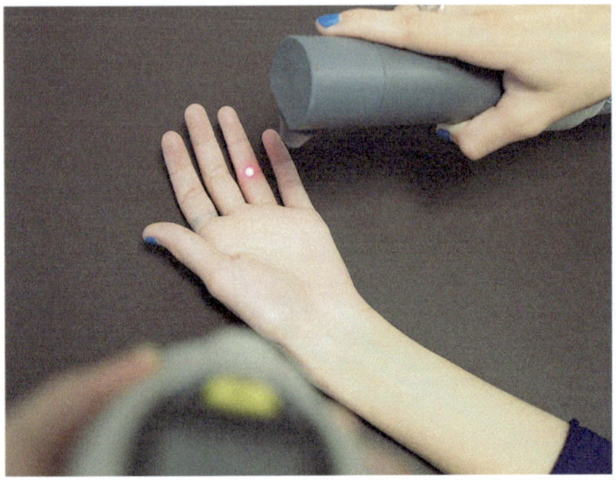

Fig. 3.4 Gaseous cryotherapy in front of the volar plate, controlling the cutaneous temperature with an infrared thermometer. (Picture by Grégory Mesplié)

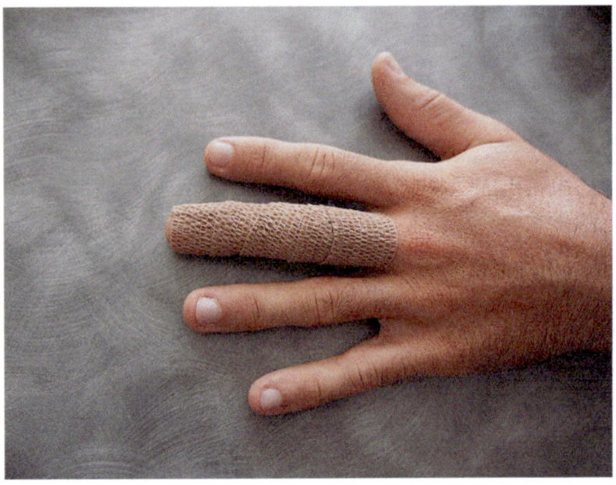

Fig. 3.5 Compressive bandage in case of important edema. (Picture by Grégory Mesplié)

➔ Progressive Recuperation of the Joint Amplitudes

- Passive mobilizations in flexion and active mobilizations in extension, then active in flexion/extension. The soft passive mobilizations in flexion relax the joint, before asking the patient to do an active exercise, which can easily lead to pain.
- Deep massages (punctiform, palpate-roll) to relax the tissues of the palmar elements of the proximal interphalangeal joint, to improve glidings between the different anatomical planes (Fig. 3.6). These techniques are realized without any inflammatory phenomena or pain.

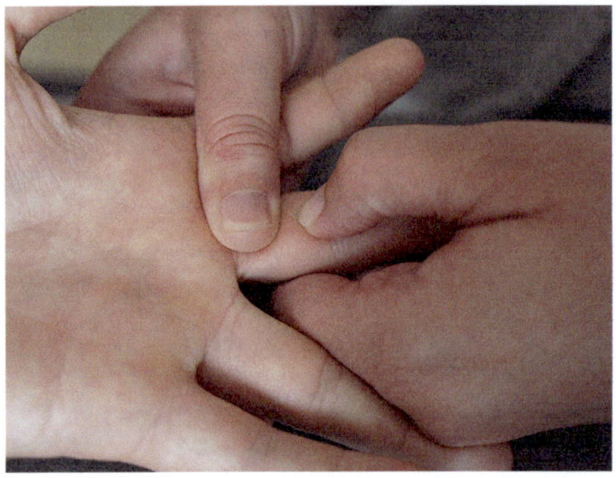

Fig. 3.6 Deep massages to relax the tissues. (Picture by Grégory Mesplié)

➔ Maintaining the Body Mapping

- Transcutaneous vibratory stimulations, varying the frequencies to solicit as many cutaneous and tendinous mechanoreceptors as possible.
- Soft manipulations exercises, soliciting the sensorimotor buckles of prehensility (Fig. 3.7).

Healing Phase (D21 to D60)

➔ Maintaining the Techniques of the Acute Phase If Necessary

If the trophic disorders and pain persist, we keep applying the techniques from the previous phase.

➔ Regaining Mobility

- *Electrostimulation*
  This technique helps regain the joint amplitudes in flexion or extension (Fig. 3.8).
  We preferably use striomotor currents (150–200 µs, 20 Hz). They are ideal for the muscles of the superior limb and stimulate the slow-twitch fibers (type 1).
  The patient associates a voluntary contraction to the electric stimulation (electro-active exercise) to stimulate the motor command, sometimes disrupted after a surgery or a prolonged immobilization.

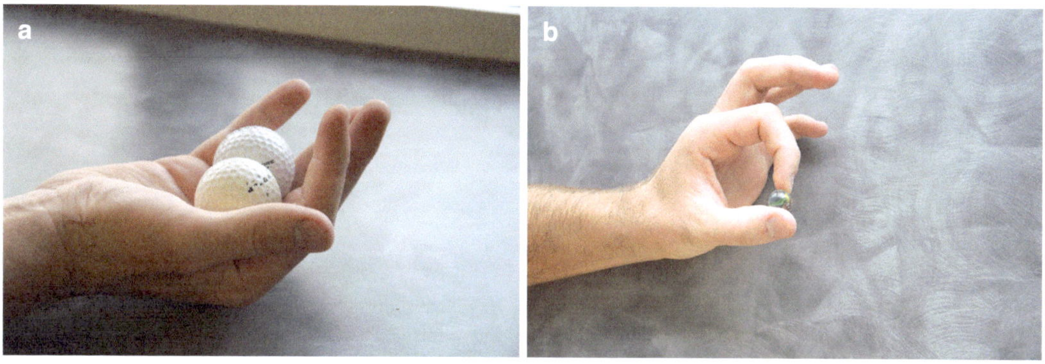

Fig. 3.7 Soft manipulations maintaining the body mapping and working on dexterity. (**a**) Exercise with golf balls (**b**) Exercise with a marble (Picture by Grégory Mesplié)

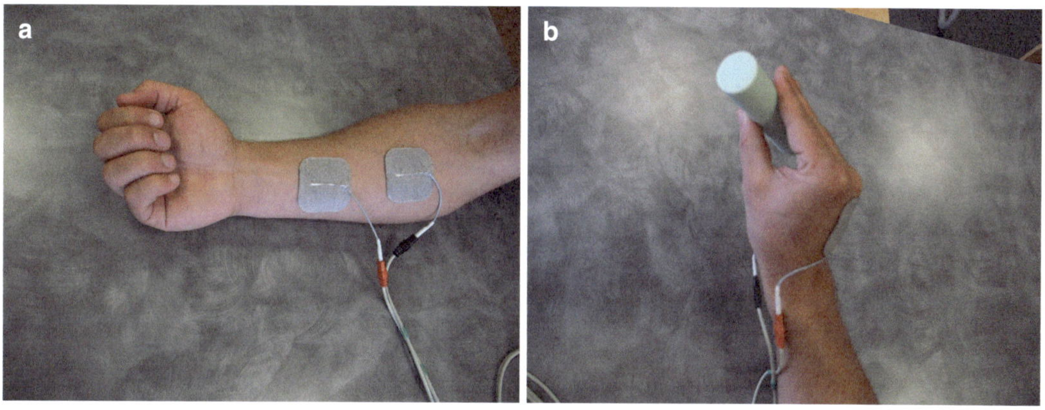

Fig. 3.8 Electro-active exercise winding the fingers, stimulating the corresponding finger flexor (**a**), and in extension of the proximal interphalangeal joint, stimulating the intrinsic muscles of the concerned finger (**b**). Example of the fourth finger on the pictures. (Picture by Grégory Mesplié)

- *Fluidotherapy*
  The fluidotherapy techniques participate in the global relaxation of the hand after this type of intervention. We ask the patient to realize flexion/extension movements and to separate the fingers, in association to the dry or wet fluidotherapy.
- *Specific Mobilizations*
  Decompression and gliding maneuvers of the digital joints allow regaining a good joint mobility, especially in the case of prolonged stiffness (see chapter "Hand and Wrist Mobilizations" in Volume 1) (Fig. 3.9).
- *Stretching of the Intrinsic Muscles*
  We must differentiate the interossei and lumbrical muscles that are not stretched the same way.
  The interossei can be stretched by positioning the hand in an extrinsic + position, reached in active or passive (Fig. 3.10).
  The lumbrical muscles are stretched only if this position is reached with the wrist in extension. This is related to the fact that the lumbrical muscles do not have an osseous proximal insertion but insert on the deep flexors that move from distal to proximal when placing the wrist in extension, allowing their stretching. Therefore, to stretch the lumbrical muscles, the wrist must be placed in extension, with the hand in the extrinsic + position.
- *Computerized Imitation Exercises*
  It consists in imitating the pictures on the screen during all the time they are on display (Fig. 3.11).

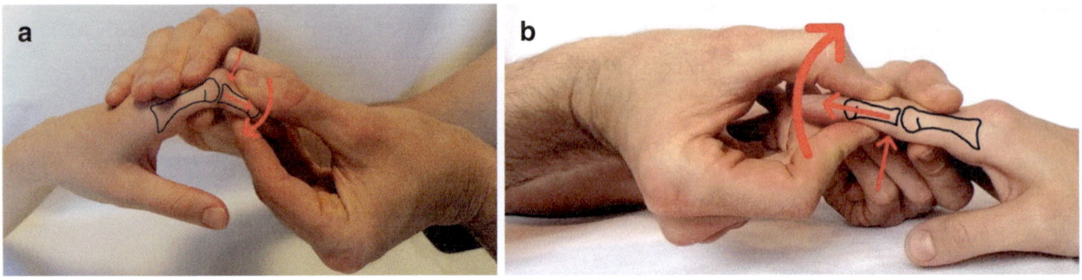

Fig. 3.9 Specific mobilizations of the proximal interphalangeal joint. The flexion is combined with a palmar gliding (**a**), and the extension with a dorsal gliding (**b**). (Picture by Josette Mesplié)

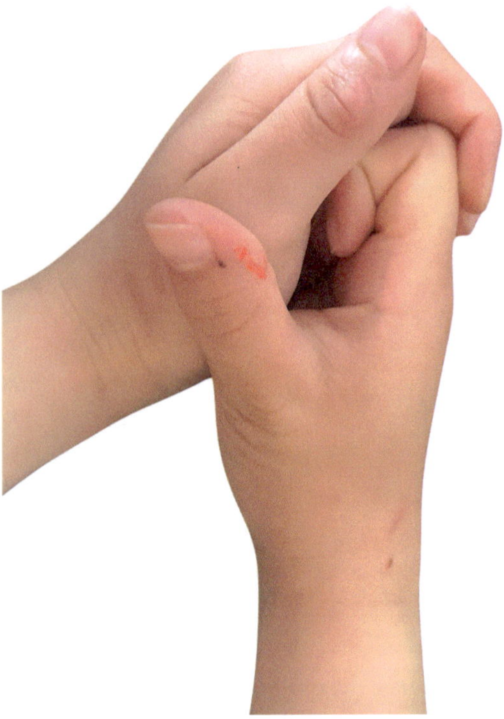

Fig. 3.10 Stretching position of the interossei. To stretch the lumbrical muscles, this posture should be performed with the wrist in extension. (Picture by Grégory Mesplié)

➔ **Prehension**

Manipulating objects improves coordination and dexterity of the operated hand more rapidly and efficiently.

Remodeling Phase (After D60)

All the previous techniques are used more intensively, so the patient can go back to his professional and sports activities. Proprioception, coordination, and dexterity are the most important things to work with in this phase.

Orthotic Treatment

Acute Phase

The orthotic treatment is composed of a tube-shaped orthosis (or "proximal interphalangeal stop") in complete extension, worn during the night, and a diurnal syndactyly with the adjacent finger (second with third fingers and fourth with fifth fingers) (Fig. 3.2).

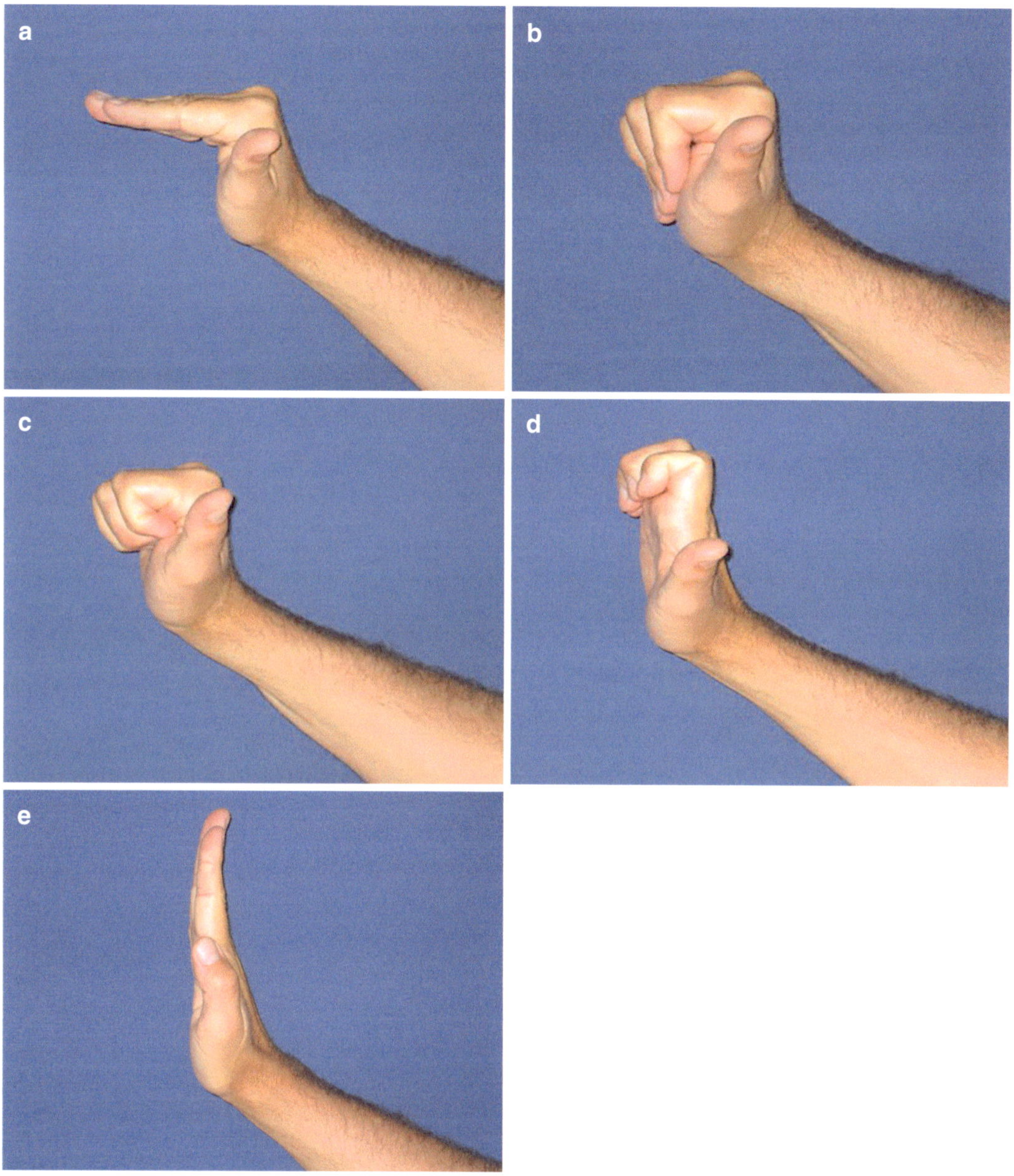

Fig. 3.11 Computerized imitation exercises. (Picture by Grégory Mesplié)

Healing and Remodeling Phases

The orthosis used during these phases helps in regaining the normal joint amplitudes.

We realize static, then dynamic orthoses depending on the evolution of the trophic disorders and ligamentous healing [10, 11] (see book 1 "HAND THERAPY - Clinical Examination and Advanced Tools for the Rehabilitation of the Wrist and Hand", part III "Common hand and wrist orthoses") (Fig. 3.12).

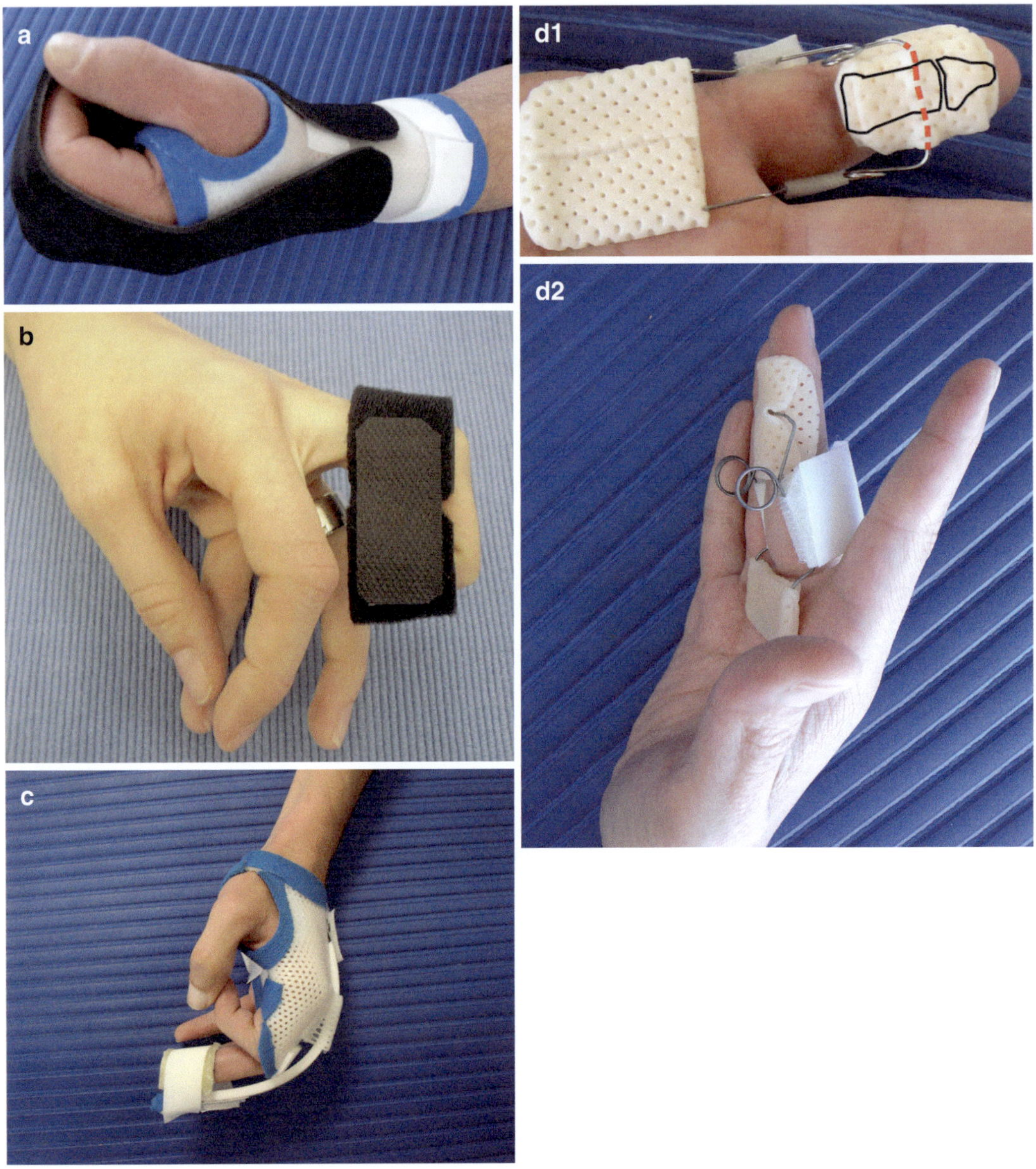

Fig. 3.12 Various dynamic orthoses, helping recover functional amplitudes. Global finger winding (**a**), selective winding of the interphalangeal joints (**b**), extension of the proximal interphalangeal joint with a Levame blade (**c**) or Capener (**d** and **d'**). (Picture by Grégory Mesplié)

Collateral Ligaments Sprains (Fig. 3.13)

The collateral ligament injuries in the proximal interphalangeal joint occur when there is a trauma bringing the proximal interphalangeal joint in valgus/varus on an extended finger (Fig. 3.14).

In case of severe sprain, X-rays can highlight a small osseous fragment on the base of the second phalanx.

A surgical reinsertion can be realized if the fragment is very voluminous, or in the case of a joint fracture, but it is even rarer than for volar plate injuries.

a

Severe collateral ligaments sprains in the proximal interphalangeal joint

	Post-trauma (A)	Relative fragility (B)	Consolidation phase (C)
REHABILITATION	**Therapeutic goals** : 1- Decrease trophic disorders 2- Decrease pain 3- Prevent stiffness 4- Prevent fonctional exclusion **Techniques:** 1- Draining massages, vacuotherapy (drainage), electrotherapy (tonolysis) 2- Cryotherapy, TENS, TVS (100Hz) 3- Passive then active mobilizations (until tension) Fluidotherapy (if no inflammation) 4- TVS (70-80Hz) and various sensory stimulations (without constraint) **Risks:** Stiffness and/or pain and/or trophic disorders if inadequate mobilizations, type 1 CRPS,	**Therapeutic goals :** 1- Same as in phase A, intensify si necessary 2- Total recovery of joint amplitudes **Techniques:** 1- Pressotherapy (drainage) (A1), manipulations of light objects (A4) 2- Electrostimulation, soft joint mobilizations (not lateral), defibrosing, vacuotherapy **Risks:** Same as phase A , functional exclusion (especially index)	**Therapeutic goals :** 1- Save as in previous phases, intensify si necessary 2- Complete functional recovery **Techniques:** 1- Postures, intrinsic stretching, electrostimulation (B2) 2- Functional activities adapted to the patient's professional and sporting needs **Risks:** Same as in phases A and B
ORTHOSIS	Syndactyly with the adjacent finger on the side of the injured ligament +/- compressive bandage	Orthosis to gain amplitude after D45 (soft tension but worn during long periods of time)	Orthosis to gain amplitude, adapting the modalities if the results are not satisfactory
	D3-D21	D21-D60	After D60

b

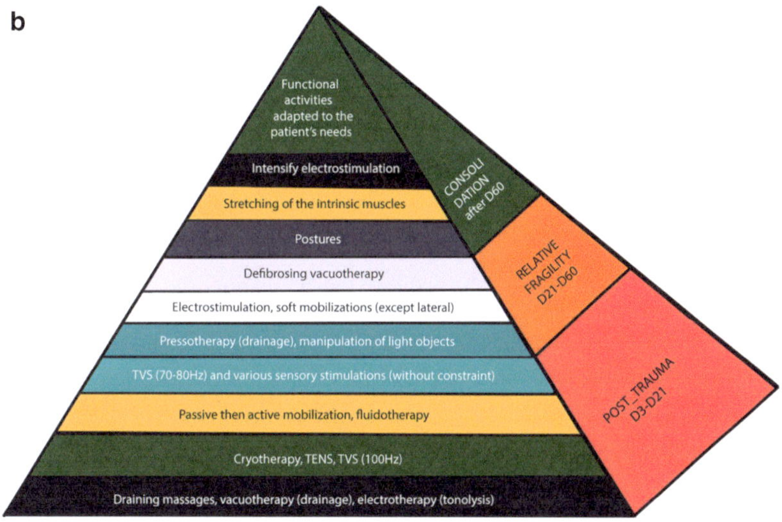

Fig. 3.13 Rehabilitation protocol (**a**) and progression pyramid (**b**) for severe collateral ligaments sprains in the proximal interphalangeal joint. (Picture by Josette Mesplié)

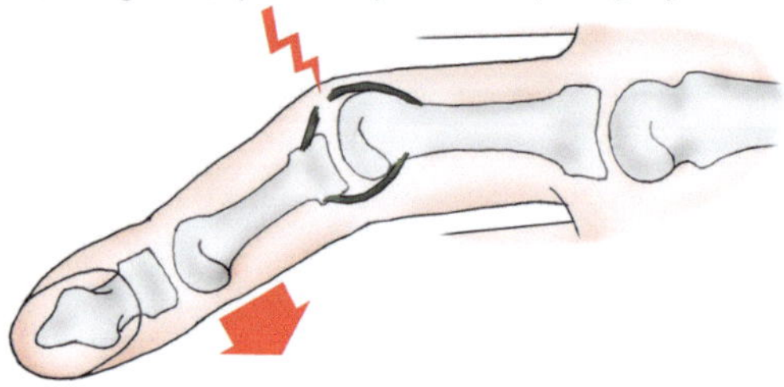

Fig. 3.14 Injury mechanism. (Picture by Josette Mesplié)

In less severe cases, the treatment is mostly orthotic, realizing a syndactyly with the finger adjacent to the damaged collateral ligament [12].

It allows the mobilization of the finger in flexion/extension while limiting the constraints in varus/valgus. This syndactyly is kept between 15 and 21 days.

In severe sprains, a tube-shaped orthosis associated to a compressive bandage can be realized for the first 3 days if the pain and trophic disorders are important.

The rehabilitation protocol uses similar techniques than the ones used in the treatment of the volar plate injuries, adapting the protocol to the anatomical particularities of the collateral ligaments of the proximal interphalangeal joint.

Dislocations

The dislocations are severe injuries of the proximal interphalangeal joint and can lead to stiffness if they are not treated well.

They can be palmar, lateral, or dorsal [13]:

- The dorsal dislocations occur when there is a trauma in hyperextension (like the one in injuries of the volar plate), sometimes combined with a varus or valgus. These dislocations lead to an avulsion of the volar plate at the level of its proximal insertion, and associated injuries of the collateral ligaments (Fig. 3.15).
- The lateral dislocations occur on an extended finger (like in the collateral ligaments sprains). They lead to a rupture of the collateral ligament and an associated injury of the volar plate (Fig. 3.16).
- The palmar dislocations are much rarer [14] and occur when there is a trauma in hyperflexion, sometimes combined with a joint torsion [13]. When there is no joint torsion, they lead to a rupture of the median strip of the extensor system and an associated injury of the principal collateral ligaments (dorsal fibers) or even the volar plate (Fig. 3.17). When associated with a torsion, an injury to the median strip of the extensor is not systematic, as one of the condyles slips between the median and lateral bands, creating an injury to the triangular ligament between the two unaffected bands [13].

The rehabilitation and orthotic treatments of the dorsal and lateral dislocations are similar to the treatments for the injuries of the volar plate with early mobilizations, a diurnal syndactyly, and a night orthosis in extension [15]. However, the treatment of the palmar dislocations is very different.

In fact, in these injuries, we realize a tubular orthosis liberating the distal interphalangeal joint if the active extension is possible after reduction. This allows the healing of the median strip. This orthosis is kept for 3 weeks straight, before starting the proximal interphalangeal joint mobilizations according to the short arc motion protocol (see Chap. 6). The orthosis is kept for 6 weeks (except during the mobilization exercises).

If the extension is impossible, the treatment is surgical to re-insert the median strip.

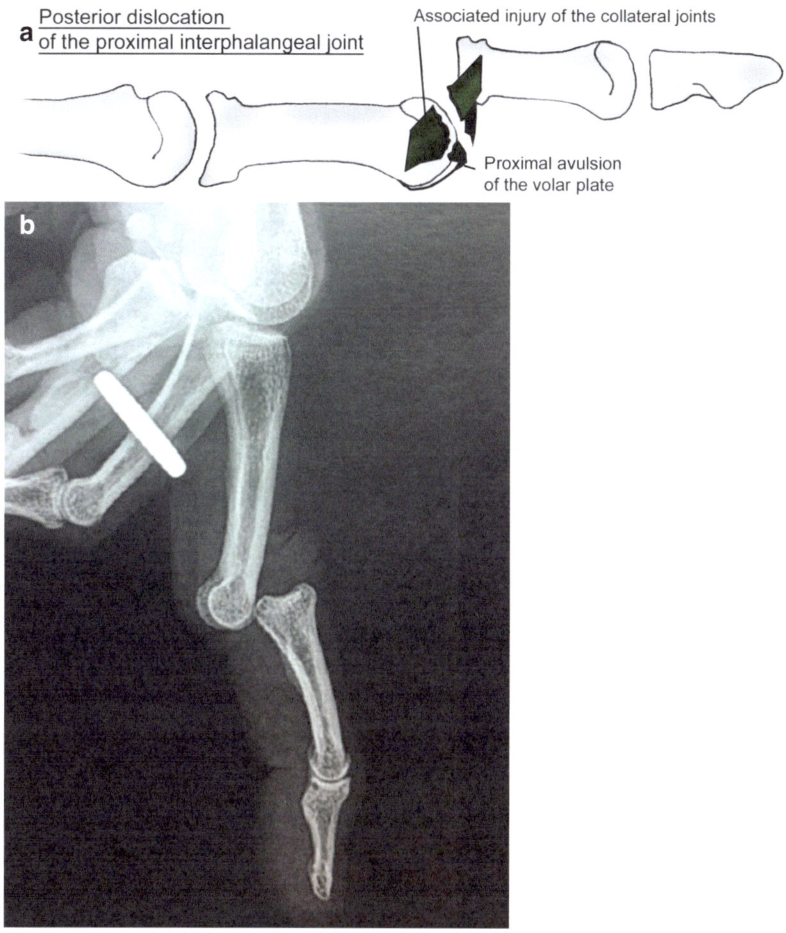

Fig. 3.15 Anatomical injuries in a dorsal dislocation (**a**) and radiography (**b**). (Picture by Josette Mesplié)

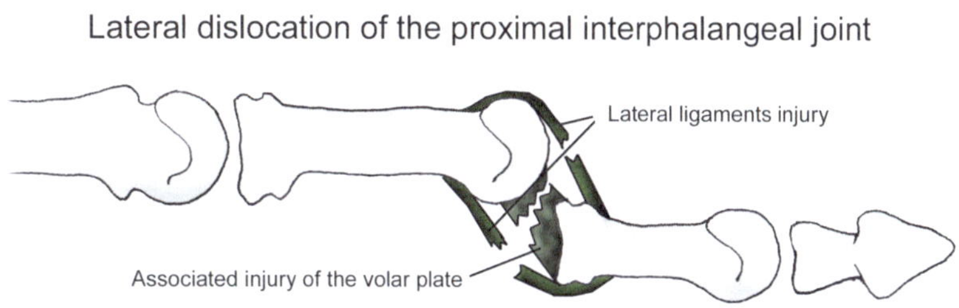

Fig. 3.16 Anatomical injuries in a lateral dislocation. (Picture by Josette Mesplié)

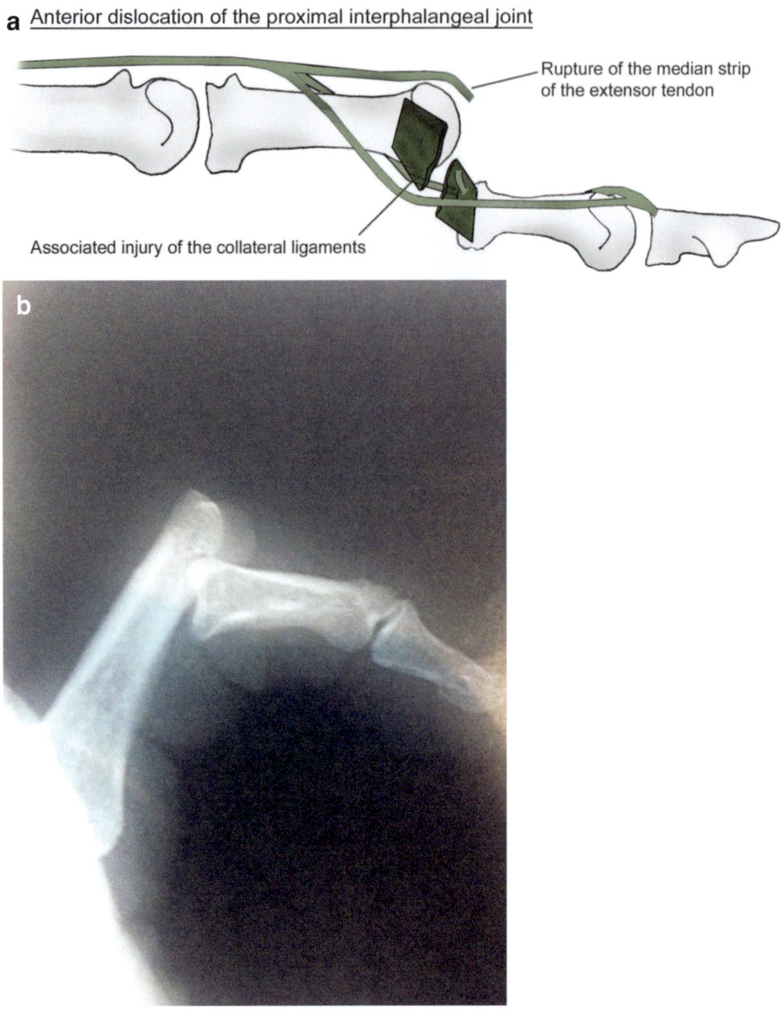

Fig. 3.17 Anatomical injuries in a palmar dislocation (**a**) and radiography (**b**). (Picture by Josette Mesplié)

The rehabilitation and orthotic treatment of palmar dislocations are therefore similar to the injuries of the extensor system in zone 3. The associated injury of the posterior fibers of the collateral ligaments and the volar plate is one more obstacle to the recovery of the mobility.

Bibliography

1. Bowers WH, et al. The proximal interphalangeal joint volar plate. I. An anatomical and biomechanical study. J Hand Surg Am. 1980;5(1):79–88.
2. Bowers WH. The proximal interphalangeal joint volar plate. II: a clinical study of hyperextension injury. J Hand Surg Am. 1981;6(1):77–81.
3. Adi M, et al. Results of conservative treatment of volar plate sprains of the proximal interphalangeal joint with and without avulsion fracture. Hand Surg Rehabil. 2017;36(1):44–7.
4. Mesplié G. Capsulo-ligamentous injuries of the proximal interphalangeal joint. In: Hand and wrist rehabilitation. Cham: Springer International Publishing; 2015. p. 217–33.
5. Glasgow C, Tooth LR, Fleming J. Mobilizing the stiff hand: combining theory and evidence to improve clinical outcomes. J Hand Ther. 2010;23(4):392–400; quiz 401.
6. Flowers KR. Reflections on mobilizing the stiff hand. J Hand Ther. 2010;23(4):402–3.
7. Douglass NP, Ladd AL. Therapy concepts for the proximal interphalangeal joint. Hand Clin. 2018;34(2):289–99.
8. Geoffroy C, Mesplié G. Les origines de la raideur de la main. Kinésithérapie, la Revue. 2020;20(222):20–3.

9. Villeco JP. Edema: a silent but important factor. J Hand Ther. 2012;25(2):153–61; quiz 162.
10. Ugurlu U, Ozdogan H. Effects of serial casting in the treatment of flexion contractures of proximal interphalangeal joints in patients with rheumatoid arthritis and juvenile idiopathic arthritis: a retrospective study. J Hand Ther. 2016;29(1):41–50; quiz 50.
11. Comer GC, Clark SJ, Yao J. Hand therapy modalities for proximal interphalangeal joint stiffness. J Hand Surg Am. 2015;40(11):2293–6; quiz 2296.
12. Freiberg A, et al. Management of proximal interphalangeal joint injuries. Hand Clin. 2006;22(3):235–42.
13. Saitta BH, Wolf JM. Treating proximal interphalangeal joint dislocations. Hand Clin. 2018;34(2):139–48.
14. Caggiano NM, Harper CM, Rozental TD. Management of proximal interphalangeal joint fracture dislocations. Hand Clin. 2018;34(2):149–65.
15. Bindra RR, Foster BJ. Management of proximal interphalangeal joint dislocations in athletes. Hand Clin. 2009;25(3):423–35.

Sprains of the Metacarpophalangeal Joint of the Thumb

4

Grégory Mesplié

Physiopathology

The metacarpophalangeal sprains are frequent in the thumb due to sports (skiing, handball, basketball, rugby, etc.) and mainly damage the medial (or ulnar) collateral ligament. The mechanism of injury creates a stress in valgus [1, 2] that puts tension on the medial collateral ligament and creates pressure on the lateral part of the metacarpophalangeal joint. It most often occurs after a fall onto the thumb in abduction. Similarly, a racket handle impacting the ulnar side of the thumb can generate forces that exceed the rupture load measured for the intact ligament at 294 N. In the case of an isolated rupture of the ulnar collateral ligament, the proximal phalanx rotates in supination around the intact radial collateral ligament. On the contrary, if the radial collateral ligament is torn, the phalanx rotates in pronation in relation to the metacarpal [1, 3].

The traumas in varus damage the lateral (or radial) collateral ligament and the ones in hyperextension damage the longitudinal palmar ligaments. Injuries with a combination of various elements often occur.

In serious sprains of the medial collateral ligament (rupture), the proximal extremity of the ligament can pass over the adductor's expansion, making the ligament's spontaneous healing impossible: it is the Stener effect [4] (Fig. 4.1).

The Stener effect can only occur if the two fascicles of the ulnar collateral ligament are injured [5].

Even if it is rarer, the same phenomenon can be observed radially, with the expansion of the external thenar muscles [6].

The varus deformity in the injuries of the radial collateral ligament is more spectacular than the valgus deformity in the injuries of the ulnar collateral ligament, due to the longitudinal orientation of the external thenar muscles and the transversal orientation of the adductor pollicis, which will have an important tendency to lead to varus in case of an injury of the radial collateral ligament (Fig. 4.2).

G. Mesplié (✉)
Institut Sud Aquitain de la Main et du Membre Supérieur (ISAMMS), Biarritz, France

G. Mesplié (ed.), *Hand Functional Anatomy and Therapy*,
https://doi.org/10.1007/978-3-031-92505-4_4

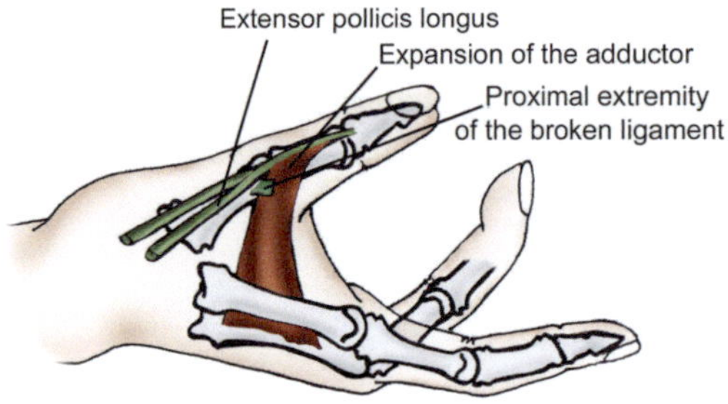

Fig. 4.1 Stener effect by interposition of the expansion of the adductor pollicis between the two parts of the broken ligament

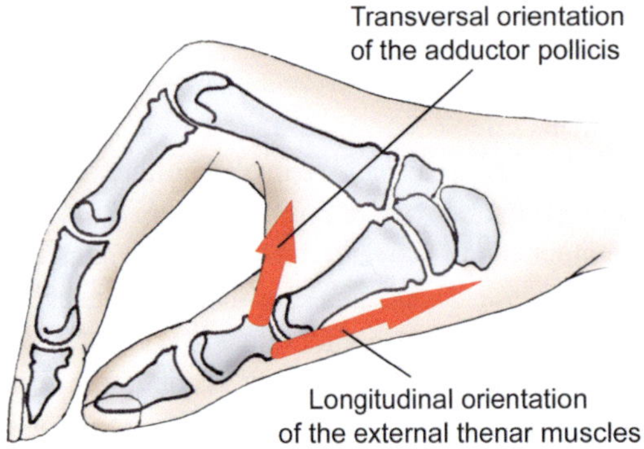

Fig. 4.2 The varus deformity in case of an injury of the radial collateral ligament is important because the adductor pollicis is transversal to the osseous lever, unlike the external sesamoid muscles

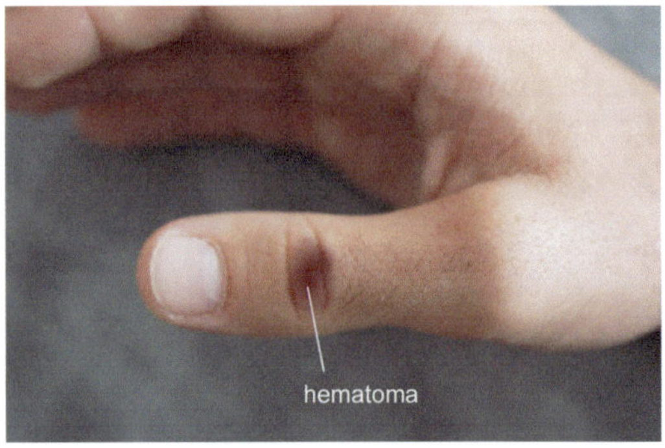

Fig. 4.3 Clinical signs leading to suspecting a Stener effect; hematoma on the dorsal side of the interphalangeal joint

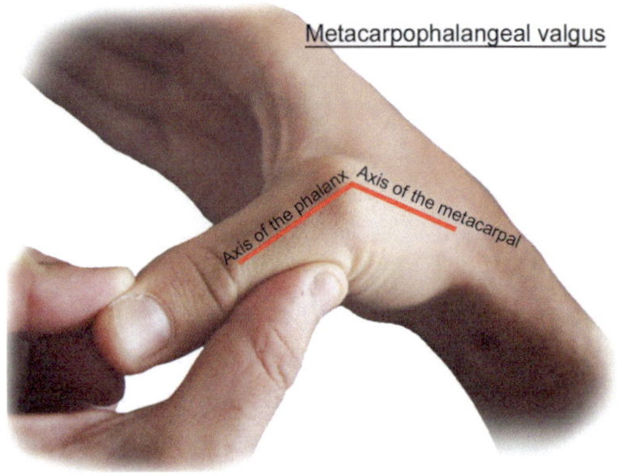

Fig. 4.4 Valgus 30% superior to the contralateral side leading us to suspect a stage 3 injury

Clinical and Paraclinical Signs

Clinical Signs

Other than the usual signs of a damaged ligament (pain when palpating and when putting it in tension, swelling, sensation of instability), we must be careful to some specific clinical signs that allow suspecting a serious sprain with a Stener effect:

- Hematoma on the dorsal part of the interphalangeal joint (highly significant) (Fig. 4.3).
- A laxity test is used to assess the level of joint laxity [7]. Grade 1 corresponds to pain when tension is applied without laxity. Grade 2 corresponds to laxity with a firm stop. Grade 3 corresponds to laxity without a stop. It is usually considered that a valgus 30% greater than the contralateral side (without a hard stop) should raise the suspicion of a stage 3 injury to the medial collateral ligament, which may be associated with a Stener effect (Fig. 4.4). When performing this test, it is important to keep the first phalanx in a neutral rotation, as pronation increases stability and may therefore hide a complete lesion of the ulnar collateral ligament, whereas supination may increase the felt instability [8]. If there is any doubt about a complete lesion, the test is performed both in 30° of flexion to test the main fascicle, and in extension to test the accessory fascicle, as the presence of a Stener effect is linked to damage to both fascicles. As the force used during the test is much lower than that of the injury mechanism, there is no risk of the maneuver creating an iatrogenic Stener effect [9].

Paraclinical Signs

The bilateral test in valgus, under a radiological control, allows obtaining a better appreciation of the angular value than the simple clinical test but is not a decisive factor in assessing the presence of a Stener effect.

The presence of a bone fragment at the level of the phalangeal insertion can be the sign of a rupture of the ligament, with a Stener effect.

Ultrasound is the examination of choice (sensitivity 88% and specificity 83%) for determining the presence of a Stener effect using the Bordet maneuver [10], which involves asking the patient to perform flexion/extension movements with the interphalangeal joint of the thumb. This movement creates a gliding from distal to proximal of the expansion of the adductor above the ligament when there is no Stener effect. Otherwise, we observe an interposition of the expansion of the adductor between the two parts of the injured ligament.

In case of doubt on ultrasound or late management, magnetic resonance imaging (MRI) is interesting [11] as it is 100% sensitive and specific [5].

Therapeutic Process and Surgical Treatment

The therapeutic approach depends on the stage of the injury, determined by the Milner et al. classification [12]:

- Stage 1: partial injury.
- Stage 2: complete injury with displacement ≤3 mm.
- Stage 3: complete injury with displacement >3 mm.
- Stage 4: Stener effect.

Forli [5] have proposed an algorithm that considers this classification, the quality of stop during the laxity test, and the associated presence of a fracture (Fig. 4.5).

In the case of a Milner et al. stage 1 and 2 sprain (partial or complete injury with displacement ≤3 mm), the treatment is conservative [13] and we propose immobilizing the joint in a functional position (without varus/valgus component), leaving the wrist and interphalangeal joint free. In the case of injury to the medial collateral ligament, the distal part of the orthosis is more important on the

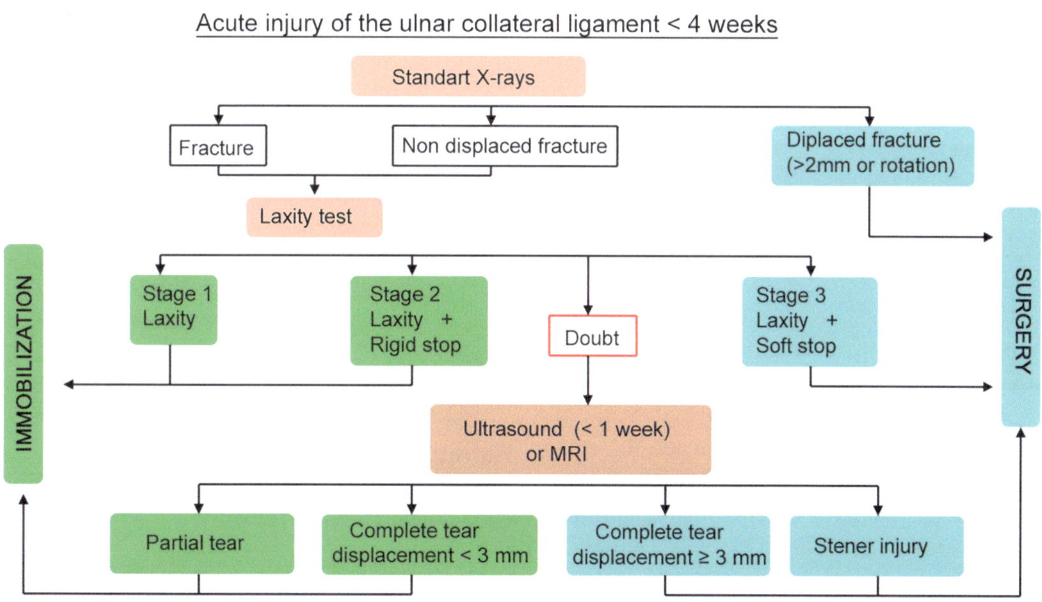

Fig. 4.5 Treatment algorithm according to Forli

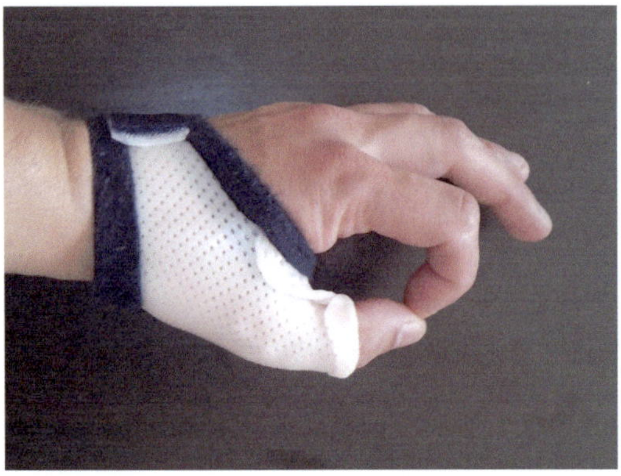

Fig. 4.6 Immobilization orthosis letting the interphalangeal joint free and opposing to varus (injury of the external collateral ligament) and valgus (injury of the internal collateral ligament) deformities of the metacarpophalangeal joint

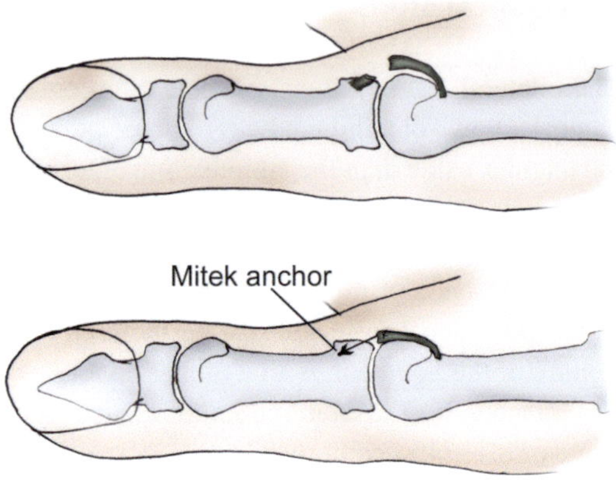

Fig. 4.7 Intraosseous anchor of the ligament in case of a serious sprain with Stener effect

radial side to prevent valgus displacement of the metacarpophalangeal joint (and the contrary in the case of injury to the lateral collateral ligament). It lets the flexion fold free to allow flexion/extension of the interphalangeal joint (Fig. 4.6).

The orthosis is realized in a thin plastic (1.6 mm) and kept for 3–4 weeks to allow the ligamentous healing.

In the case of stage 3 and 4 sprains (complete injury with displacement >3 mm or presence of a Stener effect), treatment is surgical.

Diagnosed in the acute phase, it consists in reinserting the ligament on the first phalanx using an intraosseous anchor or trans-osseous sutures, to restore good stability to the metacarpophalangeal joint (Fig. 4.7).

The injuries of the ligament itself are rare and directly sutured.

In the case of fracture (fragment >2 mm) or bone avulsion with major instability, surgery will consist respectively in reduction and pinning or removal of the small fragment (≤ 10% of the articular surface) and reinsertion of the ligament.

After reinsertion of the medial collateral ligament, a postoperative orthosis is made according to the same criteria as the ones used for benign sprains and is worn for 4 weeks at all times, then 2 weeks at night and during high-risk activities.

In the chronic phase (after 4 weeks), the ligament can no longer be repaired, and the surgical procedure will consist in reconstructing the ligament, most often using the palmaris longus [14].

After reconstruction of the medial collateral ligament, a postoperative orthosis is made using the same criteria as for benign sprains and is worn for 4 weeks at all times and for 2 weeks at night and during high-risk activities.

In cases where joint stability is not recovered, the evolution is usually negative, with instability, pain, and degenerative phenomena in the joint [15]. These developments may lead to a joint arthrodesis.

Rehabilitation and Orthoses

The metacarpophalangeal joint of the thumb is a stabilizing joint. The aim of the rehabilitation is to improve active stability of the joint, especially the muscles protecting the damaged ligament. The techniques to gain amplitude will be used very carefully during the healing period, in order not to weaken the passive stabilization structures.

In the case of surgery, ultrasounds must not be used if a metallic intraosseous anchor has been used.

Rehabilitation Protocol of Serious Medial Collateral Ligament Sprains (Postoperative) (Fig. 4.8)

From D0 to D3, an immobilization is proposed associated with a compressive bandage to limit the trophic disorders and pain inherent to this stage of healing.

a Sprains of the metacarpophalangeal joint of the thumb (surgery)

	Post-operative (A)	Relative fragility (B)	Consolidation (C)
REHABILITATION	**Therapeutic goals** : 1- Decrease trophic disorders 2- Decrease pain 3- Prevent stiffness 4- Prevent fonctional exclusion **Techniques:** 1- Draining massages and compressive bandage, vacuotherapy (drainage), electrotherapy (tonolysis) 2- Cryotherapy, TENS, TVS (100Hz) 3- Passive then active mobilizations of the free joints (until tension) 4- TVS (70-80Hz) and various sensory stimulations (without constraint) **Risks:** Stiffness and/or trophic disorders if inadequate mobilizations, type 1 CRPS,	**Therapeutic goals** : 1- Same as in phase A, intensify si necessary 2- Recovery of the metacarpophalangeal joint amplitudes 3- Progressive strenghtening of the muscles stabilizing the metacarpophalangeal joint **Techniques:** 1- Pressotherapy (drainage), vacuotherapy (scar) and defibrosing massage if the scar is closed and non-inflammatory (A1) manipulations of light objects (A4) 2- Electrostimulation, soft joint mobilizations (not lateral), 3- Electrostimulation and static contractions of the adductor pollicis (if internal collateral ligament) or external thenar muscles (if external collateral ligament) **Risks:** Same as phase A , functional exclusion (especially index)	**Therapeutic goals** : 1- Save as in previous phases, intensify si necessary 2- Complete fonctional recovery **Techniques:** 1- Intensify specific joint mobilizations, postures and electrostimulation (B2), contraints in torsion with large then finer grips, recovery of normal muscular ratios (B3) 2- Functional activities adapted to the patient's professional and sporting needs, no «high-risk» activities before D75 **Risks:** Same as in phases A and B
ORTHOSIS	Orthosis immobilizing the metacarpophalangeal joint (resting position) with the interphalangeal joint free - worn constantly except during rehabilitation	Progressively taking the immobilization orthosis off (night, light activities → more intense activity)	1- Protection orthosis for hight-risk activities (alpine) 2- Orthosis to gain amplitude if needed
	D3-D30	D30-D60	After D60

b

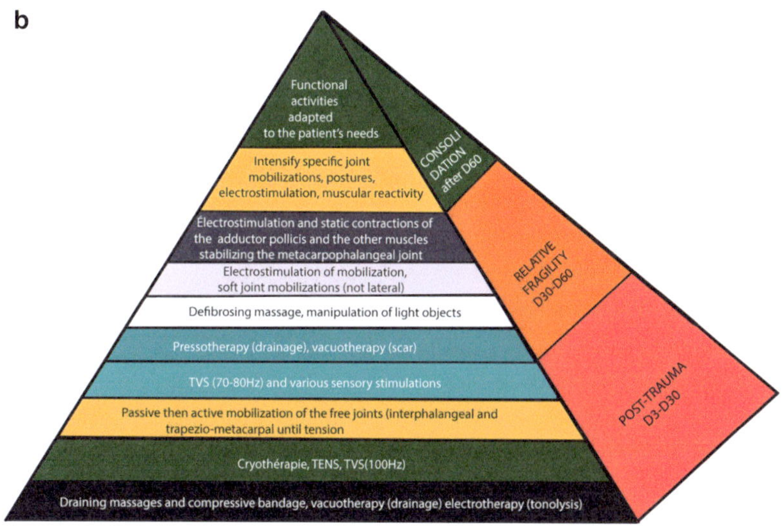

Fig. 4.8 Rehabilitation protocol (**a**) and progression pyramid (**b**)

Immobilization Phase (D3 to D30)

From D3 to D30, we must fight against trophic disorders and pain and maintain mobility in the joints adjacent to the metacarpophalangeal joint. Mobilization of the thumb's interphalangeal joint is essential at this stage to limit the risk of adherences between the ligament and the expansion of the adductor muscle, which is very common after surgery and can cause major stiffness in the thumb.

Stimulations of the thumb's pulp can be added to limit the functional exclusion (rare in the thumb).

An informed self-rehabilitation is sufficient in this phase, ideally supported by some "tip sheets."

In the case of an important inflammatory reaction, the rehabilitation can start to fight against pain and edema using the PRICE protocol:

- P for protection of the injury site throughout this whole phase, achieved by immobilization and making the patient aware of the fragility of the tissue.
- R for rest of the traumatized area, which should not be used during the entire immobilization period, apart from self-rehabilitation exercises provided by the rehabilitator.
- I for "ice" with icing of the injured area several times a day. This technique is sometimes poorly tolerated digitally and in this case should be applied proximally to the traumatized area.
- C for compression, with a compression bandage worn at night if the edema is under control, but which may be worn permanently in the opposite case. The use of a wide, stretchable, and elastic bandage in the width and length directions makes it possible to limit the thickness of the system so as not to prevent daytime mobilization.
- E for elevation of the hand for the same anti-edematous purpose.

Relative Fragility Phase (D30 to D60)

From D30 to D60, the relative fragility phase is marked by the beginning of the solicitations of the metacarpophalangeal joint, progressively reducing the immobilization. The ligament is not totally healed so it is forbidden to put important constraints on it (stress constraints).

Starting to move again in strict flexion/extension and strengthening, the stabilizing muscles of the metacarpophalangeal joint are the strong points of this phase. We keep mobilizing the adjacent joints until they are totally free.

Putting too much charge too soon on the damaged ligament leads to instability and pain.

➔ Fight Against Trophic Disorders and Pain

- Massages: trophic and analgesic goal, around the ligament healing area. This area can stay inflammatory during several months.
- Transcutaneous vibratory stimulations: 70 Hz frequency at the level of the extensor or flexor system if we want to improve the proprioceptive aspect and 100 Hz at the level of the painful areas if we want an analgesic effect.
- Depressotherapy: at the level of the healing area, privileging disto-proximal movements (Fig. 4.9).
- Electrotherapy: 1 Hz to fight against inflammatory phenomena or electro-active to regain the active amplitudes (no excessive tension).
- Compressive bandage: along the thumb, with a decreasing tension from distal to proximal.

➔ Amplitudes in Flexion/Extension

This exercise will be realized in amplitudes that do not put the surgeon's ligamentoplasty in tension, as it could lead to a joint instability by

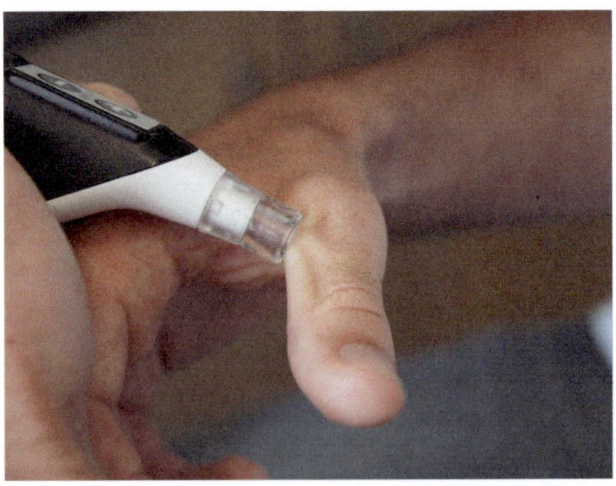

Fig. 4.9 Depressotherapy at the level of the scar area, moving disto-proximally (draining)

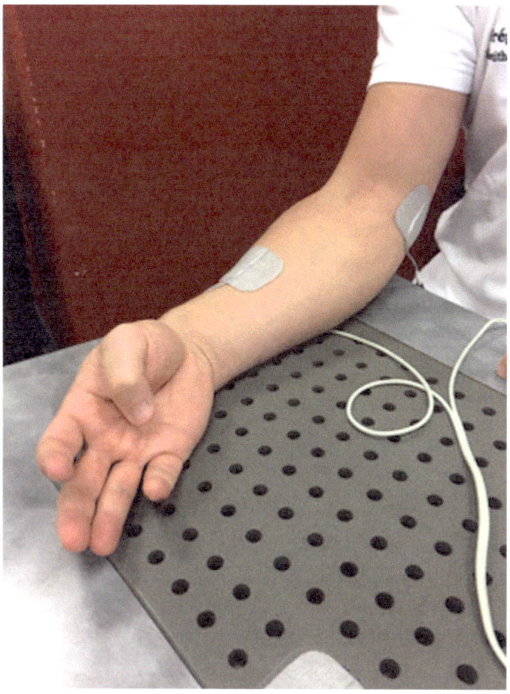

Fig. 4.10 Examples of active electrostimulations with of the interphalangeal joint in flexion

relaxing the stabilizing elements repaired during the surgery.

The mobilizations must never be realized with strength and must stay painless. We do not make any specific mobilization in this phase.

The techniques used are as active as possible to allow the patient to control the tension put on the hypo-extensible tissues.

The use of active electrostimulation can be considered (Fig. 4.10).

➔ Proprioceptive Abilities

It is important to propose a coherent evolution for the exercises depending on the healing phase, in order not to disturb the consolidation process. The recovery stage of the proprioceptive abilities must also be considered so that the patient does not develop compensative pathologies such as tendinopathies or reflex contractures.

- *Perception of joint position (Hagert's stage 3)*

It is defined as the ability to precisely reproduce a given joint angulation [16].

The rehabilitation of this perception is done in three steps. In the first step, the therapist places the patient's wrist in a defined joint position and controls the joint amplitude with a goniometer.

In the second step, the wrist is placed in another position, indifferently. In the third step, the patient must place his forearm in the first position [16, 17].

The exercise is realized with the patient's eyes closed to avoid any visual afference.

This test is highly correlated with the hand's sensorimotor abilities [17] and must therefore be done before any evolution of the rehabilitation protocol—especially before Hagert's stage 5.

- *Kinesthesia (Hagert's stage 4)*

It is defined as the ability to detect a passive movement. The therapist realizes the movement while the patient keeps his eyes closed and tells him when he perceives the movement.

This exercise is easy to realize at the physiotherapy office or at home but does not allow a precise analysis regarding the patient's perception threshold.

Using an arthromotor device allows analyzing more precisely the movement speed and the studied angular sector.

A laser can also be a very helpful tool to improve conscious proprioceptive abilities. The patient must follow trajectories becoming increasingly complex, going faster and faster.

- *Conscious neuromuscular rehabilitation (Hagert's stage 5)*

Several strengthening modes have been described to improve neuromuscular abilities. They help increase the basic muscle tone and therefore the joint's dynamic stability [18].

We ask the patient to realize isometric contractions with a low intensity during 6 s. Thirty repetitions or less are done, considering that it must not create any pain or secondary trophic disorder.

The first function of the metacarpophalangeal joint of the thumb is to allow a good stability during the grips between fingers and thumb and during the cylindrical grasps with a full palm.

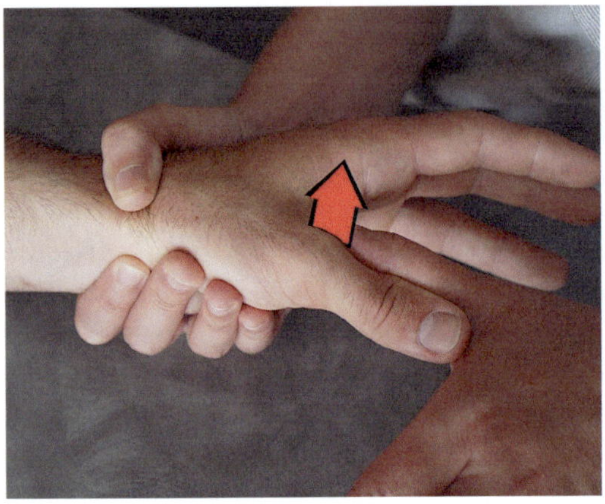

Fig. 4.11 Manual strengthening of the adductor pollicis

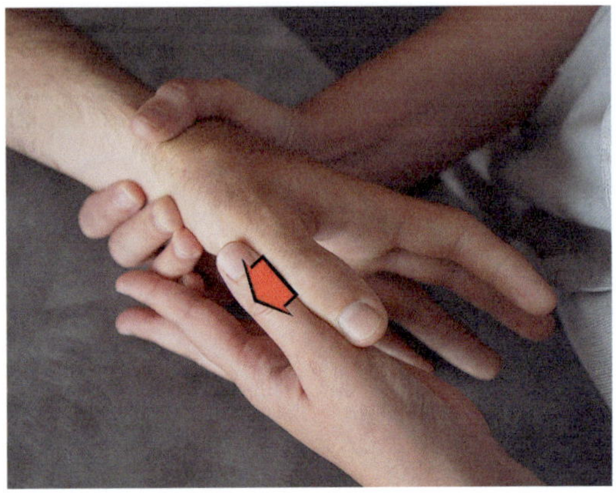

Fig. 4.12 Manual strengthening of the external sesamoid muscles

Therefore, strengthening the muscles participating in this function is the key element of this rehabilitation.

The muscle strengthening is mostly for the internal ones in the ulnar collateral ligament injuries.

However, it is essential to do a global stabilization work in the joint, in order not to create a muscular imbalance, which is a pathogenic source.

- *Adductor pollicis*

We fix the first metacarpal with the proximal hand and put a resistance with the pulp of the distal hand's thumb at the level of the ulnar side of the first phalanx, as close as possible to the joint (especially before the end of the healing process), to limit the shear forces on the joint (Fig. 4.11).

- *External sesamoid muscles*

The same modalities are applied than for the internal sesamoid muscles, except for the resistance, which is placed at the level of the radial side of the first phalanx. This exercise must not create a valgus in order not to put excessive constraints on the operated ligament (Fig. 4.12).

- *Synergic exercise for the external and internal sesamoid muscles*

We ask for a clamping between the pulp of the thumb and the radial side of the second phalanx, controlling the full extension of the interphalangeal joint of the thumb.

Using a pinch can provide a visual feedback of the contraction's intensity (Fig. 4.13).

NB: the interphalangeal flexion is a sign of compensation by the flexor pollicis longus and must therefore be avoided.

- *Electrostimulation*

In theory, in the case of a medial collateral ligament injury, it should be necessary to place the electrodes exclusively on the muscular group we want to strengthen (adductor pollicis).

In practice, we obtain a co-contraction of the internal and external sesamoid muscles regardless of the stimulated muscular group, as the antagonist muscles contract to fight against the movement created by the electrical stimulation.

Therefore, we ask the patient to maintain the initial position during the electric stimulation to obtain a co-contraction of the internal and external sesamoid muscles (Fig. 4.14).

It is therefore a global strengthening technique for the metacarpophalangeal joint.

- *Coordination and dexterity*

We realize exercises that improve coordination and dexterity of the thumb and hand.

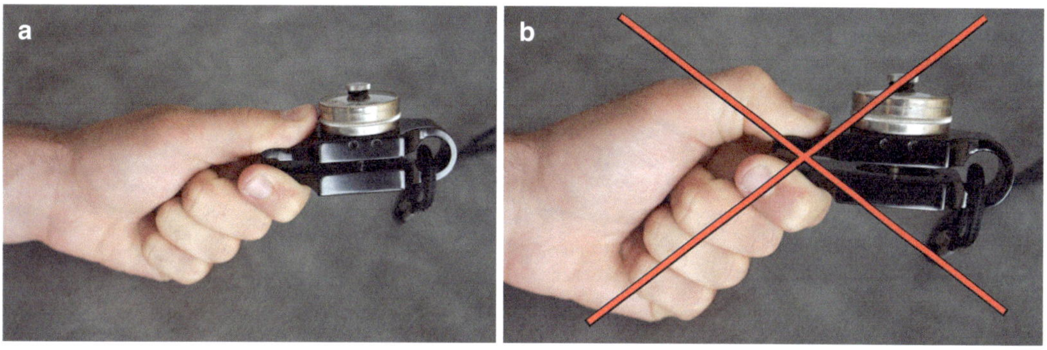

Fig. 4.13 Instrumental strengthening of the tip-to-side pinch using a pinch (**a**), without an interphalangeal flexion, which is a sign of a flexor pollicis longus contraction (**b**)

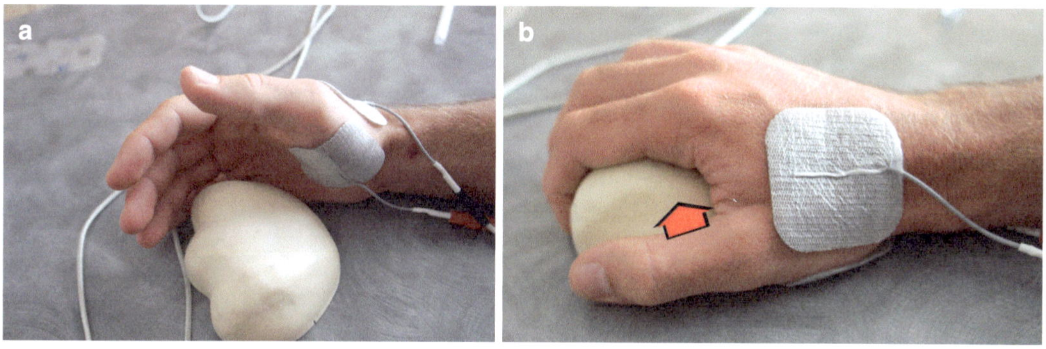

Fig. 4.14 Active electrostimulation of the sesamoid muscles. Placement of the electrodes (**a**). The patient must squeeze the hand-rest during the active phase, without soliciting the flexor pollicis longus (**b**)

Consolidation Phase (After D60)

The ligament is healed and can stand more important constraints.

The goal of this phase is the complete recovery of the patient's abilities. High-risk activities, such as sports that may induce valgus stress on the joint, are not permitted before D75.

➔ Full Recovery of the Joint Amplitudes

- *Specific mobilizations.*

These techniques, used after the healing of the damaged ligament, allow regaining the joint glidings that are essential for the proper functioning of the joint.

The metacarpophalangeal joint of the thumb is a condylar joint where the head of the first metacarpal and the base of the proximal phalanx face each other. It has flexion/extension and abduction/adduction movements [19]. However, the mobility in the frontal plane is limited because the collateral ligaments ensure the lateral stability of the joint both in flexion for the main fascicles and in extension for the accessory fascicles. In addition to these movements, there is an automatic axial rotation movement, which is essential for understanding the prehension opposing the fingers' pulps with the thumb's pulp. Thus, the

Table 4.1 Summary table of movement associations depending on the mobilization of the metacarpophalangeal joint of the thumb

	Mobilization in flexion	Mobilization in extension
Antero-posterior glidings	Anterior	Posterior
Axial rotations	Pronation	Supination

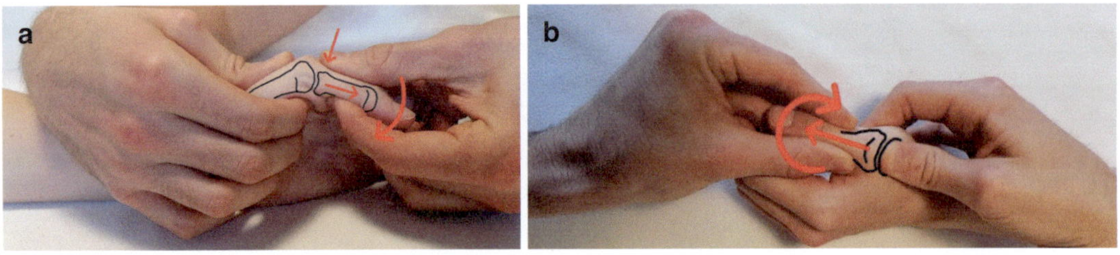

Fig. 4.15 Specific mobilization of the metacarpophalangeal joint, combining it with a slight decoaptation

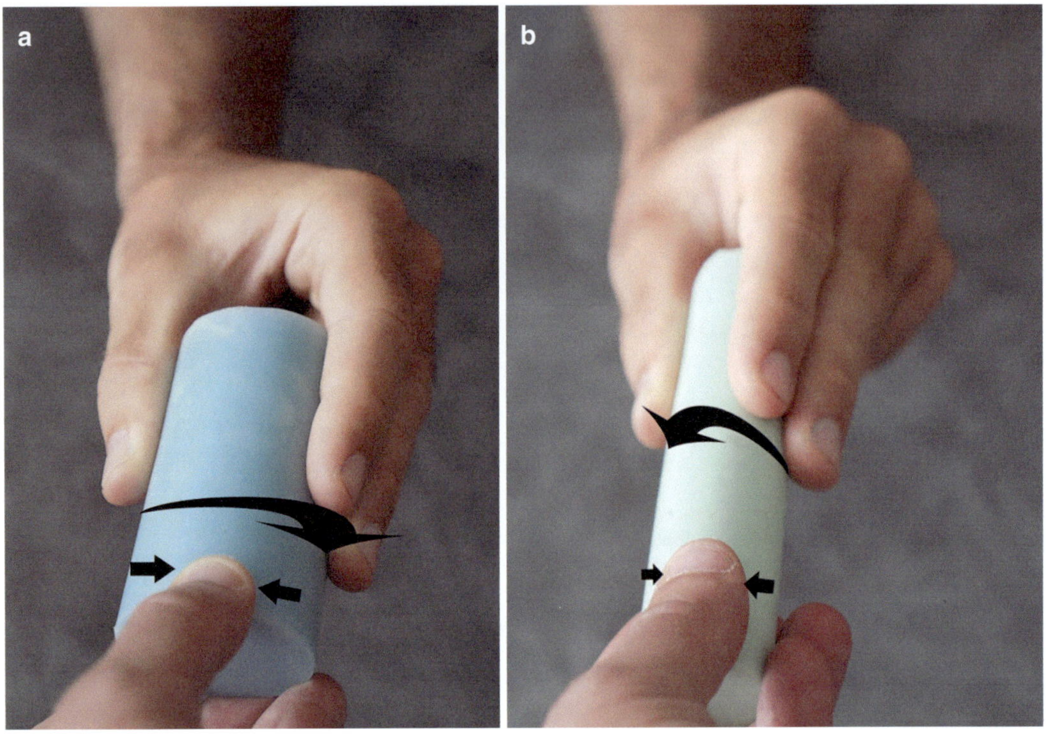

Fig. 4.16 Rotatory stability with a silicon cylinder, progressively decreasing the diameter of the cylinder (**a** and **b**)

first phalanx pronates during flexion and supinates during extension. This joint also complies with the concavity rule (Table 4.1). A gentle axial traction allows decoaptation, which facilitates the mobilization of the joint surfaces.

With one hand, the therapist fixes the first metacarpal, and with the other hand he/she holds the first phalanx and realizes mobilizations in flexion and extension, combining them with accessory mobilizations. The distal hand can also apply a decoaptor traction for an easier manipulation (Fig. 4.15).

- *Full recovery of proprioceptive abilities*

We intensify the techniques described in phase 2 to regain muscular ratios comparable with the healthy side.

The use of a silicon (or other) cylinder allows a solicitation of the internal sesamoid muscles, appealing to their component of anti-pronation rotatory stabilization (Fig. 4.16).

- *Functional recovery*

These exercises will be realized according to the multidirectional stresses imposed on the metacarpophalangeal joint and adapted to each patient's professional and sports activities.

Rehabilitation Protocol After Benign and Medium Sprains (No Surgery)

We will use the same techniques, adapting them to the healing time of a benign sprain (3–4 weeks). The rehabilitation phases are mainly the same, but the techniques can be intensified earlier if there is no trophic disorder or pain.

It should be noted that in the lateral collateral ligament sprains, we strengthen the external thenar muscles more, as they have an anti-varus and anti-supination role (and therefore protect the lateral collateral ligament).

Orthotic Treatment

Immobilization Phase

We realize an orthosis with thin thermoformable plastic (1.6 mm), keeping the interphalangeal joint free.

Its molding at the level of the metacarpophalangeal joint opposes the varus or valgus deformities [20].

It must be worn all the time and allows the patient to take baths (Fig. 4.6).

Resuming Sports Activities and Career

An "alpine" orthosis can be made when the patient gets back to work and sports activities (Fig. 4.17).

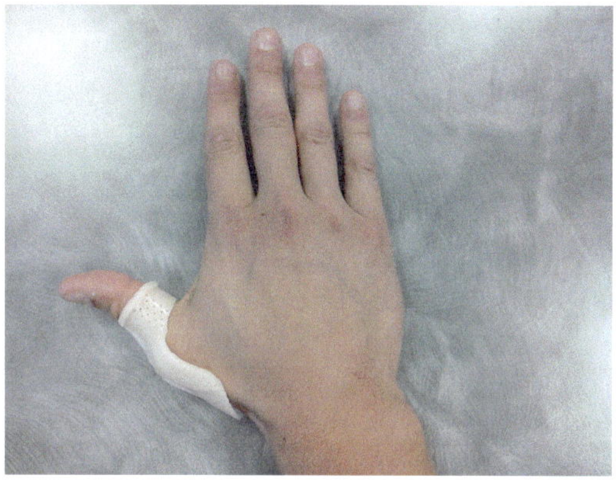

Fig. 4.17 Alpine orthosis made to return to sports and professional activities and associated to strapping

Dynamic Orthoses

A global winding dynamic orthosis of the thumb or an analytical dynamic orthosis of the metacarpophalangeal joint can be made after 8 weeks if there is a persisting stiffness.

It is worn shortly (15 min maximum), under the pain threshold, but repeatedly during the day.

A commissural opening orthosis can also be made if there is a deficit of movement when spreading the thumb. It is worn during the night and can be associated with a silicon sheet placed on the scar if it is inflammatory (Fig. 4.18).

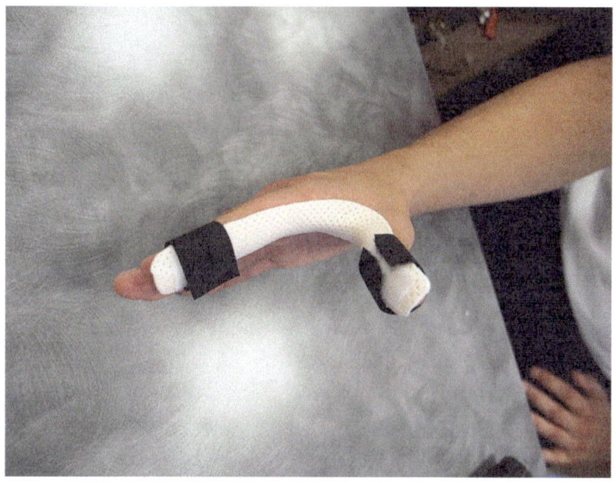

Fig. 4.18 Commissural opening orthosis associated to a silicon pad if the scar is inflammatory

Bibliography

1. Lee AT, Carlson MG. Thumb metacarpophalangeal joint collateral ligament injury management. Hand Clin. 2012;28(3):361–70, ix-x.
2. Mesplié G. Sprains of the metacarpophalangeal joint of the thumb, in hand and wrist rehabilitation. Springer; 2015. p. 173–88.
3. Firoozbakhsh K, et al. A study of ulnar collateral ligament of the thumb metacarpophalangeal joint. Clin Orthop Relat Res. 2002;403:240–7.
4. Johnson JW, Culp RW. Acute ulnar collateral ligament injury in the athlete. Hand Clin. 2009;25(3):437–42.
5. Forli A, et al. Recent and chronic sprains of the first Metacarpo-phalangeal joint. Orthop Traumatol Surg Res. 2022;108(1S):103156.
6. Doty J, Rudd J, Jemison M. Radial collateral ligament injury of the thumb with a Stener-like lesion. Orthopedics. 2010;33(12):925.
7. Riou P. Les entorses du ligament collatéral ulnaire de l'articulation métacarpo-phalangienne du pouce dans les accidents de sport de glisse en montagne. Kinésithérapie scientifique. 2014;2014(560):7–14.
8. Mayer SW, Ruch DS, Leversedge FJ. The influence of thumb metacarpophalangeal joint rotation on the evaluation of ulnar collateral ligament injuries: a biomechanical study in a cadaver model. J Hand Surg Am. 2014;39:474–9.
9. Adler T, et al. Can clinical examination cause a Stener lesion in patients with skier's thumb?: a cadaveric study. Clin Anat. 2012;25(6):762–6.
10. Bordet B, Borne J, Pialat J. Échographie de l'entorse du ligament collatÉral ulnaire (LCU) de l'articulation mÉtacarpo-phalangienne (MCP) du pouce: une nouvelle manoeuvre dynamique pour visualiser l'effet Stener. J Radiol. 2009;90:217–20.
11. Hergan K, Mittler C, Oser W. Pitfalls in sonography of the gamekeeper's thumb. Eur Radiol. 1997;7:65–9.
12. Milner CS, Manon-Matos Y, Thirkannad SM. Gamekeeper's thumb–a treatment-oriented magnetic resonance imaging classification. J Hand Surg Am. 2015;40(1):90–5.
13. Avery DM 3rd, Inkellis ER, Carlson MG. Thumb collateral ligament injuries in the athlete. Curr Rev Musculoskelet Med. 2017;10(1):28–37.
14. Catalano LW 3rd, et al. Results of surgical treatment of acute and chronic grade III [corrected] tears of the radial collateral ligament of the thumb metacarpophalangeal joint. J Hand Surg Am. 2006;31(1):68–75.
15. Patel S, et al. Collateral ligament injuries of the metacarpophalangeal joint of the thumb: a treatment algorithm. Strategies Trauma Limb Reconstr. 2010;5(1):1–10.
16. Hagert E. Proprioception of the wrist joint: a review of current concepts and possible implications on the rehabilitation of the wrist. J Hand Ther. 2010;23(1):2–16. quiz 17
17. Karagiannopoulos C, et al. Responsiveness of the active wrist joint position sense test after distal radius fracture intervention. J Hand Ther. 2016;29(4):474–82.
18. Riemann B, Lephart S. The sensorimotor system, part 1: the physiologic basis of functional joint stability. J Athl Train. 2002;37(1):71–9.
19. Leversedge FJ. Anatomy and pathomechanics of the thumb. Hand Clin. 2008;24(3):219–29. v
20. Gil JA, et al. Efficacy of a radial-based thumb metacarpophalangeal-stabilizing orthosis for protecting the thumb metacarpophalangeal joint ulnar collateral ligament. J Hand Ther. 2019;32(1):80–5.

Digital Pulley Rupture

5

Denis Gerlac and Alexandra Forli

In the space of a few decades, the frequency of injuries of finger pulleys has increased significantly. This is attributable to the popularity of a relatively recent sport: climbing, especially indoor climbing. What was once a recreational activity has now become a high-level competitive sport. The difficulty of the climbing paths, which is necessary to select the elite, has forced athletes and most amateurs to develop their musculature to be able to grip holds that have become smaller and smaller over the years.

Unfortunately, the pulleys suffer from this increase in muscular strength, especially when it is obtained over short periods of time. Studies tend to show that when the finger flexor muscles are strengthened, the strength of the pulleys does not increase as quickly as the development of muscle power, and the muscles become more powerful than the pulleys too quickly. The latter suffer from this sudden overload which strains them.

D. Gerlac (✉)
IUD Hand Rehabilitation and Orthopaedic Devices, Echirolles, France

A. Forli
Unité Chir Plastique, Chirurgie de la Main, Hôpital Michallon, Grenoble, France
e-mail: AForli@chu-grenoble.fr

History

The first descriptions of pulley rupture in rock climbing date back to the 1990s. Two of them are well known: the first, by N.J. Barton, was reported by S. Bollen [1]. It involved a young climber who, after feeling his foot rip from the support on which it was resting, abruptly shifted his body weight onto the hand from which he was suspended, in order not to lose his balance and fall. But at the same moment he felt a violent pain under his fingers that caused him to let go of his grip and fall.

The second description was French, by Y. Tropet [2] in Besançon. In the same way, it concerned a 21-year-old climber who felt one of his fingers "crack" during a traction effort while climbing.

The important thing to remember is that after these traumas, both climbers benefited from treatment. The first had a conservative treatment, and the second a surgical treatment (repair of the A2 pulley using the A. Kapandji method). According to both authors, after consolidation, both climbers recovered their previous abilities and were able to resume climbing.

Anatomy and Biomechanics

Lined with synovial fluid, the pulleys guide the flexor tendons and keep them pressed against the skeleton [3–5]. Through transmission elements,

G. Mesplié (ed.), *Hand Functional Anatomy and Therapy*,
https://doi.org/10.1007/978-3-031-92505-4_5

the pulleys are positioned in series on the palmar surface of the phalanges. Together, they form an osteofibrous tunnel known as the digital canal. This way, when the strength of the flexor muscles is expressed, the "hollow of the hand" remains free to grasp an object.

Usually, on a long finger, there are eight pulleys: five annular (A1 to A5) and three cruciform (C1 to C3) (Fig. 5.1). The A2 and A4 pulleys are the longest and thickest. They are also the strongest. They insert directly on the inferior and lateral surfaces of the diaphyses of the proximal and intermediate phalanges, whereas the odd-numbered pulleys (A1, A3, and A5) insert on the respective palmar plates of the metacarpophalangeal joint, the proximal interphalangeal joint, and the distal interphalangeal joint [2]. The cruciform pulleys, referred to as accessories, are inserted between A2 and A3 for C1, between A3 and A4 for C2, and between A4 and A5 for C3.

In mechanical terms, the A2 and A4 pulleys are by far the most important. Their presence is essential for a good finger winding [3, 5–9].

The results of research into the breaking strength of these two pulleys need to be clarified, as they vary from one study to another. Some find A2 to be stronger than A4, others the opposite, and finally one study concludes that the strengths of these two pulleys are equal [10]. What is clear is that A2 must be able to withstand the solicitations from two muscles, the flexor digitorum superficialis and the flexor digitorum profundus, whereas A4 is constrained only by the flexor digitorum profundus tendon.

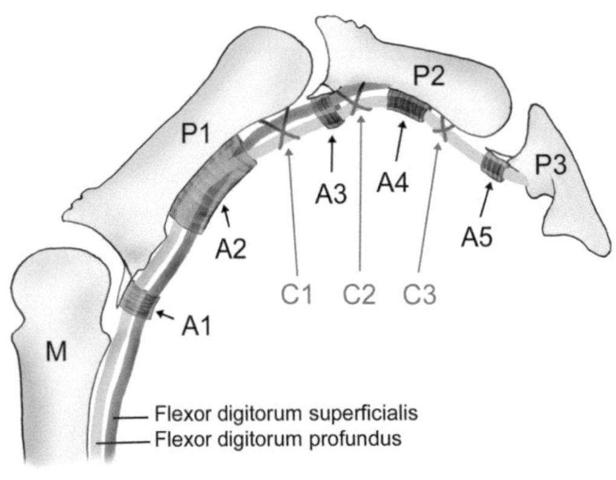

Fig. 5.1 Anatomy of the digital pulleys, annular (from A1 to A5) and cruciform (from C1 to C3), which together form the digital canal that holds and guides the flexor tendons (flexor digitorum superficialis and flexor digitorum profundus) on the palmar side of the skeleton

From a biomechanical point of view, the loss of pulleys leads to the formation of a "bowstring." This phenomenon generates a reduction in the tendon course, which translates into a loss of grip strength and a reduction in digital mobility [4, 6, 10, 11].

Etiopathogenesis

Climbing as a sport, which has been growing steadily in recent years, remains the main cause of these injuries [5, 8, 12, 13], far ahead of other causes [8]—sports (rugby, judo, windsurfing, etc.) [4, 14] or others [15–17].

Statistically, the ring finger is the most frequently injured finger, followed by the middle finger [11, 13, 16–18]. The other fingers are rarely concerned by this injury.

A2 and A4 are the most frequently injured pulleys [4, 11, 13, 18–20].

Physiopathology

It is always the same mechanism that traumatizes the pulley [7]: overloading. It is commonly referred to as a pathology of repeated microtraumas, the last of these traumas causing the rupture!

The arched position (Fig. 5.2) is the source of the problem. This posture places the proximal interphalangeal joint in a 90–100° flexion and the distal interphalangeal joint in extension [8]. In this configuration, the flexors exert a pull on the A2, A3, and A4 pulleys (whose role is to prevent the "bowstring") that is far greater than the mechanical resistance they can provide. This gradually or suddenly causes an injury that may even lead to rupture (Fig. 5.3) [18].

The injury mechanism occurs in two modes: the first is static, the second dynamic.

In the static mode, the accident occurs when the hand, already exerting an effort, must now

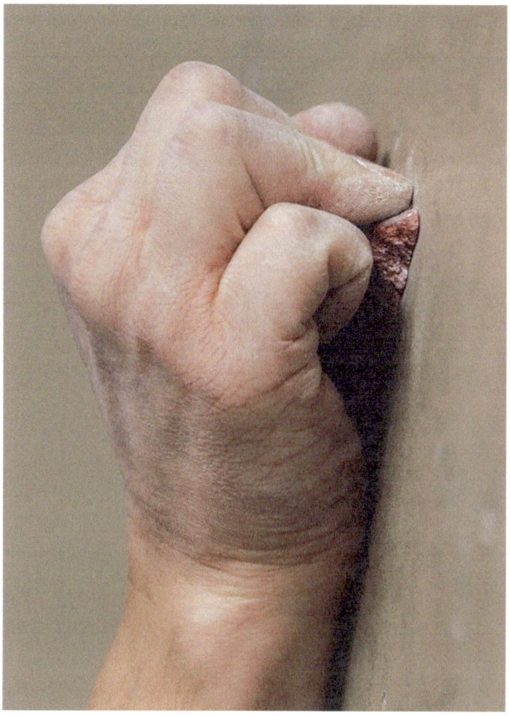

Fig. 5.2 Arched position

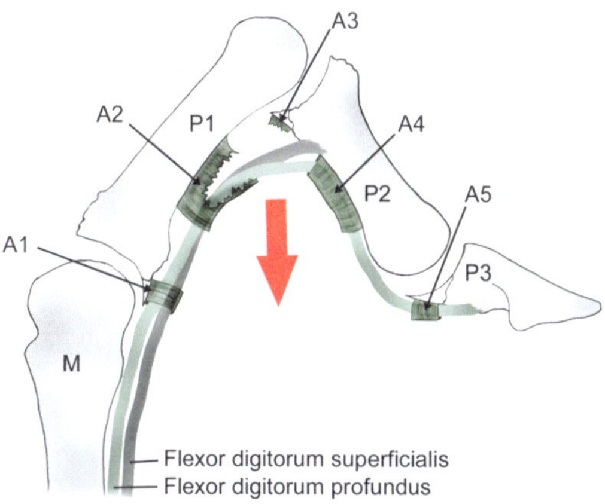

Fig. 5.3 Physiopathology of the rupture of pulleys in an arched position

endure further stress. For example, in climbing, this happens when the feet slip off their supports, transferring the load (body weight) to the fingers.

In the dynamic mode, the hand, rushing to grab a hold, finds itself badly adjusted when it contacts with its objective. For example, still in climbing, during a "throwing" maneuver, the climber, even when stretched out to his full length and unable to reach the hold above him, chooses, to continue his ascent, to take an impulse on his legs and "throws" himself towards the hold. Once he has grabbed it but cannot grip it well enough, despite the energy developed by the flexors to hold on to the wall, it is during the eccentric part of the contraction that the injury occurs [18].

Diagnosis

Signs suggesting a pulley rupture are essentially clinical.

When questioning the patient, we find:

- Excessive traction of the finger flexors, usually on a finger in an arched position (metacarpophalangeal joint and proximal interphalangeal joint flexion, associated with distal interphalangeal joint extension).
- An audible snap (80% of cases).
- Moderate initial pain, except for that perceived as "flashing" at the moment of cracking. Pain usually appears with a delay after a few minutes' rest.

During the assessment, there is:

- Swelling, with or without bruising. Swelling is late and progressive, often of moderate size. Ecchymosis is not systematic.
- Loss of full finger flexion and loss of full extension as well (persistence of a small flessum of the proximal interphalangeal joint).
- If the rupture is total, the presence of a "bowstring," formed by the protrusion of the tendon when an effort is made to flex the finger against resistance. If the rupture is partial, the "bowstring" does not always show.

Confirmation of the diagnosis is obtained through imaging (MRI or ultrasound) performed with the finger performing a flexion against resistance. These exams show the "bowstring" or the loss of congruence between the tendons and the concavity of the phalanges. A space has been created between the two structures.

Severity of Injury

In 2006, V. Schöffl established a classification of this pathology [13], based on the type of injury (inflammation, sprain, partial rupture, total rupture) and the number of injured pulleys. It has four stages that define the level of severity:

- Grade 1: sprain (distension) of pulley.
- Grade 2: complete rupture of A4 or partial rupture of A2 or A3.
- Grade 3: complete rupture of A2 or A3.
- Grade 4: multiple ruptures (A2/A3 or A2/A3/A4) or simple rupture of A2 or A3 combined with trauma of the lumbricals or the collateral ligaments.

Treatment

Two types of treatment are available for pulley injuries: conservative therapy and surgery. Unfortunately, there is no place here for therapeutic abstention, as it would seriously compromise the functionality of the finger, allowing pain to persist and worsening the risk of injuries.

According to Schöffl in a study on the evaluation of the hand strength recovered after surgery, surgical treatment should only be done in grade 4 of his score [13]. However, this rule is not absolute, especially in the case of high-level climbers who do not wish to stop for too long and, above all, wish to recover a maximum of functional ability (strength, mobility, indolence, etc.). In Grenoble, for example, Schöffl's grade 3 is also operated on, and M. Bouyer has shown that surgical reconstruction of the pulley allows climbers to return to their previous level, with hands that are pain-free and just as powerful as before [12].

Conservative Treatment

This treatment is usually aimed at grades 1, 2, and 3 [8, 21], but in recent years some grade 4 patients with no "bowstring" have also benefited from it, with generally very good results [13, 22].

Based on complete rest of the finger throughout the healing process, it includes wearing a thermoplastic protective ring and rehabilitation [4, 23].

Protective Ring (Fig. 5.4)

Its goal is to bring the edges of the tear together and allow the pulley to heal.

Made of thermoplastic, it is circular and closed for greater strength and should be long enough to cover the entire diaphysis of the affected phalanx.

M. Schneeberger's study shows that an orthosis that is too short and placed on the proximal part of the phalanx is less effective, especially for bowstring correction [24]. If we compare this

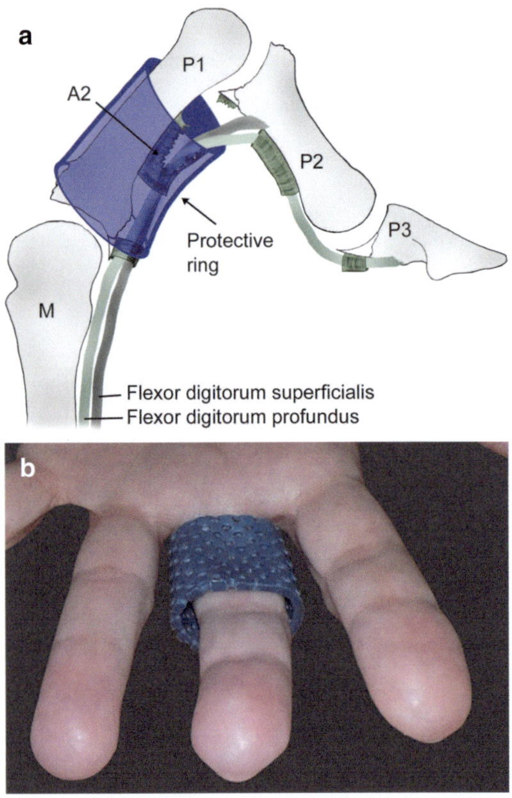

Fig. 5.4 (**a**, **b**) Protective ring: its length must cover the entire length of the pulley to allow proper healing. A flat part must be made to reproduce the concavity of the phalanx, without forgetting to create lateral spaces to avoid compressing the vasculo-nervous bundles

study with that of N.J. Barton (1969), who wanted to define the best theoretical location for a pulley [25], we find similarities. Both authors conclude that the ideal position for a reflection pulley (natural or thermoplastic) is at the level of the interphalangeal joints (proximal or distal). This is where the bowstring effect is most attenuated.

The ring must be tight enough from front to back to keep the tendon close to the skeleton, and loose enough laterally to avoid compressing the vasculo-nervous elements. To this end, the ring is made with a flat part on the palmar side to meet these specifications.

As the swelling decreases, the circumference of the ring should be adjusted to the diameter of the finger.

W.J. Warme has shown that strapping has no mechanical interest: it cannot prevent the flexor tendons from moving away from the phalanges during a bowstring effect [14]. It is therefore not recommended for therapeutic purposes [12, 26, 27]. It does, however, provide psychological security and analgesia. In this context, A. Schweizer stresses the importance of the strapping width. He has shown that the wider it is, and the closer it is to the proximal interphalangeal joint, the more effective it is [28]. The H-shaped strapping described by V. Schöffl [29], placed under the proximal interphalangeal joint, seems to correspond perfectly to these recommendations. Moreover, without wishing to make an analogy, it resembles the result of N.J. Barton's study on the optimal location of a pulley (seen before).

Rehabilitation

It should be started early [7, 22, 30] and has two phases, one before and one after healing.

From D0 to D45: Healing Phase

It involves the use of a protective ring, which must be worn continuously, 24 h a day, whether the rupture is complete or partial. This is followed by rehabilitation, which includes fighting against edema and maintaining joint mobility. The aim is to avoid the formation of capsuloligamentous retractions and, secondarily, tendinous adherences.

The fight against edema is carried out using the RICE protocol. The acronym stands for: rest, ice, compression, elevation. With the help of draining massages, a Coheban® compression bandage, declive postures, and the application of cryotherapy, edema can be well resorbed.

Joint mobility is maintained through passive and active mobilizations. These mobilizations are always made under with the ring, and active mobilizations must be performed without resistance (Figs. 5.5 and 5.6). During these mobilizations, attention must be paid to the proximal and distal interphalangeal joints. It is important to prevent a possible flessum in the first joint and a loss of flexion in the second.

After D45: Functional Recovery Phase

Healing is acquired, so resistance can be gradually introduced. However, at the beginning of this period, there may still be some degree of inflammation. In this case, it is prudent to delay the introduction of resistances until the inflammation has completely disappeared.

The ring is kept for another 45 days (adapting its diameter to the circumference of the finger if necessary).

Climbing can only be resumed after D90 and only gradually. During this phase of functional recovery, the patient should be introduced to the importance of physical preparation (warm-up, recovery, diet, etc.) and taught to stretch his/her muscles, especially the interosseous, lumbrical, extensor, and flexor muscles of the fingers (Fig. 5.7).

Another notion: the finger flexor muscles are very powerful. When they come into action with the proximal interphalangeal joint in 90° of flexion, they are likely to generate an anterior glide of the middle phalanx relative to the proximal phalanx (Fig. 5.8). This is all the more true as the distal end of the intermediate phalanx is immobilized by the grip during climbing.

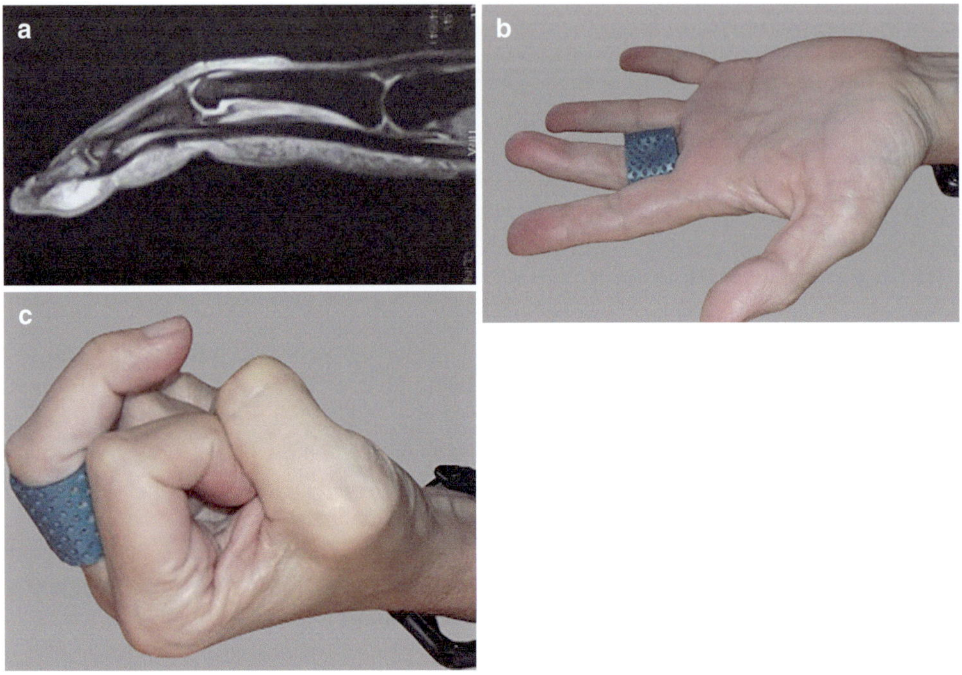

Fig. 5.5 (**a-c**) Injury of the A2 pulley: conservative treatment with early mobilization with a rigid ring

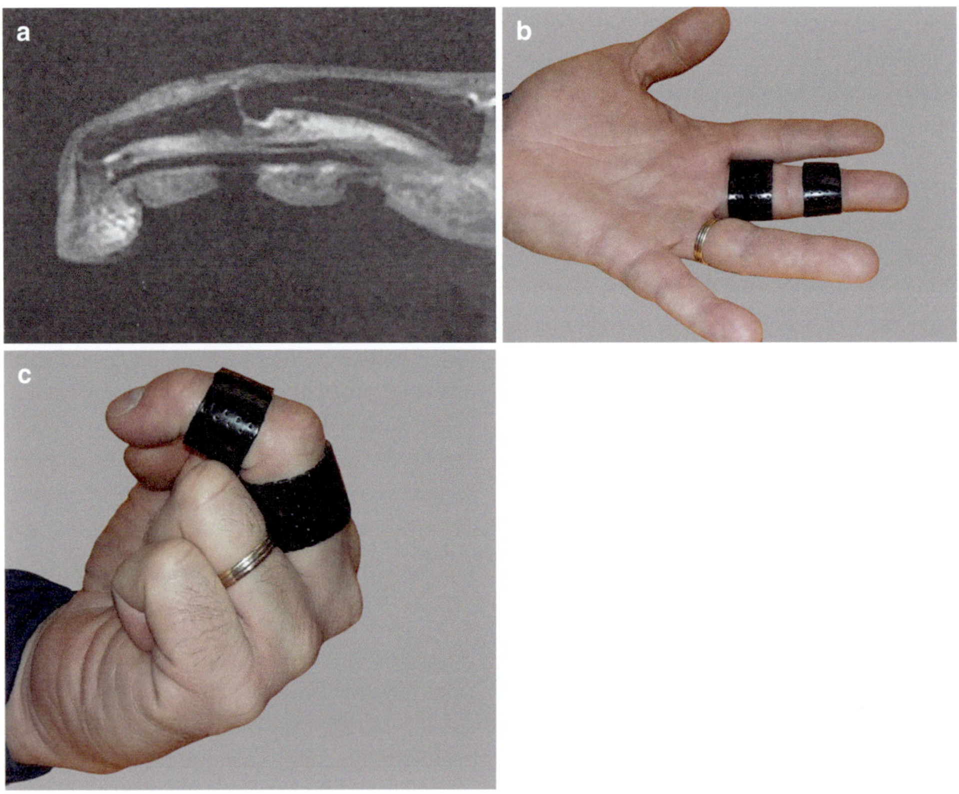

Fig. 5.6 (**a-c**) Injuries of the A2, A3, and A4 pulleys: conservative treatment with early mobilization with two rigid protective rings for A2 and A4

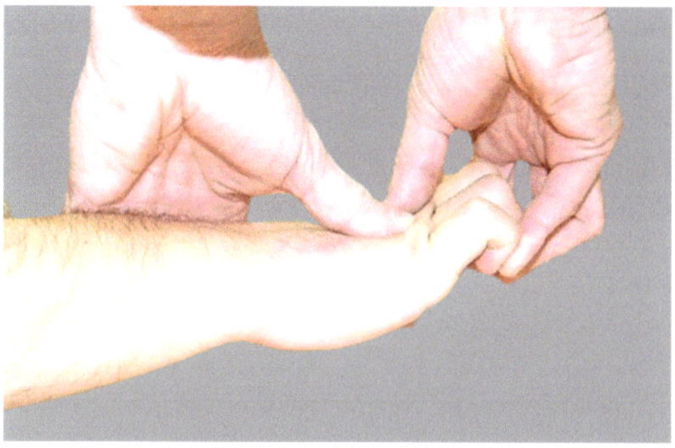

Fig. 5.7 Stretching of the interossei (extension of the metacarpophalangeal joints + flexion of the proximal interphalangeal joints + flexion of the distal interphalangeal joints)

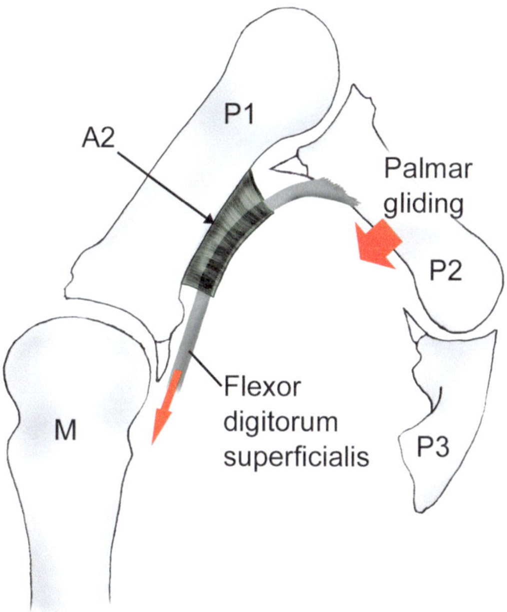

Fig. 5.8 The tonus of the flexor digitorum superficialis can generate an anterior (palmar) gliding of the base of the second phalanx relative to the first phalanx

Gradually, if nothing is done to counteract this gliding, the joint range of motion in flexion will be limited by the formation of a premature abutment of the volar plate against the proximal phalanx. This palmar advancement of the base of the intermediate phalanx is evidenced by a loss of mobility in active flexion. It is itself objectified by a loss of contact between the pulp of the distal phalanx and the pulp of the proximal phalanx when the patient is asked to place his fingers in a hook position (extension of the first phalanx combined with flexion of the second and third phalanges) (Fig. 5.9).

This "decentering" can be corrected by a reverse glide (posterior glide). In practice (Fig. 5.10), the finger to be treated is positioned with the proximal interphalangeal joint in a 90° flexion. The therapist places the intermediate phalanx of his own index against the base of the intermediate phalanx (palmar side). With the thumb of the same hand, he/she produces a counter-pressure on the dorsal, distal part of the intermediate phalanx. In this position, all that is required is a slight pull of around 300 g with the index to reharmonize the joint centering. This posterior gliding is sometimes accompanied by a small, audible click. It has no therapeutic value, nor is it a pejorative factor. At most, it can be used to show that the phalanx has "moved back," and joint "recentering" can be verified by repeating the initial test (Fig. 5.11).

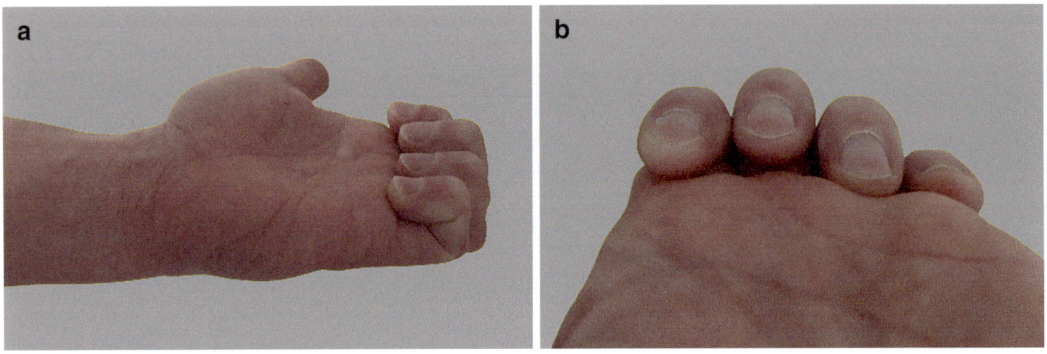

Fig. 5.9 (**a**, **b**) Loss of flexion in the third finger, linked to the palmar gliding of the second phalanx relative to the first phalanx

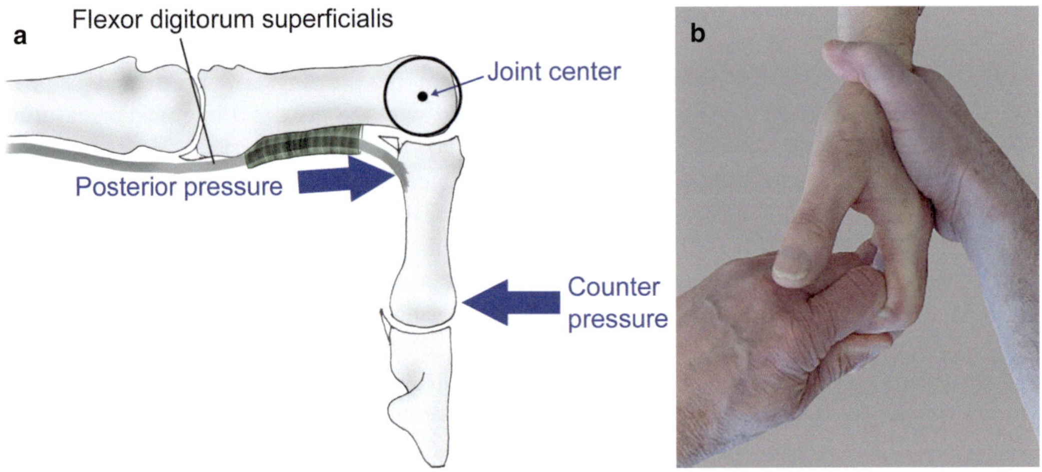

Fig. 5.10 (**a**, **b**) Principle of off-center correction. Slide the base of the second phalanx (from palmar to dorsal), producing a concomitant counter-pressure on the back of the distal end of the second phalanx

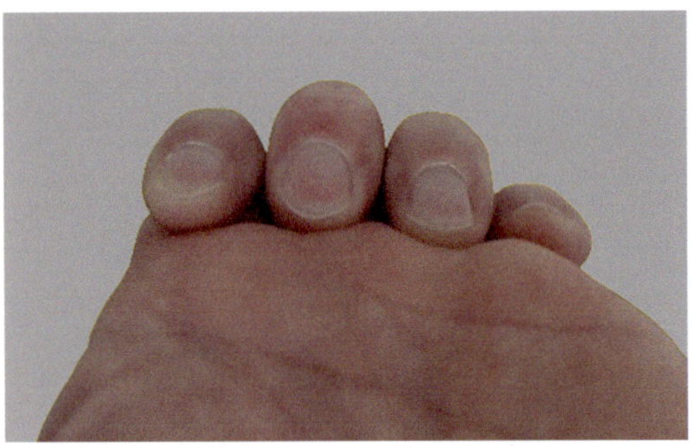

Fig. 5.11 After correction, the pulp of the third phalanx contacts with the pulp of the first phalanx again

Surgical Treatment

There are several methods for repairing or rebuilding a pulley [31]. Whatever the method, the goal of the surgery is to correct the "bowstring" and restore joint mobility and grip strength [12]. The literature indicates that this type of surgery is in fact infrequent and above all rather difficult to perform. The risk of losing a few degrees of mobility exists [7, 12, 15].

Surgical treatment is usually reserved only for competitive climbers and stage 4 injuries with a "bowstring" effect [11, 13].

Surgery is also required when an avulsed pulley has become lodged in the space between the tendon and the phalanx. In this case, the pulley has no chance of healing. This phenomenon can be compared to the Stener effect in sprains of the ulnar collateral ligament in the metacarpophalangeal joint of the thumb.

Different Surgical Repair Methods

Whatever the technique, surgical repair (direct suture or reconstruction of the injured pulley) is ambulatory, under local anesthesia and pneumatic tourniquet at the root of the limb, or under WALANT (Wide Awake Local Anesthesia No Tourniquet) for some teams.

The approach uses a Brüner incision centered on the injured pulley (proximal phalanx for A2 and intermediate phalanx for A4) and extended beyond the folds proximally and distally.

Direct Suture

Description

A direct suture [32] requires rapid, semi-emergency management, with only a few days for the edges to become viable before retraction of both ends of the ruptured pulley occurs, compromising direct suturing. It consists in suturing the two edges (radial and ulnar) of the pulley, more or less associated with an enlargement plasty, using an overlock or separate stitches with PDS 5/0 or 4/0 (poly P-dioxanone, Ethicon) absorbable monofilament thread.

Advantages

A direct suture eliminates the need to remove a graft for pulley reconstruction, making the procedure simpler, faster, and less invasive while preserving the original pulley and its properties.

Disadvantages

A direct suture requires rapid management before the stumps are retracted. In the case of pulley stump retraction, the resulting tissue loss does not allow direct suturing. Direct suturing is performed on pathological tissue resulting from an overload on the pulley, which can make the repair fragile.

Plasty

There are several techniques for reconstructing the osteofibrous annular pulley, depending on the choice of graft and its fixation or path.

Reconstruction Using the Lister Technique [33]

➔ **Description**

This is the technique of choice in our department. Scar tissue that is mechanically non-functional is excised until good-quality pulley grooves are obtained on each side of the digital canal. The neo-pulley is reconstructed using a graft harvested from the dorsal carpal ligament, at the level of the middle third of the fourth compartment, through a dorsal and transverse approach to the wrist (Fig. 5.12). The height of the harvested graft is approximately 15 mm, which corresponds approximately to the average height of A2 (16.8 mm according to Doyle) [34].

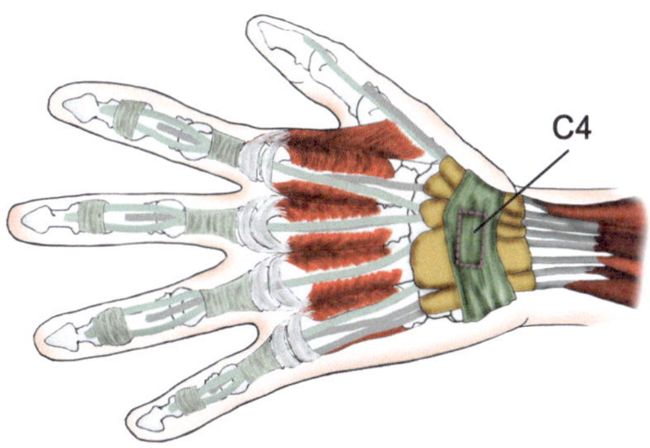

Fig. 5.12 Harvest of the middle third of the dorsal carpal ligament at the level of C4

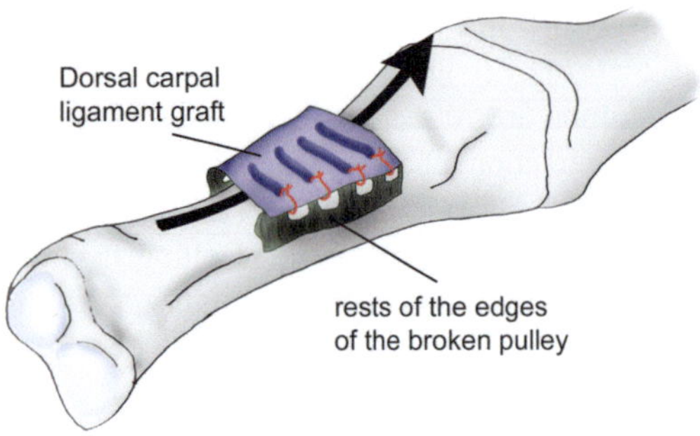

Fig. 5.13 Suturing the dorsal carpal ligament graft to the edges of the pulley

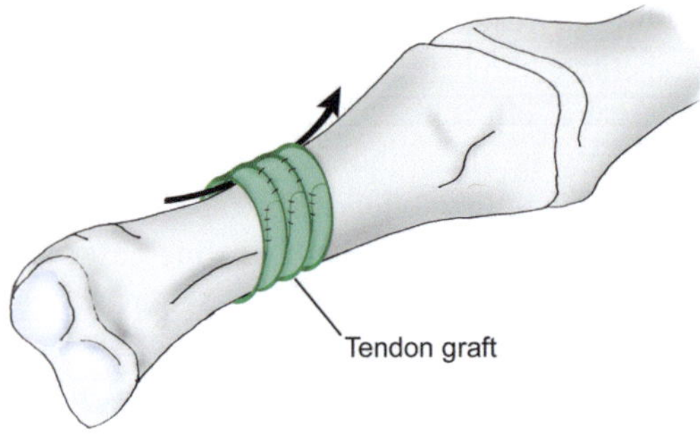

Fig. 5.14 Bunnell technique

The graft is placed in such a way that its fibers are perpendicular to the flexor tendons, and its synovial side is placed against the tendons to promote their gliding. The graft is secured to the edges with separate U-shaped stitches using PDS 4/0 (poly P-dioxanone, Ethicon) absorbable monofilament (Fig. 5.13). The suture is made maintaining the flexor tendons flat at the bottom of the digital canal, i.e., with the finger in a flexed position, to relieve the neo-pulley of any constraints from the flexor tendons. At the end of the suture, the absence of conflict between the neo-pulley and the flexor tendons is checked in flexion and extension.

If several pulleys are repaired, the palmaris longus or the contralateral dorsal carpal ligament is used.

➔ Advantages

The dorsal carpal ligament has the following advantages:

- It is synovialized (on its deep surface) like the pulleys it replaces, so when put in contact with the flexor tendon it eliminates friction and the risk of adherences by recreating a true gliding plane.
- It is an annular structure, and as its transverse fibers are positioned perpendicular to the tendon path, it offers greater resistance to the risk of longitudinal tearing.

Finally, the time required for repair does not affect the decision or the quality of the result.

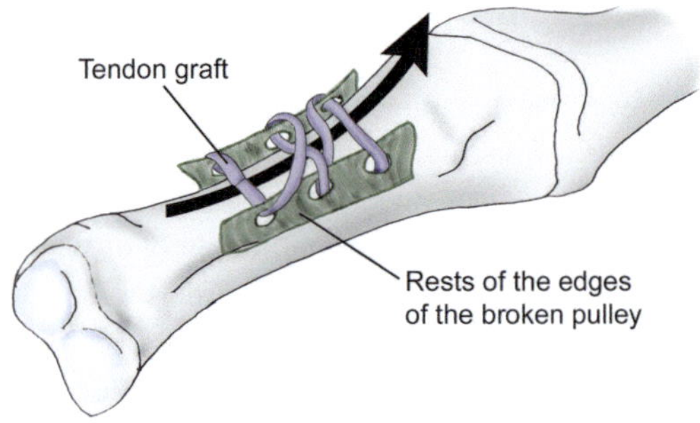

Fig. 5.15 Kleinert technique

➔ Disadvantage

Harvesting the graft from the dorsal carpal ligament involves a second surgery site, the complications of which may be wrist stiffness and/or pain linked to adherences, or even in extreme cases, “bowstrings” of the extensors from the fingers to the wrist.

Other Techniques

Other surgical techniques have been described for the repair of digital pulleys, using other types of graft (palmaris longus, flexor digitorum superficialis, plantaris, etc.):

- Bunnell’s technique [35] (Fig. 5.14) uses a graft of the palmaris longus or the extensor digiti minimi, wrapped around the phalanx and passed dorsally between the bone and the extensor tendon.
- Kleinert’s technique [36] (Fig. 5.15) fixes the same type of tendon graft (usually palmaris longus) by suturing it to the remaining edges of the pulley in the form of a lacing.

Rehabilitation

Rehabilitation after surgery is now well codified [4, 12, 37]. This is true for the surgeons with experience in this procedure. However, for other surgeons, who rarely operate pulleys, it remains at the experimental stage [21].

Here too, rehabilitation begins at an early stage [37]. This is essential to prevent tendon adherences and capsuloligamentous retraction, especially in the proximal interphalangeal joint. The danger is that flessum may set in on this joint. This flessum, in addition to impairing the mobility of the proximal interphalangeal joint, would have repercussions on the mobility of the distal interphalangeal joint, as these two joints are intimately linked by the oblique retinacular ligaments.

Rehabilitation is organized around two phases, one before healing and the other after.

From D0 to D45: Healing Phase

This involves wearing two orthoses (Fig. 5.16), which are made the day after surgery.

One is a long dorsal orthosis, made with the wrist flexed at 30° and the metacarpophalangeal joints flexed at 30° [4, 12]. The goal of this orthosis is to rest the flexor system and secure the repair. The other is a digital protection ring placed at the level of the repaired pulley(s). The long dorsal splint is worn for 45 days (24 h a day), while the ring is worn for 90 days [4, 12].

During this phase, rehabilitation aims to fight against the edema and maintain the capsuloligamentous flexibility and tendon glidings. In practice, for these last two elements, passive, analytical (Duran-type), and global mobilizations are performed (within the limits allowed by the orthosis). We then move on to gentle active mobilization (Fig. 5.17), following a sequence of pro-

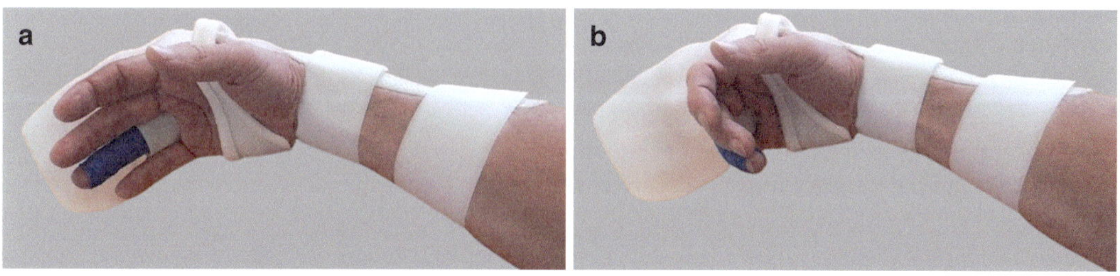

Fig. 5.16 (**a**, **b**) After surgery, a protective ring is prescribed, as well as a long dorsal protective orthosis

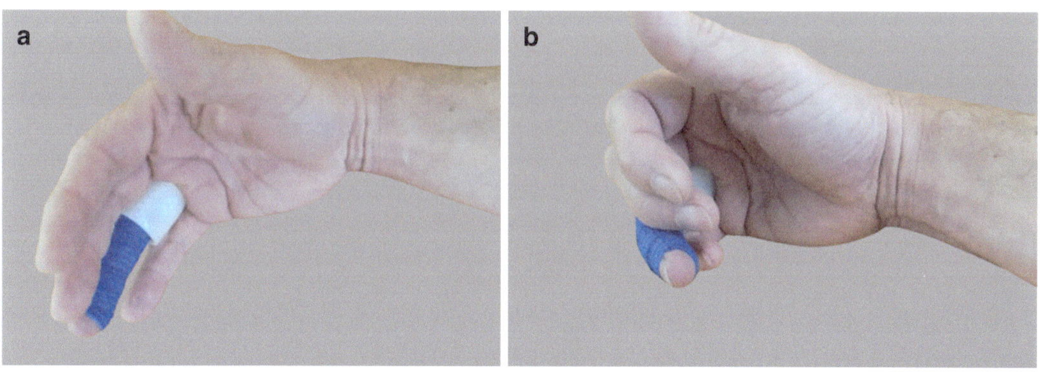

Fig. 5.17 (**a**, **b**) Early active mobilization after a surgical repair of the A2 pulley

gressive stresses: we start by performing a few "held-placed" movements, then a few active-assisted movements, and finally a few active movements without resistance. Of course, the ring must always be worn during these exercises.

After D45: Functional Recovery Phase

It is similar to the second phase of conservative treatment, to which we add the progressive recovery of the extension of the fingers and wrist. We keep mobilizing the tissues, and resistance is introduced progressively. To help quantify this progression, a Jamar® -type force clamp (Fig. 5.18) can be used during static exercises. Based on the maximum value measured on the healthy side, the patient is asked to perform lower-intensity (percentage) grasps with the recovering hand. During the first week of this second phase, we do not go higher than 20%. The resistance is then increased by 20% each week if the patient is pain-free.

For dynamic exercises, once the patient's range of motion has been regained, a 2 kg barbell can be used, and the patient is asked to perform an eccentric contraction with the flexor muscles by unwinding the wrist and fingers, followed by a concentric mobilization to flex the fingers and then the wrist (Fig. 5.19).

We gradually increase the resistance by adding weights to the barbell.

Climbing may not be resumed until after 90 days post-surgery and then only very gradually in terms of duration and intensity.

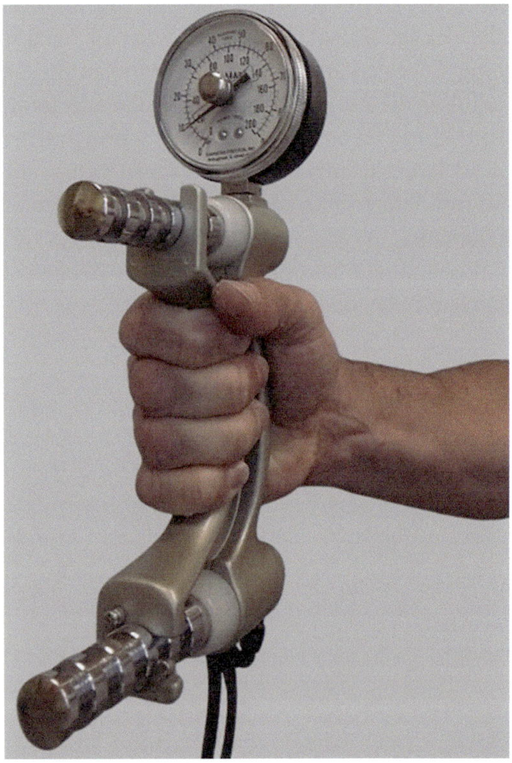

Fig. 5.18 A Jamar®-type force clamp is used to calibrate strength recovery

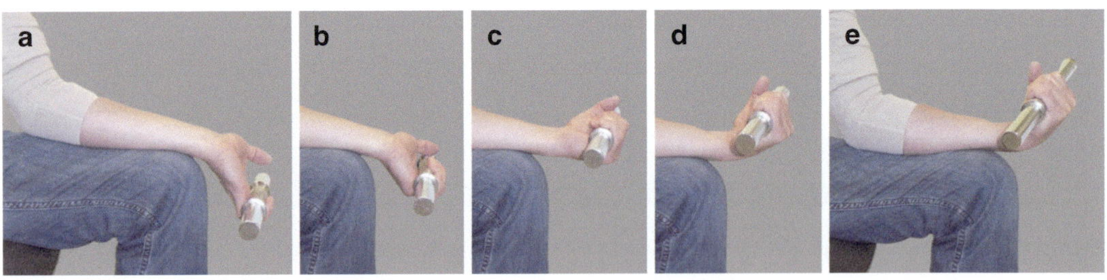

Fig. 5.19 Active mobilization of the fingers' flexors against progressive resistance, in a concentric (A to E) then eccentric (E to A) way

Conclusion

Conservative treatment is now the preferred option for treating finger pulley injuries. Surgery is still the exception rather than the rule and is reserved for extensive lesions involving several pulleys and for top-level sportsmen and women.

Overall, pulley restoration, which was relatively rare just a few years ago [21, 38], remains a surgical challenge today [21, 39]. The quality of the results often depends on the expertise of the treatment team [4].

Conservative treatment, based on wearing a thermoplastic ring combined with rehabilitation, provides excellent results if the healing times are respected.

As for the future of this pathology, it will depend very much on the prophylactic education given to climbers. It has been shown that a lack of warm-up and an inappropriate physical preparation are the main causes of ruptures [29]. It is therefore essential to explain to climbers the importance of a good physical preparation and a good warm-up if we want to see a decrease in this pathology [4, 18, 25].

Bibliography

1. Bollen SR. Injury to the A2 pulley in rock climbers. J Hand Surg (Br). 1990;15:268–70.
2. Tropet Y, Menez D, Balmat P, Pem R, Vichard PH. Closed traumatic rupture of the ring finger flexor tendon pulley. J Hand Surg. 1990;15A:745–7.
3. Lin GT, Cooney WP, Amadio PC, An KN. Mechanical properties of human pulleys. J Hand Surg Br. 1990;15(4):429–34.
4. Moutet F. Flexor tendon pulley system: anatomy, pathology, treatment. Chir Main. 2003;22:1–12.
5. Roloff I, Schöffl V, Vigouroux L, Quaine F. Biomechanical model for the determination of the forces acting on the finger pulley system. J Biomech. 2005;39:915–23.
6. Peterson WW, Manske PR, Bollinger BA, Lesker PA, McCarthy JA. Effect of pulley excision on flexor tendon biomechanics. J Orthop Res. 1986;4(1):96–101.
7. King EA, Lien JR. Flexor tendon pulley injuries in rock climbers. Hand Clin. 2017;33:141–8.
8. Crowley T. The flexor tendon pulley system and rock climbing. J Hand Microsurg. 2016;04(01):25–9.
9. Bollen SR. Soft tissue injury in extreme rock climbers. Br J Sports Med. 1988;22:145–7.
10. Marco RA, Sharkey NA, Smith TS, Zissimos AG. Pathomechanics of closed rupture of the flexor tendon pulleys in rock climbers. J Bone Joint Surg. 1998;80(A):1012–9.
11. Zafonte B, Rendulic D, Szabo RM. Flexor pulley system: anatomy, injury, and management. J Hand Surg Am. 2014;39(12):2525–32.
12. Bouyer M, Forli A, Semere A, et al. Recovery of rock climbing performance after surgical reconstruction of finger pulleys. J Hand Surg Eur. 2016;41(4):406–12.
13. Schoffl VR, Einwag F, Strecker W, et al. Strength measurement and clinical outcome after pulley ruptures in climbers. Med Sci Sports Exerc. 2006;38(4):637–43.
14. Warme WJ, Brooks D. The effect of circumferential taping on flexor tendon pulley failure in rock climbers. Am J Sports Med. 2000;28:674–8.
15. Arora R, Fritz D, Zimmermann R, et al. Reconstruction of the digital flexor pulley system: a retrospective comparison of two methods of treatment. J Hand Surg Eur Vol. 2007;32(1):60e66.
16. Schöffl VR, Jüngert J. Closed flexor pulley injuries in nonclimbing activities. J Hand Surg Am. 2006;31:806–10.
17. Leung KH, Ho PC. A rare cause of thumb boutonniere deformity: flexor pulley rupture. J Orthop Trauma Rehabil. 2012;16:75–7.
18. Martinoli C, Bianchi S, Cotten A. Imaging of rock climbing injuries. Semin Musculoskelet Radiol. 2005;9:334–45.
19. Schöffl V, Popp D, Küpper T, et al. Injury trends in rock climbers: evaluation of a case series of 911 injuries between 2009 and 2012. Wilderness Environ Med. 2015;26(1):62–7.
20. Vigouroux L, et al. Estimation of finger muscle tendon tensions and pulley forces during specific sport-climbing grip techniques. J Biomech. 2006;39:2583–92.
21. Dy CJ, Daluiski A. Flexor pulley reconstruction. Hand Clin. 2013;29:235–42.
22. Scott K, Dulle D, Garcia G, Flug JA, Chhabra A. Multiple flexor tendon pulley ruptures in a division 1 collegiate football player. Orthop Rev (Pavia). 2019 Dec 2;11(4):8316.
23. Moutet F, Guinard D, Gerard P, Mugnier C. Subcutaneous rupture of long finger flexor pulleys in rock climbers. 12 case reports. Ann Chir Main Memb Super. 1993;12:182–8.
24. Schneeberger M, Schweizer A. Pulley ruptures in rock climbers: outcome of conservative treatment with the pulley-protection splint-a series of 47 cases. Wilderness Environ Med. 2016;27:211–8.
25. Barton NJ. Experimental study of optimal location of flexor tendon pulleys. Plast Reconstr Surg. 1969;43:125–9.
26. Voulliaume D, Forli A, Parzy O, Moutet F. Surgical repair in flexor tendon pulley rupture in high level rock climbing. Chir Main. 2004;23:243–8.
27. Dykes B, Johnson J, San Juan JG. Effects of finger taping on forearm muscle activation in rock climbers. J Electromyogr Kinesiol. 2019;45:11–7.

28. Schweizer A. Biomechanical effectiveness of taping the A2 pulley in rock climbers. J Hand Surg Br. 2000;25:102–7.
29. Schöffl I, Einwag F, Strecker W, Hennig F, Schoffl V. Impact of taping after finger flexor tendon pulley ruptures in rock climbers. J Appl Biomech. 2007;23(1):52e62.
30. Ginszt M, Ginszt A, Berger M, Gawda P, Tarkowski Z. Finger flexor pulley injury of sport climbers—literature review. Pol Ann Med. 2016;23(2):191–4.
31. Widstrom CJ, Johnson G, Doyle JR, Manske PR, Inhofe P. A mechanical study of six digital pulley reconstruction techniques: Part I. Mechanical effectiveness. J Hand Surg Am. 1989b;14:821–5.
32. Philip L. Rééducation apres suture directe d'une poulie rompue chez le grimpeur de haut niveau. Mémoire DIU rééducation et appareillage après chirurgie de la main 2019. https://www.sfrm-gemmsor.fr/file/medtool/webmedtool/gemmtool01/botm0206/pdf00001.pdf
33. Lister GD. Reconstruction of pulleys employing extensor retinaculum. J Hand Surg. 1979;4:461–4.
34. Doyle JR. Anatomy of the finger flexor tendon sheath and pulley system. J Hand Surg Am. 1988;13:473–84.
35. Boyle JH. In Bunnell's surgery of the hand. 5th ed. Philadelphia: JB Lippincott; 1970. p. 403–4.
36. Kleinert HE, Bennett JB. Digital pulley reconstruction employing the always present rim of the previous pulley. J Hand Surg. 1978;3:297–8.
37. Clark TA, Skeete K, Amadio PC. Flexor tendon pulley reconstruction. J Hand Surg Am. 2010;35(10):1685–9.
38. Dy CJ, Lyman S, Schreiber JJ, Do HT, Daluiski A. The epidemiology of reoperation after flexor pulley reconstruction. J Hand Surg Am. 2013;38(9):1705e1711.
39. Mehta V, Phillips CS. Flexor tendon pulley reconstruction. Hand Clin. 2005;21(2):245–51.

Part III

Tendon Injuries of the Hand

6 Injuries of the Extensor Tendons

Grégory Mesplié

The extensor system is composed of an extrinsic system and an intrinsic system that work in synergy during the digital extension.

It is extra-synovial, except at the level of the extensor retinaculum where it is surrounded by a synovial sheath allowing its lubrication and nutrition [18] (Fig. 6.1).

The tendons are flat, composed of longitudinal fibers and located directly under the skin.

Their treatment depends on the injured area.

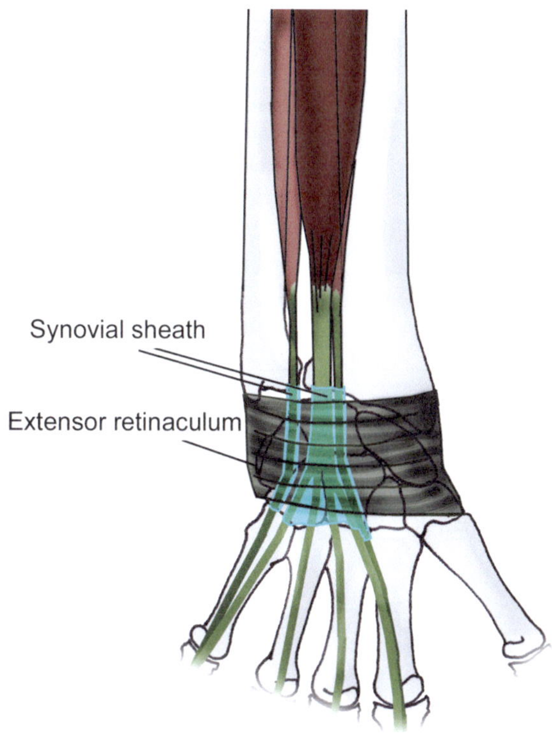

Fig. 6.1 Synovial sheath of the extensor system, allowing its lubrication and nutrition

G. Mesplié (✉)
Institut Sud Aquitain de la Main et du Membre Supérieur (ISAMMS), Biarritz, France

G. Mesplié (ed.), *Hand Functional Anatomy and Therapy*,
https://doi.org/10.1007/978-3-031-92505-4_6

Classification

The International Federation of Societies for Surgery of the Hand made a classification allowing us to study their physiology depending on their topography (Fig. 6.2).

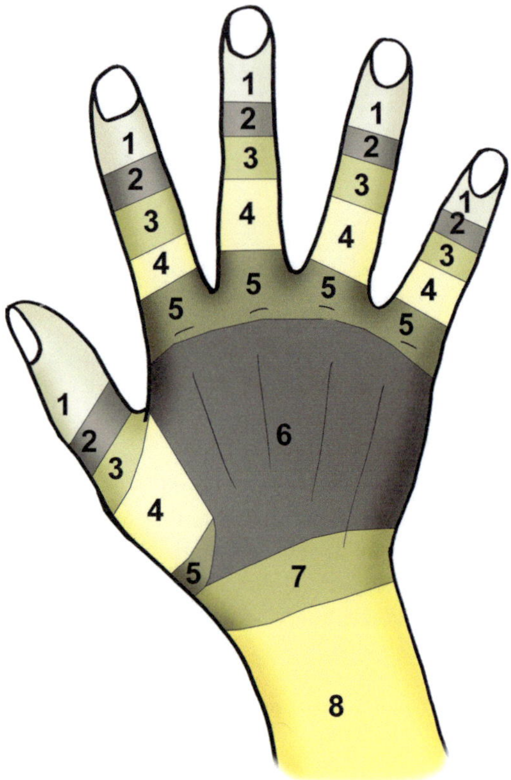

Fig. 6.2 Topographic classification of the extensors

Fingers

Zone 1

It is the area where the lateral strips end; they come together and insert on the base of the dorsal side of the distal phalanx. The tendon is not vascularized much at this level.

The injuries at this level lead to a mallet finger, characterized by a drop in flexion of the distal phalanx (Fig. 6.3).

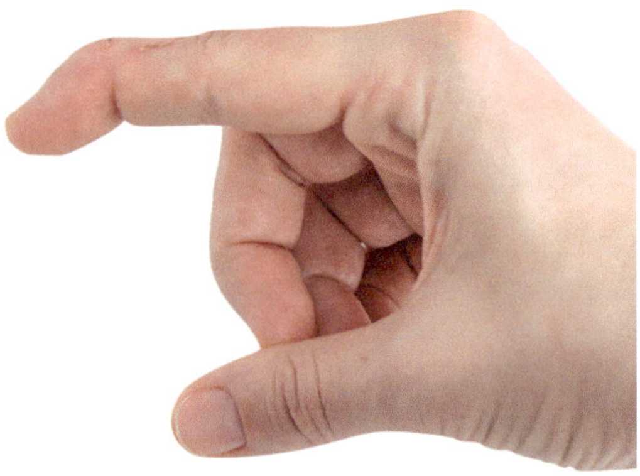

Fig. 6.3 Mallet finger

These deformities can evolve into a swan-neck deformity, especially when the volar plate of the proximal interphalangeal joint is slack (Fig. 6.4).

Zone 2

In this zone we find the lateral strips, next to the diaphysis of the second phalanx. The deformity is the same as in zone 1, but there can be an associated injury of the oblique retinacular ligament, leading to a faster swan-neck deformity especially if the volar plate of the proximal interphalangeal joint is slack.

Zone 3

Next to the proximal interphalangeal joint, it is the area of trifurcation of the extensor system, forming the two lateral strips and the median strip ending on the base of the second phalanx.

An isolated injury of the median strip leads to a boutonnière deformity (Fig. 6.5). The lateral strips go to palmar, putting the proximal interphalangeal joint in flexion and the distal interphalangeal joint in extension.

Zone 4

It is the zone next to the diaphysis of the first phalanx, at the level of the dorsal expansion of the interossei.

Zone 5

It is the zone next to the metacarpophalangeal joint. At this level, the extensor tendons are stabilized on the metacarpals by the sagittal strips that insert on both sides of the tendon, on the interglenoidal ligaments (Fig. 6.6).

These stabilizing elements are tensed when the metacarpophalangeal is flexed and relaxed when it is extended.

An injury in the radial sagittal strip leads to a dislocation of the extensor tendon in the ulnar intermetacarpal area, as the extensor system is decentered relative to the axis of the metacarpophalangeal joints. Therefore, the injuries of the ulnar sagittal

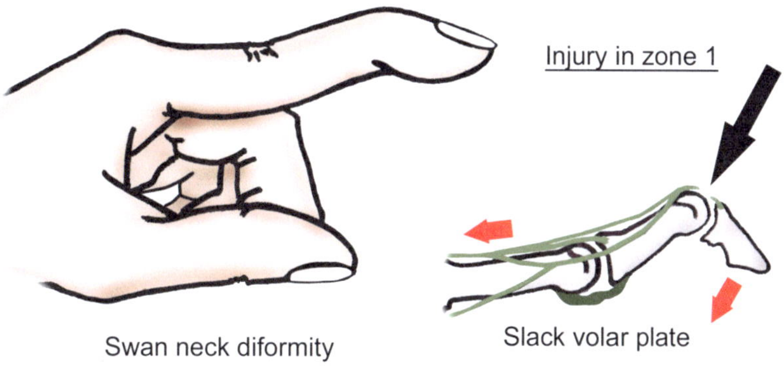

Fig. 6.4 Swan-neck deformity after a mallet finger badly treated. The tension normally applied on the second and third phalanges is now only applied on the second phalanx. In case of slackness of the proximal interphalangeal joint, this excess of tension leads to a joint in hyperextension

Fig. 6.5 Boutonnière deformity

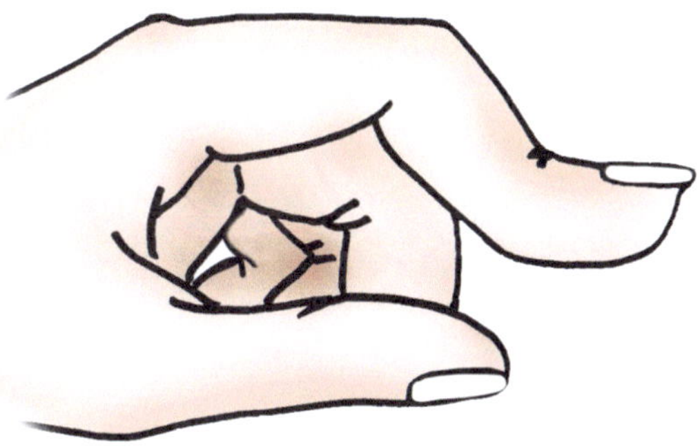

strip do not lead to a dislocation of the extensor tendon in the radial inter-metacarpal area (Fig. 6.7).

Zone 6

The extensor tendons pass along the dorsal side of the metacarpals. At this level, there are some inter-tendinous junctions that connect the extensor tendons.

If there is an injury above the inter-tendinous junctions, the extension deficit will be small, because it is partly compensated by the adjacent tendons (Fig. 6.8).

Zone 7

The tendons slide in the synovial sheath next to the extensor retinaculum. Unlike the extensor indicis, the extensor digiti minimi has its own sheath (Fig. 6.9).

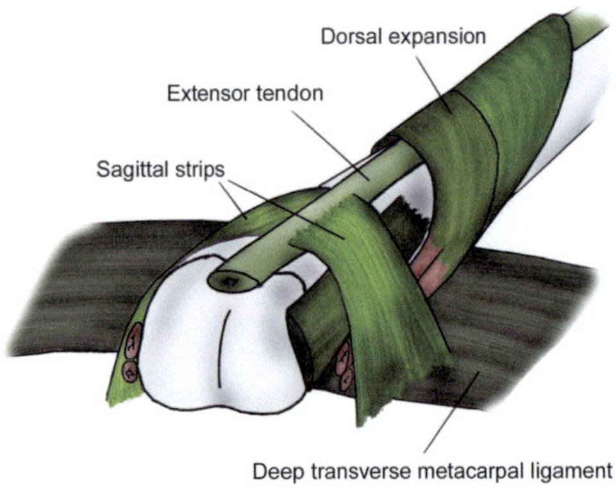

Fig. 6.6 At the level of the metacarpophalangeal joints, the sagittal strips stabilize the extensor tendons in the frontal plane

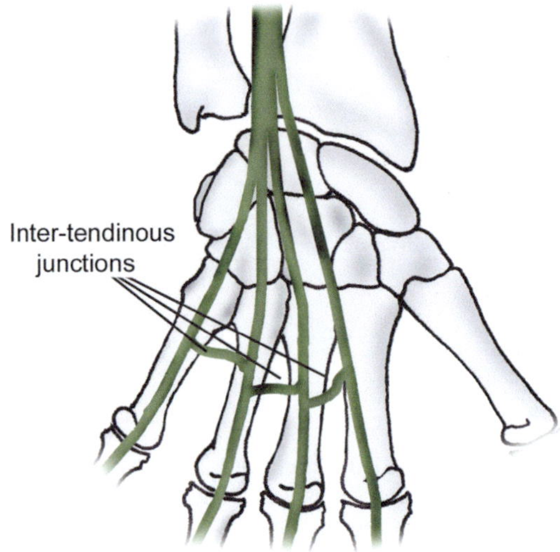

Fig. 6.8 Inter-tendinous junctions in zone 6

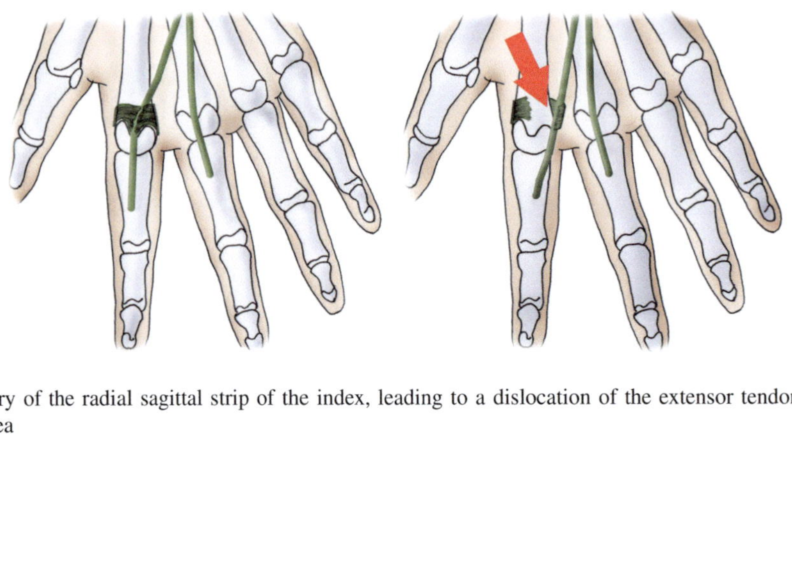

Fig. 6.7 Injury of the radial sagittal strip of the index, leading to a dislocation of the extensor tendon in the inter-metacarpal area

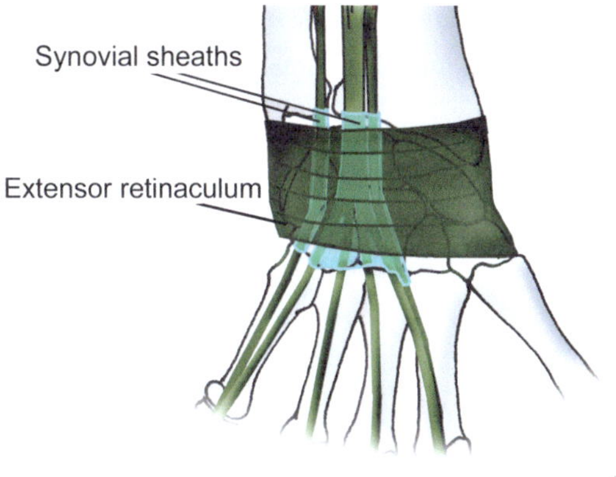

Fig. 6.9 Unlike the extensor indicis, the extensor digiti minimi has its own sheath

Zone 8

It is the zone above the extensor retinaculum, until the myotendinous junction.

Thumb

The extensor system of the thumb also depends on an extrinsic system made by the extensor pollicis brevis and the extensor pollicis longus, and an intrinsic system made by the sesamoid muscles. The abductor pollicis brevis and the flexor pollicis brevis form the radial part of the dorsal expansion, and the adductor pollicis forms the ulnar part.

The extensor tendons of the thumb pass through six zones, four of which are specific to the thumb and are preceded by the letter T (thumb): TI, TII, TIII, TIV. Two zones are shared with the extensors of the fingers: zones VII (wrist) and VIII (forearm).

Physiopathology

There are two types of injuries of the extensor system:

- Subcutaneous rupture: the most frequent are at the level of the distal interphalangeal joint (leading to a mallet finger) and the proximal interphalangeal joint (leading to a boutonnière deformity). We can also observe this injury at the level of the metacarpophalangeal joint after a punch that causes a rupture of the sagittal strip and a dislocation of the extensor in the inter-metacarpal area. In the thumb, the injury is most often in the extensor pollicis longus at the level of the Lister tubercle, where the muscle changes its direction (Fig. 6.10).
- Open traumas: they most often affect the index or the thumb. Their severity depends on the nature of the device that has damaged the extensor system and on the associated injuries. Wounds are the most frequent injuries of the extensor tendons, which are very superficial, located subcutaneously on the dorsal surface of the hand and wrist, and are therefore very exposed in the event of an injury. In traumas by crushing, the dorsal abrasions and infectious factors worsen the functional prognosis.

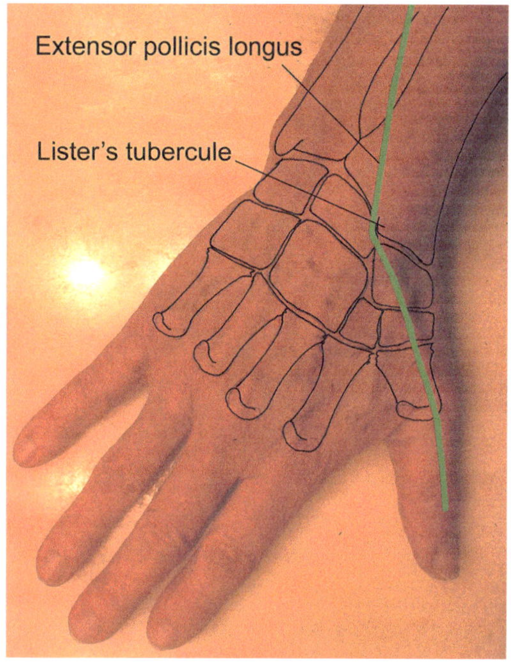

Fig. 6.10 Lister's tubercle is an "at-risk" zone for the extensor pollicis longus, as it changes direction at this level, increasing the stresses to which it is subjected

Clinical and Paraclinical Signs

Several clinical tests make it possible to determine an injury of the extensor system:

- Extensor pollicis longus: hand lying flat on the table, we ask the patient to lift the thumb from the table (Fig. 6.11).
- Extensor pollicis brevis: we ask the patient to realize an extension of the metacarpophalangeal joint against resistance.
- Extensor indicis and extensor digiti minimi: we ask the patient to make a selective extension of the index and the little finger ("make horns") (Fig. 6.12).
- Extensor digitorum: the patient must be able to realize a selective extension of the phalanges against resistance. If there is an injury above the inter-tendinous junctions, a relative compensation can be realized by the adjacent extensor tendons.
- Median strip: the active extension of the distal interphalangeal joint can only be realized with the proximal interphalangeal joint in extension. The tension of the median strip during the flexion of the proximal interphalangeal joint relaxes the lateral strips, making them ineffective on the distal interphalangeal joint. If active extension of the distal interphalangeal joint is possible with the proximal interphalangeal joint in flexion, this indicates a rupture of the median strip. This phenomenon is the physiological basis of the Elson test (Fig. 6.13).

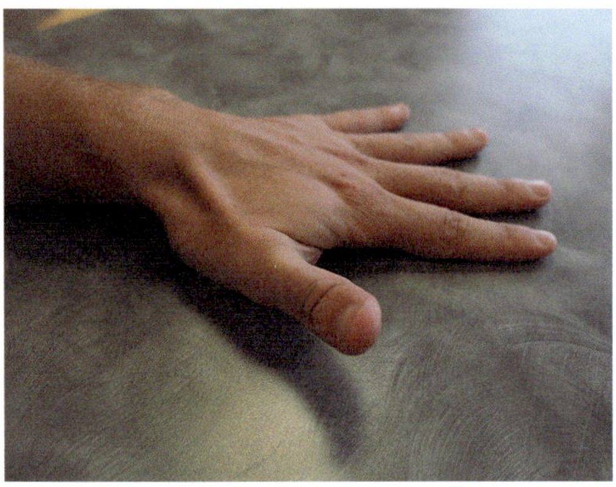

Fig. 6.11 If the patient cannot lift the thumb off the table, the extensor pollicis longus is probably broken

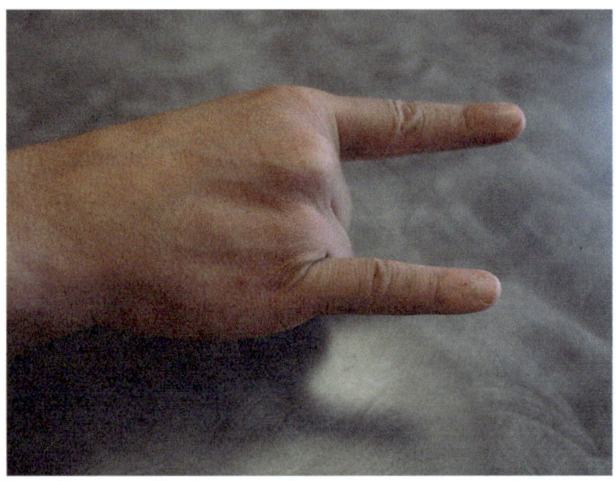

Fig. 6.12 "Horns" test verifying the integrity of the extensor indicis and extensor digiti minimi

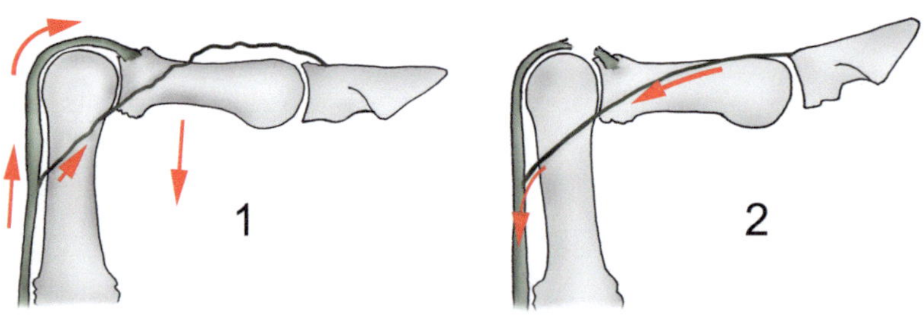

Fig. 6.13 Elson test: if the median strip is broken, the flexion of the proximal interphalangeal joint does not relax the lateral strips. The lateral strips keep their efficiency and can realize an extension of the distal interphalangeal joint

- Lateral strips: the active extension of the distal interphalangeal joint is impossible in extension of the proximal interphalangeal joint, indicating a lesion of the lateral strips.

If there is any doubt about all these injuries, an ultrasound may be performed to confirm or refute the diagnosis.

Therapeutic Process and Treatments

The therapeutic process for this type of injuries depends on the affected area.

Zones 1 and 2

The cause of a mallet deformity is usually a blow to the fingertip that causes sudden flexion and pulls the lateral strips of the extensor system [1, 2]. Active extension of the distal interphalangeal joint is impossible, as the lateral strips responsible for its extension are injured.

In a retrospective study of mallet fractures in 42 patients, 74% of fractures involved the dominant hands, while only 26% involved the nondominant hands. Over 90% of injuries occurred in the three ulnar fingers [3].

Mallet fingers can be tendinous or, more rarely, bony. There are three types of injury [4] (Fig. 6.14):

- Type I: simple rupture of the tendon near its distal insertion. The X-ray does not reveal any abnormality. In practice, the proximal end of the tendon recedes by 2 to 4 mm towards the neck of the second phalanx, depending on whether the rupture is complete or incomplete.
- Type II: a bone tear at the base of the distal phalanx, which is sometimes tiny and involves less than a third of the joint surface. It is usually separated from its original site by a space of 2 to 3 mm, due to the flessum of the phalanx. In this case, the extensor system is not retracted.

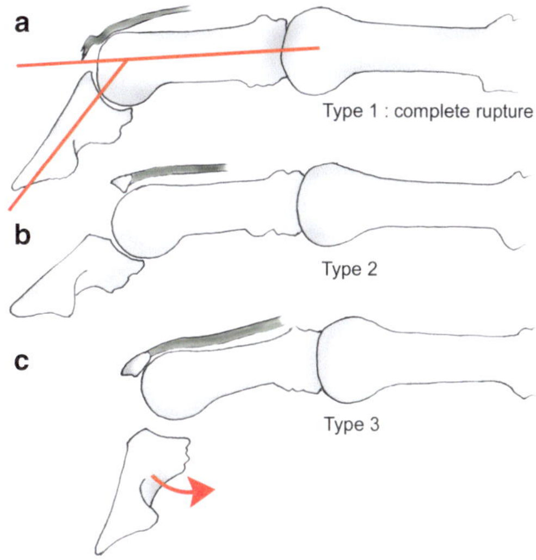

Fig. 6.14 Types of mallet fingers

- Type III: large bone tear, often greater than a third of the joint surface and accompanied by a palmar subluxation of the distal interphalangeal joint.

The treatment is usually conservative (types 1 and 2) [5–8], but surgery is necessary in the case of a bony mallet finger when the bone fragment represents more than a third of the joint surface with or without palmar subluxation of the distal phalanx (type 3) [1]. It will then be reduced and fixed with an arthroplasty pin.

For the period of strict immobilization, we prefer to use a stack orthosis made of thin microperforated plastic (1.6 mm) (Fig. 6.15).

A dorsal tile that frees the pulp can also be proposed, especially in damages to the index, where the risk of functional exclusion is greater.

Strict immobilization is maintained for 6–8 weeks after surgery and 8 weeks in the case of conservative treatment, with monitoring of the orthosis and weekly bandage changes. Whether after surgery or not, this period is followed by 2 weeks during which the patient wears the orthosis at night.

Bastien and Rouzaud [9] recommend starting the immobilization at D20, especially in the case of marked inflammatory phenomena, to significantly optimize the chances of successful treat-

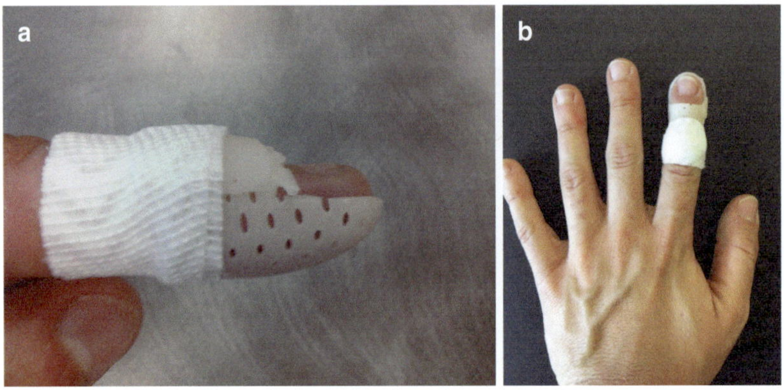

Fig. 6.15 Stack orthosis

ment (13 times greater chance of obtaining a good or excellent result) [9].

D0 to D45–60 (After Surgery) or D60 (Conservative Treatment)—Immobilization (Fig. 6.16)

Aside from the advice of self-mobilization of the proximal interphalangeal joint, the rehabilitation is not essential from D1 to D60, but we do ask the patient to come in for a control of the orthosis once a week to limit the risks associated with this type of treatment (cutaneous state, observance of the instructions, etc.).

Physiologically, the active mobilization of the proximal interphalangeal joint does not tense the lateral strips of the extensor system (Fig. 6.17). It is essential in this phase to avoid stiffness.

D45–60 (After Surgery) or D60 (Conservative Treatment) to D90—Fragility

This phase corresponds to the end of the immobilization; we must regain the mobility of the distal interphalangeal joint in flexion while maintaining the active extension lock.

The goals of the rehabilitation during this phase are:

➔ Fight Against Trophic Disorders and Pain

- Massages: trophic and analgesic goals, around the tendinous healing area. This area can stay inflammatory during several months.
- Transcutaneous vibratory stimulations: 70 Hz frequency on the extensor system if we want to improve the proprioceptive aspect or 100 Hz on the painful areas if we want an analgesic effect (Fig. 6.18).
- Depressotherapy: on the healing area, preferring disto-proximal movements of the head (Fig. 6.19).
- Electrotherapy: 1 Hz to fight against inflammation or electro-active to regain the active amplitudes (without excessive tension).

➔ Progressive Recovery of the Joint Amplitudes

- Recovery of the active and passive amplitudes of the proximal interphalangeal joint: this exercise is not always necessary, as it is part of the self-rehabilitation exercises proposed to the patient during the immobilization phase.
- Fluidotherapy: hot if there is no inflammation, to improve viscoelasticity of the tissues and therefore mobility.
- Active exercise for the flexion of the distal interphalangeal joint, active-assisted then active extension: the flexion of the distal interphalangeal joint is realized actively only to limit the risks of excessive tension on the tendinous callus. In the first sessions, the patient returns to the extension position with passive and active-assisted movements, then with a simple active movement when the active extension locking is reached (Fig. 6.20). Evans [10] suggests limiting flexion to 25° the

a **Subcutaneous injuryof the extensors in zones 1-2 / Mallet-finger**

	Immobilization (A)	Relative fragility (B)	Consolidation (C)
REHABILITATION	**Therapeutic goals** : 1- Tendon healing 2- Maintain the mobility of the proximal interphalangeal joint **Techniques:** 1- Learning the protection rules during the maintenance of the orthosis (+control by the orthotist once a week) 2- Self-mobillizations of the proximal interphalangeal joint **Risks:** Bad tendon healing, stiffness of the proximal interphalangeal joint	**Therapeutic goals** : 1- Same as in phase A, intensifying the techniques si necessary 2- Recover active amplitudes in the distal interphalangeal joint 3- Fight against potential trophic disorder 4- Maintain the body mapping **Techniques:** 1- Specific and global mobilizations of the proximal interphalangeal joint (A2) 2- Active exercice in flexion (< 25° before D60) of the distal interphalangeal joint returning to extension with an active-assisted movement, then simple active exercice (depending on the locking in extension) Exercice with the proximal interphalangeal joint flexed, then extended. Increase of the flexion of the distal interphalangeal joint of 10°/week if no lag. Electrostimulation. 3- Trophic massages, fluidotherapy, depressotherapy around the scar. 4-Manipulations of light objects, TVS (70-80Hz) **Risks:** Distension or inflammation of the tendinous callus if the exercices in flexion are too intense	**Therapeutic goals** : 1- Intensify the techniques from the 2 previous phases if necessary 2- Complete functional recovery **Techniques:** 1- Specific joint mobilizations, increasing the electrostimulation's electric intensities, and stretching the intrinsic muscles (B1) 2- Functional activities adapted to the patient's professional and sporting needs, **Risks:** Same as in phase B
ORTHOSIS	Immobilization orthosis worn all the time with the distal interphalangeal joint between 0° and 15° of hyperextension Stack or dorsal tile	Stack orthosis worn during the night until D75 if necessary	Orthosis to gain amplitude if limitation of articular origin
	D0-D60	D60-D90	After D90

b

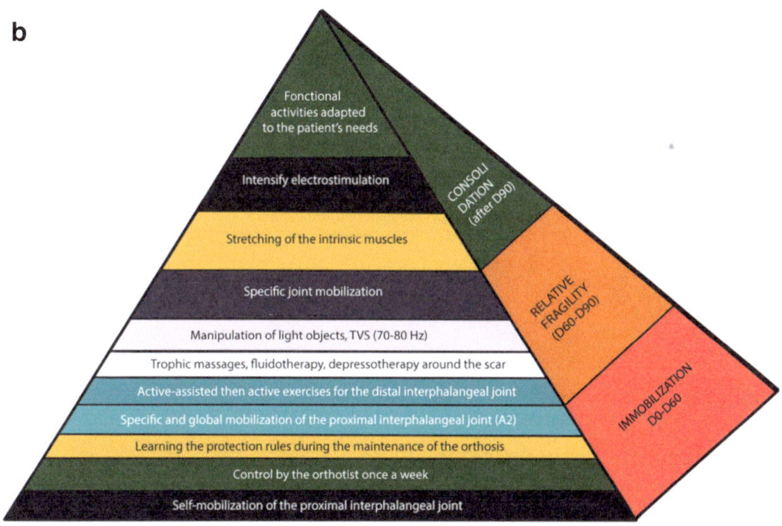

Fig. 6.16 Rehabilitation protocol (**a**) and progression pyramid (**b**) after mallet finger

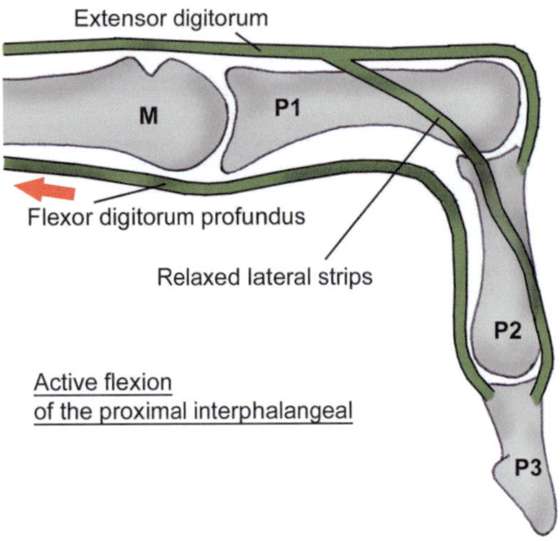

Fig. 6.17 The mobilization of the proximal interphalangeal joint puts the median strip in tension, which leads to a relaxation of the lateral strips

week following the removal of the orthosis, then increasing this amplitude by 15° per week if active extension is maintained.

- Specific mobilizations of the proximal interphalangeal joint: realized if there still is stiffness in the joint (loss of the intra-articular glidings) (see chapter "Hand and Wrist Mobilizations" in Volume 1 (Fig. 6.21).

➔ Maintaining the Body Mapping

The "blinding" of the finger pulp for 2 months, related to the Stack orthosis, can lead to a perturbation in the body mapping (until functional exclusion of the concerned finger).

These disorders essentially concern the index, which is rarely concerned by this type of injuries [9] and are treated by stimulating the mechanore-

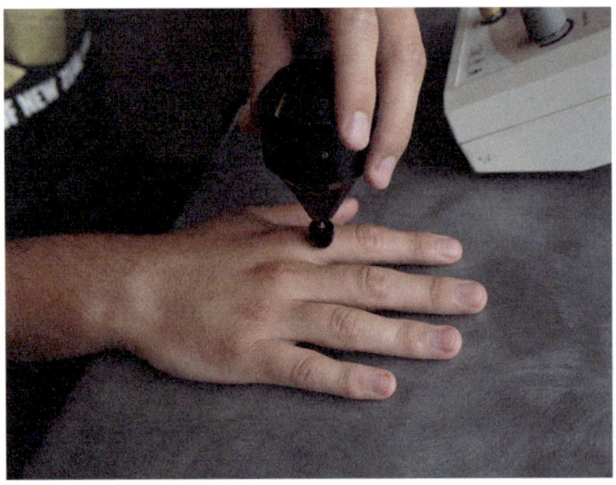

Fig. 6.18 Transcutaneous vibratory stimulation with a proprioceptive or analgesic effect, depending on the frequency

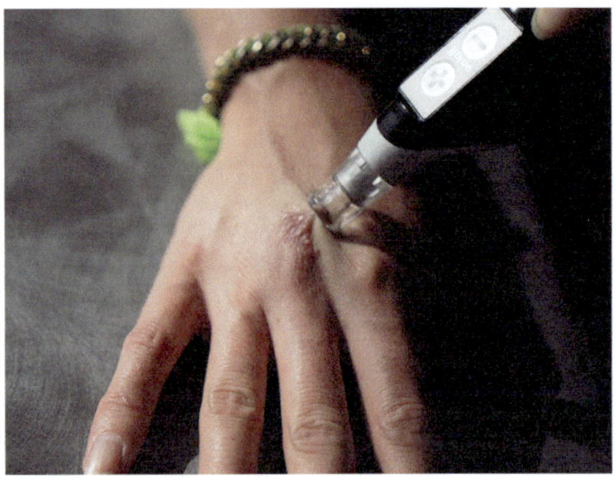

Fig. 6.19 Depressotherapy to relax the scar and fight against the edema

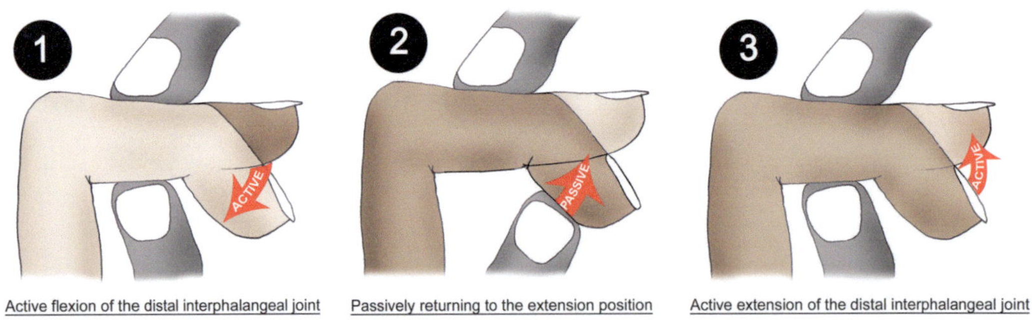

Fig. 6.20 Progressive mobilizations to limit the constraints on the tendinous callus

ceptors of the pulp of the concerned finger and working with simple and complex grips.

Recognizing this trouble is an essential element in the treatment success (Fig. 6.22).

After D90 (Solidity)

This phase corresponds with the patient going back to doing all his sports and professional activities.

The rehabilitation is focused on the complete rehabilitation of the joint amplitudes, the strength of the hand and wrist, the complex grips, the proprioception, and the digital dexterity.

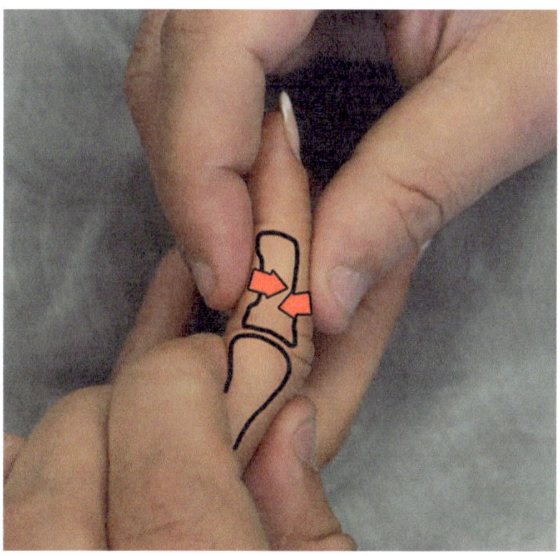

Fig. 6.21 Specific mobilizations of the proximal interphalangeal joint

➔ Specific Mobilizations of the Proximal and Distal Interphalangeal Joints

Regaining the intra-articular glidings is essential in the good recuperation of the amplitudes and the decrease of the resistances to movement. These glidings are realized in all the planes, without pain or tension on the tendinous callus (see chapter "Fractures of Metacarpals and Phalanges").

➔ Stretching the Intrinsic Muscles

These stretchings are realized if the Finochietto test is positive, meaning there is a retraction of the intrinsic muscles.

We stretch the interossei passively placing the hand in the "extrinsic +" position.

To stretch the lumbrical muscles, this position must be combined with an extension of the wrist to put tension of the flexor digitorum profundus (where the lumbrical muscles have their proximal insertion) (Fig. 6.23).

➔ Recovery of Proprioceptive Abilities

Rebalancing the muscular ratios, especially between the extrinsic and intrinsic systems, is realized, comparing the healthy side with dynamometers (Fig. 6.24). It is combined with an exercise for dexterity and coordination, adapted to the patient's functional needs.

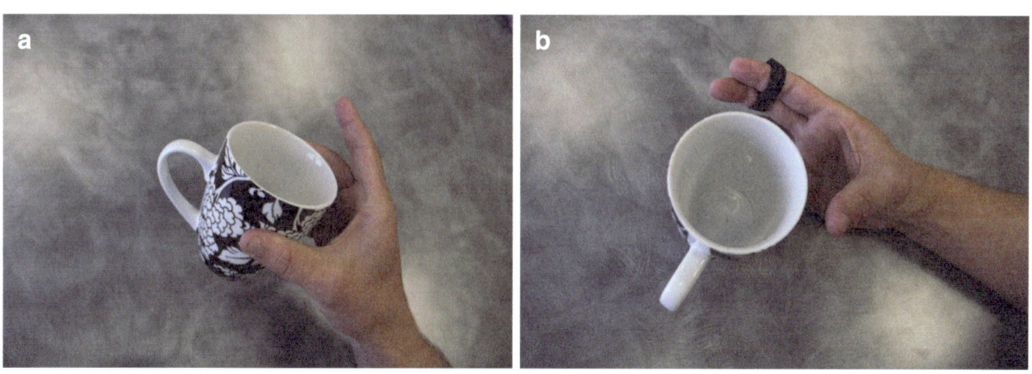

Fig. 6.22 Functional exclusion of the index (rare but must be carefully monitored) (**a**). Syndactyly participating in the reintegration of the index in the grips (**b**)

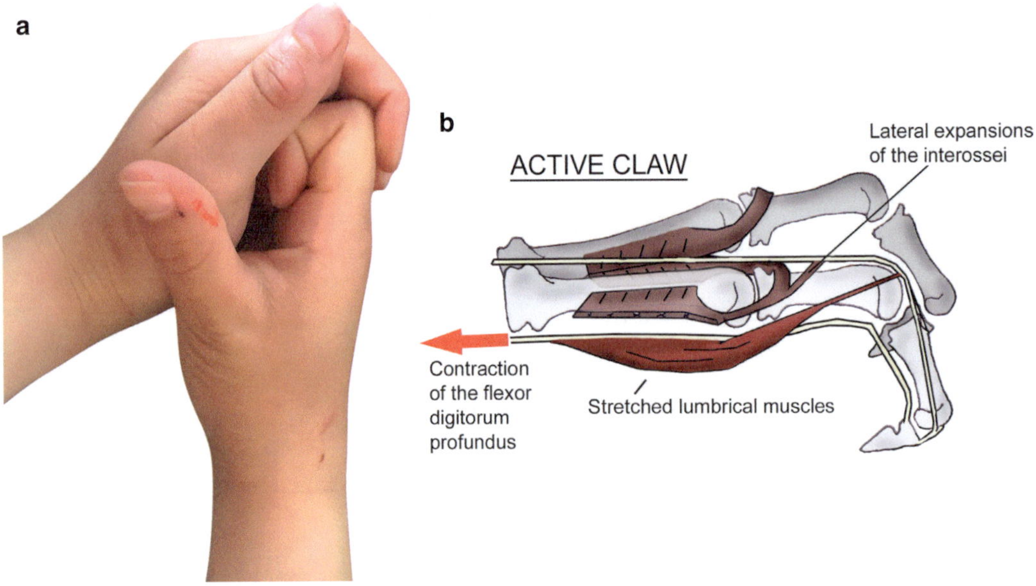

Fig. 6.23 The stretching of the interossei is done passively placing the hand in the extrinsic + position. To stretch the lumbrical muscles, we need to place the wrist in extension

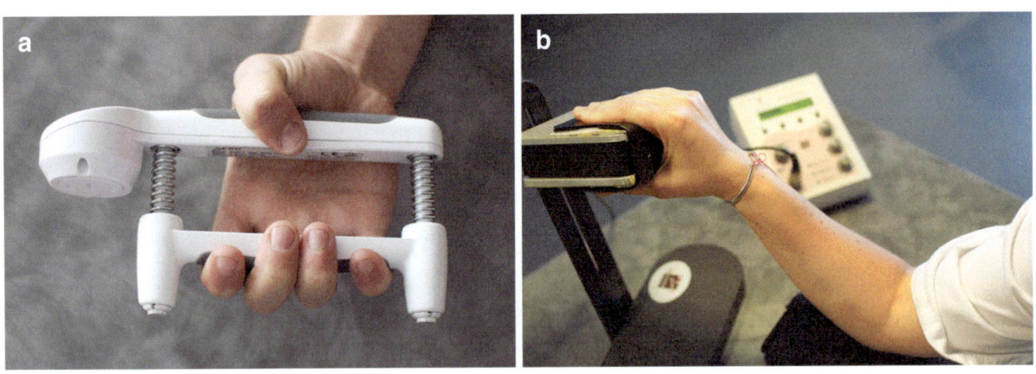

Fig. 6.24 Using dynamometers allows evaluating eventual muscular unbalances (here between the extrinsic (**a**) and intrinsic (**b**) forces)

Complications

Even if the results are good or excellent in 91% of cases when the treatment is carried out properly [9], some complications can occur. After the initial treatment, the most frequent complication is a lack of active extension of the distal interphalangeal joint. In these cases, a tenodermodesis may be proposed; this consists of suturing the skin and tendon together (the tendon is only 0.7 mm long at this level) to recover the extension of the distal interphalangeal joint.

It is also possible to repeat the same orthotic treatment, with more satisfactory results than when the treatment is carried out in the acute phase (93% good or excellent results) [9, 11].

In cases of chronic mallet finger, Fowler's tenotomy can be proposed. Its goal is to rebalance the extensor system by partially cutting the insertion of the median strip at the base of the middle phalanx, thus transmitting increased tension from the extensor force to the terminal tendon [12].

A "swan-neck" deformity may occur because the rupture of the lateral strips causes the distal interphalangeal joint to fall into flexion and creates excessive tension on the median strip, which may cause the proximal interphalangeal joint to hyperextend, especially in lax subjects [13]. When this deformity occurs in the acute phase of the mallet finger, it is essential to use an orthosis that immobilizes the distal interphalangeal joint in extension and the proximal interphalangeal joint in 50° of flexion. This position allows the lateral strips to be recentered and the balance of the extensor and retinacular systems to be restored [13, 14]. The orthosis is worn for 8 weeks (+ 2 weeks at night) and allows the proximal interphalangeal joint to be mobilized under the orthosis so as not to compromise the healing of the relaxed elements [15].

The same protocol can be used in cases of swan-neck deformity in chronic mallet fingers, when they are not stiffened.

Zone 3

These injuries correspond with a damage of the median strip of the extensor system (Fig. 6.25). An associated injury to one or both lateral strips is possible and will modify the rehabilitation protocol, considering the elements described in the previous paragraph.

They occur during forced flexion, palmar dislocation, or direct impact on the dorsal surface of the proximal interphalangeal joint [16].

A boutonnière deformity only occurs in cases of palmar subluxation of the lateral strips, due to the combined damage to the median strip, the triangular ligament, and the transverse and oblique fibers of the interossei [17].

In the presence of an isolated median strip injury, the boutonnière deformity is not present in the acute phase, and the diagnosis is made by a positive Elson maneuver (Fig. 6.26), confirmed by an ultrasound assessment in case of doubt.

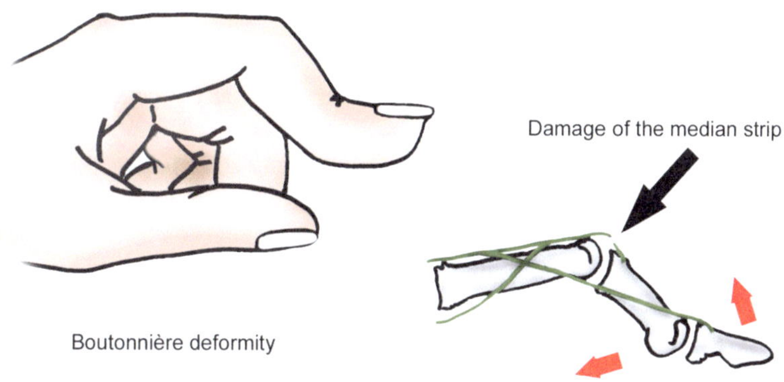

Fig. 6.25 The injuries in zone 3 correspond with a damage of the median strip

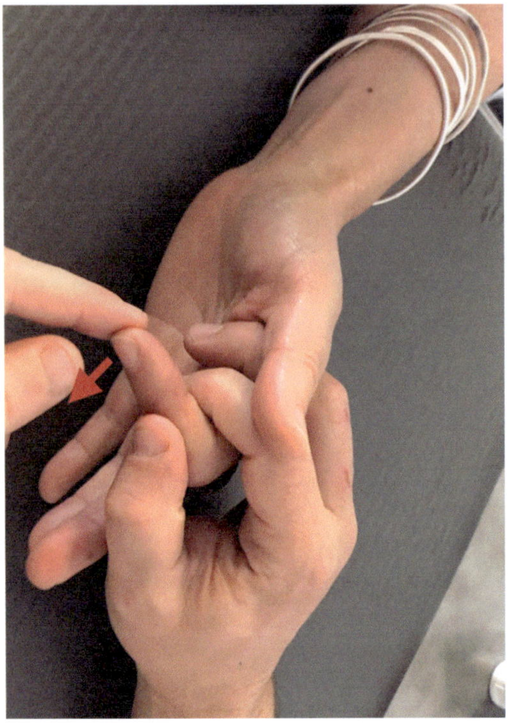

Fig. 6.26 Elson test: if the median strip is broken, the flexion of the proximal interphalangeal joint does not relax the lateral strips. The lateral strips keep their efficiency and can realize an extension of the distal interphalangeal joint

No Surgery (Fig. 6.27)

In non-surgical subcutaneous injuries, we immobilize the proximal interphalangeal joint strictly in extension, leaving the distal interphalangeal joint free, by realizing a tube-shaped orthosis with a thin (1.6 mm) micro-perforated plastic. This orthosis is controlled every week to check the pressure points and adapt it to the trophic evolution of the damaged finger (Fig. 6.28).

➔ D0 to D45 (Immobilization)

As for the subcutaneous injuries in zones 1 and 2, the rehabilitation is not necessary and only consists in a regular control of the orthosis and self-rehabilitation advice.

The analytic flexion of the distal interphalangeal joint tenses the lateral strips but not the median strip (Fig. 6.29); therefore, it is encouraged in this phase.

It also puts in tension the oblique retinacular ligament, which tends to retract and fix the boutonnière deformity.

➔ D45 to D90 (Fragility)

In this phase, we stop the immobilization, keeping the orthosis during the night for 15 days.

The rehabilitation goals in this phase are:

- *Fight against trophic disorders and pain*

The techniques used are identical to the ones used in the injuries in zones 1 and 2.

- *Progressive recovery of the joint amplitudes*
  - Fluidotherapy: hot, used if there is no inflammation, to improve viscoelasticity of the tissues and therefore mobility.
  - Regain the active and passive amplitudes of the distal interphalangeal joint: this exercise is not always necessary, as it is part of the self-rehabilitation exercises proposed to the patient from D0 to D45.
  - Active exercise for the flexion of the proximal interphalangeal joint, active-assisted then active extension: the flexion of the proximal interphalangeal joint is realized only actively to limit the risks of excessive tension on the tendinous callus. Returning in extension is a passive movement, and active-assisted in the first sessions, then a simple active movement when the active extension locking is reached (Fig. 6.30).
  - Specific mobilizations of the distal interphalangeal joint: realized if the stiffness persists in the distal interphalangeal joint.

➔ After D90 (Solidity)

Like in the subcutaneous injuries in zones 1 and 2, in this phase the patient goes back to doing his work and sports activities. The rehabilitation is focused on the complete recovery of the joint amplitudes, the strength, the complex grips, and the proprioception.

The techniques used are comparable to the ones used in zones 1 and 2.

Subcutaneous injury of the extensors in zone 3 – Boutonnière deformity without surgery

a	Immobilization (A)	Relative fragility (B)	Consolidation (C)
REHABILITATION	**Therapeutic goals** : 1. Tendon healing 2. Maintain the mobility of the distal interphalangeal joint **Techniques:** 1. Learning the protection rules during the maintenance of the orthosis (+ control by the orthotist once a week) 2. Self-mobilizations of the distal interphalangeal joint **Risks:** Bad tendon healing, stiffness of the distal interphalangeal joint	**Therapeutic goals** : 1. Same as phase A, intensifying the techniques if necessary 2. Recover active amplitudes in the proximal interphalangeal joint 3. Fight against potential trophic disorder 4. Maintain the body mapping **Techniques:** 1. Specific and global mobilizations of the distal interphalangeal joint (A2) 2. Active exercise in flexion (< 30° before D45) of the proximal interphalangeal joint returning to extension with an active-assisted movement, then simple active exercise (depending on the locking in extension). Exercise with the metacarpophalangeal joint extended and the wrist at 30° of flexion (at D45). Increase of the flexion of the proximal interphalangeal joint of 15°/week if no lag. Electrostimulation. 3. Trophic massages, fluidotherapy, depressotherapy around the scar 4. Manipulations of light objects, TVS (70-80 Hz) **Risks:** distension or inflammation of the tendinous callus if the exercises in flexion are too intense	**Therapeutic goals** : 1. Intensify the techniques from the 2 previous phases if necessary 2. Complete functional recovery **Techniques:** 1. Specific joint mobilizations, increasing the electrostimulation's electric intensities (B1), and stretching the intrinsic muscles. 2. Functional activities adapted to the patient's sporting and professional needs **Risks:** Same as in phase B
ORTHOSIS	Immobilization orthosis worn all the time with the proximal interphalangeal joint in extension (distal interphalangeal joint free)	Orthosis worn during the night until D60 if necessary	Orthosis to gain amplitude if limitation of articular origin
	D0-D45	D45-D90	After D90

b

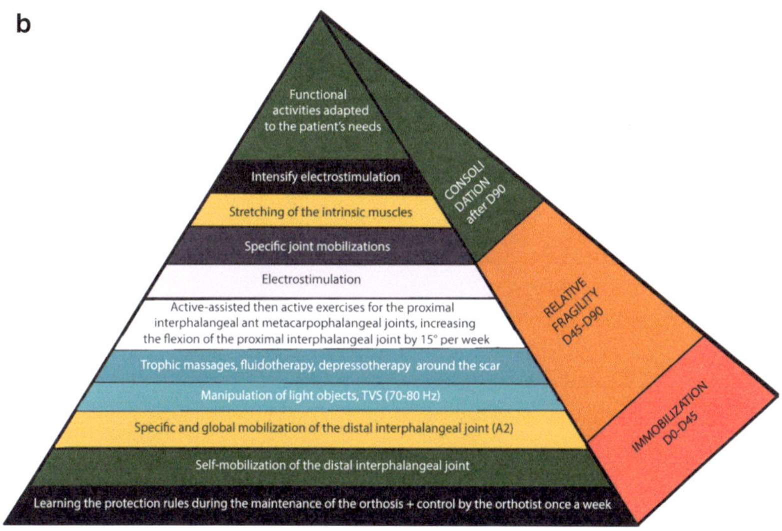

Fig. 6.27 Rehabilitation protocol (**a**) and progression pyramid (**b**) for injuries in zone 3 without surgery

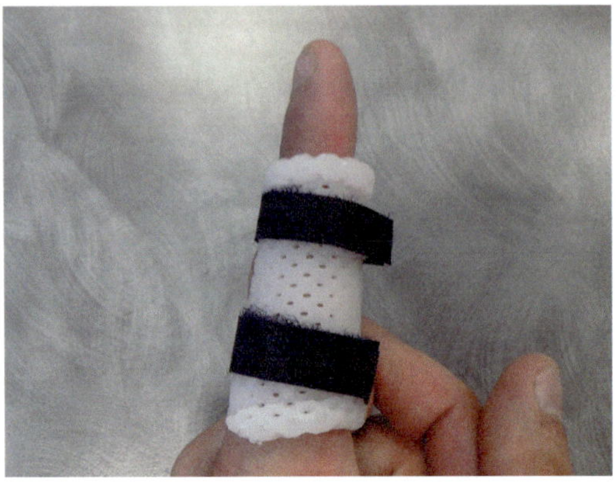

Fig. 6.28 Tube-shaped orthosis leaving the distal interphalangeal joint free

After Surgery (Fig. 6.31)

In the case of surgery, usually using a transosseous reinsertion device (metal or resorbing anchor), it is possible to start the mobilization in the protected sector from D3 using the Short Arc Motion (SAM) protocol [10, 18, 19].

This protocol is based on the fitting of a rehabilitation orthosis in addition to the tubular immobilization orthosis, which is worn permanently for 6 weeks except during the mobilization exercises.

The gutter-shaped rehabilitation orthosis allows mobilization of the proximal interphalangeal joint within a range of 0–30° for the first

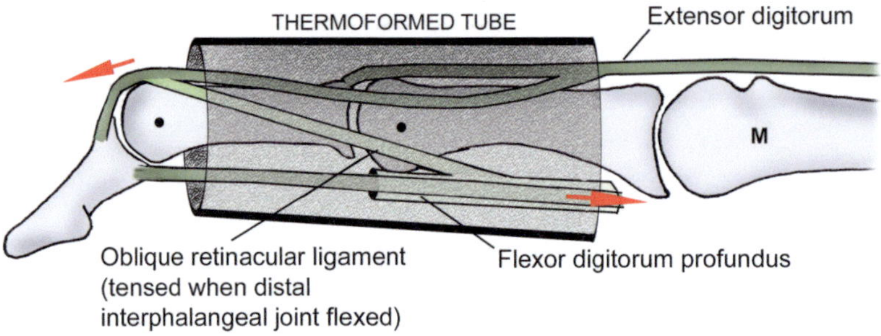

Fig. 6.29 The flexion of the distal interphalangeal joint tenses the lateral strips, which relaxes the median strip

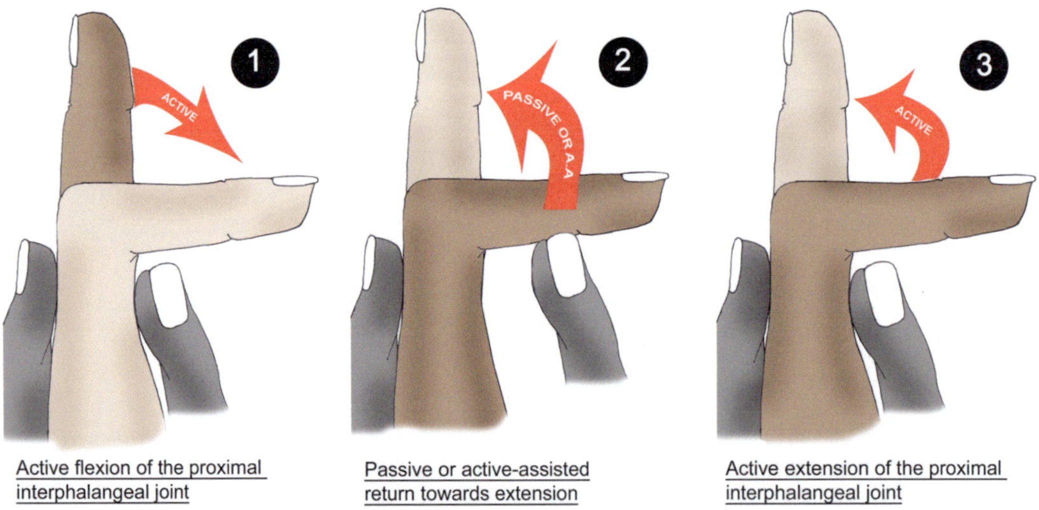

Fig. 6.30 Progressive mobilizations to limit the constraints on the median strip

a **Extensor injuries in zone 3 with surgery – Modified Short Arc Motion (SAM)**

	Fragility (A)	Relative fragility (B)	Consolidation (C)
REHABILITATION	**Therapeutic goals** : 1. Tendon healing 2. Maintain the mobility of the distal interphalangeal joint 3. Progressive recovery of the amplitudes of the proximal interphalangeal joint **Techniques:** 1. Learning the protection rules 2. Self-mobilizations of the distal interphalangeal joint 3. Flexion of the proximal interphalangeal joint, with the metacarpophalangeal joint in flexion and the wrist in 30° of extension: 0-30° for 3 weeks, then increasing by 15°/week if no lag (10 repetitions / hour) **Risks:** Distension or inflammation of the tendinous callus if the exercises in flexion are too intense	**Therapeutic goals :** 1. Same as phase A, intensifying the techniques if necessary 2-. Fight against potential trophic disorder 3-. Maintain the body mapping **Techniques:** 1. Specific and global mobilizations of the distal and proximal interphalangeal joints, electrostimulation if no lag (A2-A3) 2. Trophic massages, fluidotherapy, depressotherapy around the scar 3. Manipulations of light objects, TVS (70-80 Hz) **Risks:** Same as in phase A	**Therapeutic goals :** 1. Intensify the techniques from the 2 previous phases if necessary 2. Complete functional recovery **Techniques:** 1. Stretching the intrinsic muscles and intensifying electrotherapy (B1) 2. Functional activities adapted to the patient's sporting and professional needs **Risks:** Same as in phase B
ORTHOSIS	1. Since D1, immobilization orthosis worn all the time except during rehabilitation with the proximal interphalangeal joint in extension (distal interphalangeal joint free) + compressive bandage 2. Gutter-shaped orthosis allowing 30° (for the rehabilitation), then modified depending on the evolution	Orthosis worn during the night until D60 if necessary	Orthosis to gain amplitude if limitation of articular origin
	D3-D45	D45-D90	After D90

b

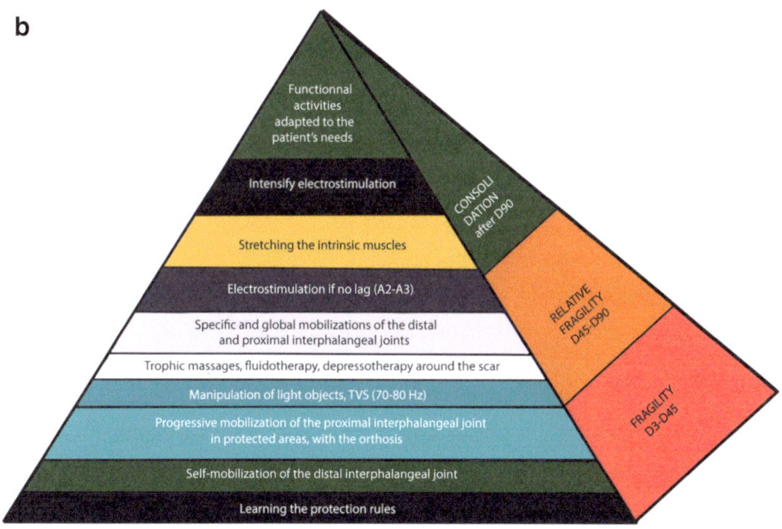

Fig. 6.31 Rehabilitation protocol (**a**) and progression pyramid (**b**) for injuries in zone 3 with surgery (Short Arc Motion protocol)

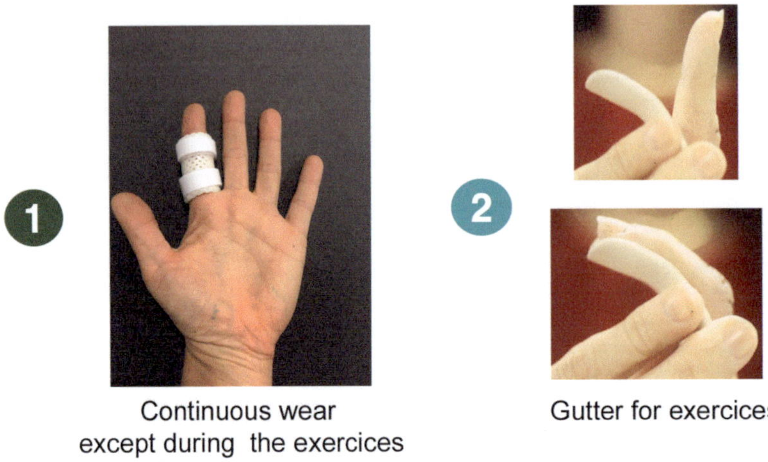

Fig. 6.32 In the Short Arc Motion protocol, two orthoses are made, one to be worn all the time during the day and the other for mobilizations in protected areas

3 weeks, up to 40° between the third and fourth weeks, 60–70° between the fourth and sixth weeks, and then through the full range after the sixth week [18, 20] (Fig. 6.32).

Mobilization exercises with the orthosis are performed with the wrist flexed to 30° and the metacarpophalangeal joints in extension to reduce the stress on the median strip [10].

Complications

The most frequent complication of this type of injury is a boutonnière deformity, which is treated differently depending on its stage [13]. In stage 1, the deformity is flexible, and the treatment is identical to that proposed for an acute injury (6 weeks of orthosis with extension of the proximal interphalangeal joint, then 15 days at night). The distal interphalangeal joint is free in the orthosis to allow the gliding of the lateral strips and the oblique retinacular ligament.

When the boutonnière deformity is fixed (stages 2, 3, and 4), it must first be softened before any other treatment, ranging from orthotic treatment (stage 2), tenotomy or tendon grafting (stage 3), to arthroplasty or arthrodesis of the proximal interphalangeal joint (stage 4). The orthosis used and the way in which it is worn following these treatments are identical to those proposed in the case of an injury to the median strip in the acute phase or the flexible boutonnière deformity (stage 1).

Zones 4–8

Injuries in these areas are always treated surgically. Although no orthosis has been shown to be superior to others, there is evidence of the benefits of implementing a rehabilitation protocol allowing early mobilization in a protected area [21]. In our practice, we prefer to use a relative motion orthosis (RMO) because it allows active mobilization in a protected area and, unlike dynamic orthoses, does not require regular adjustment and monitoring [22]. This orthosis places the wrist in 25° extension and the metacarpophalangeal joint of the affected finger in 15–20° extension in relation to the other fingers

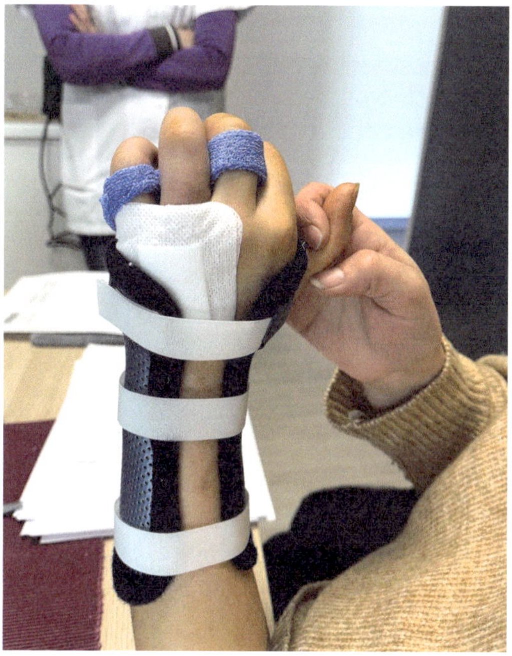

Fig. 6.33 The relative motion orthosis (RMO) protects the extensor suture in zone 4–8 by placing the wrist in 25° of extension and the metacarpophalangeal joint of the affected finger in 15–20° of extension relative to the adjacent fingers

while allowing it to be flexed (Fig. 6.33). This wrist position, combined with the limited amplitude of the metacarpophalangeal joint of the injured finger, considerably limits the tension on the suture [23]. Making a thermoformable plastic yoke allows it to be adapted to each finger (Fig. 6.34).

At a surgical level, the technique must be adapted to the injured area.

In zone 4, the extensor tendon becomes thicker and wider, which allows the use of 4/0 slow resorption threads. Care should be taken to look for associated lesions of the dorsal expansion of the interossei at the lateral edges of the extensor tendons.

In zone 5, the extensor tendon is repaired using multi-strand stitches, combined with a peripheral overlock. The difficulty in this case will be to maintain the sagittal balance of the tendon to avoid dislocation of the tendon in the intermetacarpal area.

In zone 6, the extensor tendons become rounder than in the fingers. In the event of a wound, there is generally no retraction of the proximal edge, which is retained by the intertendinous juncta. The sutures are made using a slow-resorbing 4/0 thread.

In zone 7, the tendon will be repaired using a multi-strand stitch with a slow-resorbing 4/0 thread (Kessler or Tsuge), combined with a peripheral suture with a thinner 5 or 6/0 thread. At the end of the suture, care must be taken to ensure that there is no conflict with the extensor retinaculum, and a Z-plasty of the retinaculum may be needed.

In zone 8, injuries are rare, and the repair involves a conventional suture using a slow-resorbing 4/0 thread.

For the thumb, repair of the tendons will follow the same rules as for the similar zones in the fingers. Immobilization of the interphalangeal joint of the thumb for a rupture of the terminal strip in zone 1 may require the use of an arthrorise pin, given the difficulty of immobilizing this joint on its own.

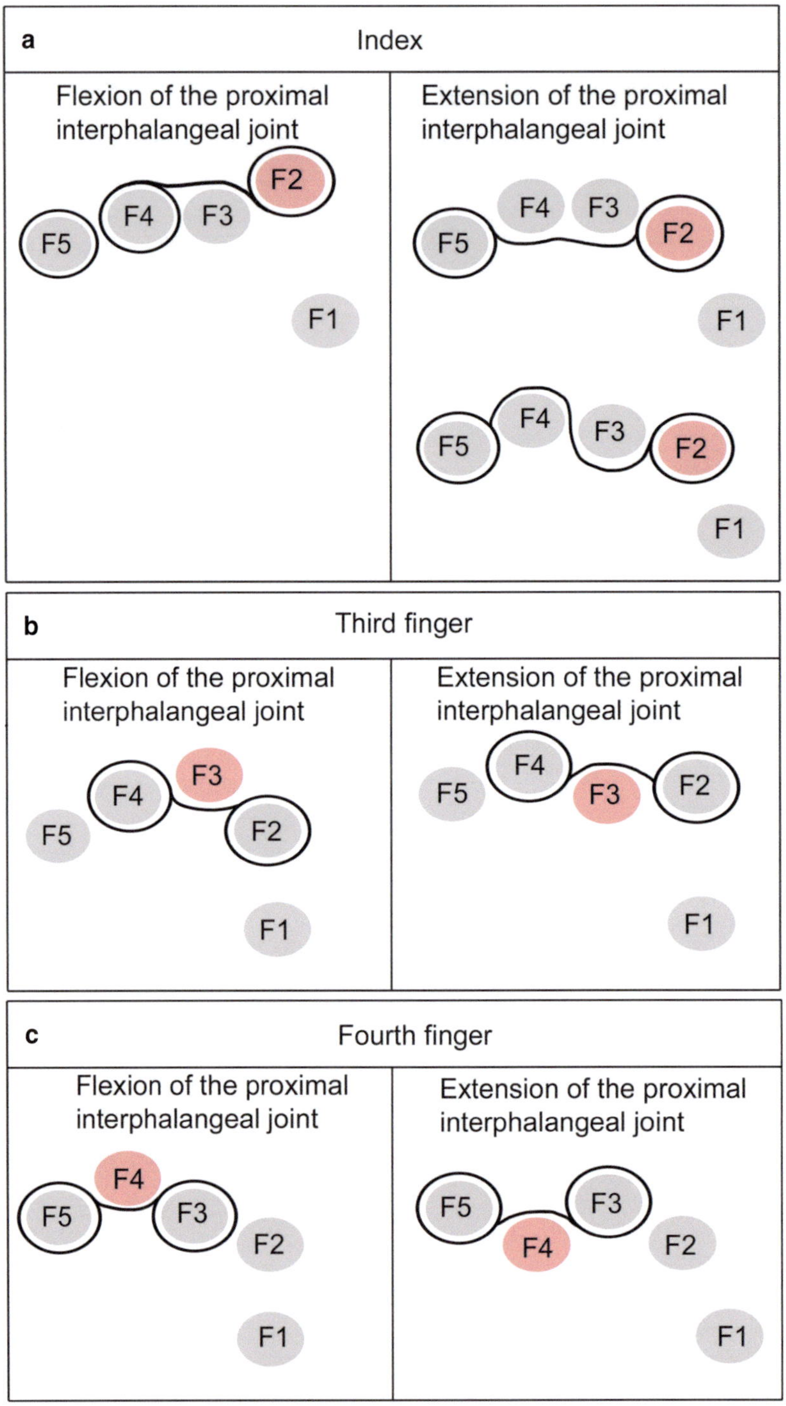

Fig. 6.34 Practical techniques for making a yoke on any affected finger

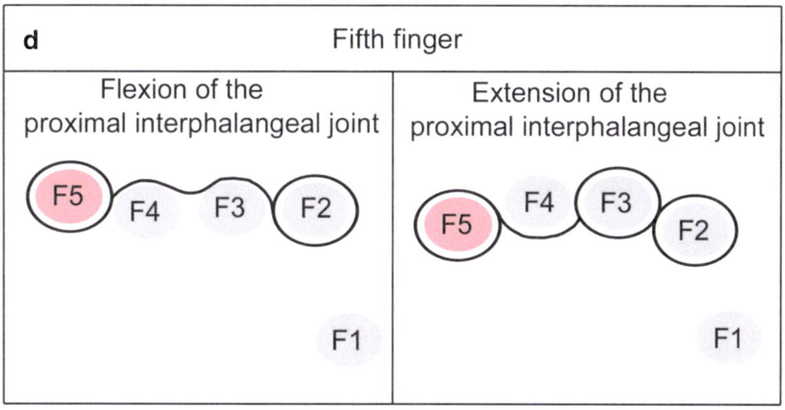

Fig. 6.34 (continued)

Rehabilitation Protocol (Fig. 6.35)

From D0 to D3, a strict immobilization orthosis is used combined with a compression bandage. This combination limits the risk of maintaining trophic phenomena and pain while waiting for the RMO orthosis to be made, allowing self-mobilization in a protected area to begin [23, 24].

➔ **From D3 to D21 (Immobilization)**

This phase must improve tendon healing and limit trophic disorders and pain while avoiding adherences around the scar.

The orthosis must be worn all the time, except during the dressing replacement and the rehabilitation.

- *Fight against trophic disorders and pain*
  - Transcutaneous vibratory stimulations with a 70 Hz frequency next to the extensor system if we want to improve the proprioceptive aspect or 100 Hz next to the painful areas if we want an analgesic effect.
  - Electrotherapy 100 Hz (TENS) to fight against pain or 1 Hz to fight against trophic disorders.
  - Analgesic or draining massage, staying away from the wound (risk of sepsis).
- *Mobility in protected area.*

These exercises are carried out in an RMO orthosis, without tension and without carrying even light loads. Movements are performed regularly, without tension or pain.

➔ **From D21 to D45 (Fragility)**

We keep fighting against trophic disorders and pain, if necessary, but the priority goal is to fight against stiffness, which is closely related to fibrosis around the scar. The “wrist” module of the RMO orthosis is removed, except during “high-risk” activities. The yoke is kept on permanently until D35, then only during “high-risk” activities until D50 [25].

- *Recovery of active amplitudes.*
  - Fluidotherapy: hot if there is no inflammation and the scar has closed, to increase the tissue viscoelasticity and therefore improve mobilization.
  - Massage around the scar and defibrosing depressotherapy to fight against adherences if the vitro-pressure test is longer than 2 s [26] (Fig. 6.36).
  - From D35: active electrostimulation if the lock in extension has been acquired in joints distal to the injury. These exercises are realized in flexion and in extension (Fig. 6.37).
  - Active mobilizations in extension and global flexion: the patient stops when he feels tension. These exercises are also realized by the patient outside the sessions, as often as pos-

a **Injuries of the extensors in zones 4 to 8**

	Immobilization (A)	Relative fragility (B)	Consolidation (C)
REHABILITATION	**Therapeutic goals** : 1. Decrease pain 2. Decrease trophic disorders 3. Progressive recovery of the amplitudes in a protected area 4. Prevent functional exclusion **Techniques:** 1. TENS and TVS (100 Hz) 2. Draining massages and compressive bandage, scar massage then depressotherapy when the scar is closed and if it is not inflammatory, ultrasounds after the scar is closed (not validated) 3. Complete mobilization of the finger in protected areas thanks to the ICAM orthosis: wrist in 25° of extension and metacarpophalangeal joint in 15-20° of extension relative to the other fingers (if no lag) 4. TVS (70-80 Hz) and various sensory stimulations (without constraint) **Risks:** Distension or inflammation of the tendinous callus if the exercises in flexion are too intense	**Therapeutic goals :** 1. Same as in phase A, intensify if necessary 2. Recovery of the active mobility 3. Recovery of coordination and dexterity **Techniques:** 1. Pressotherapy, scar massages and mobilizations 2. Passive analytical mobilization of all the joints in all their amplitudes (in a position that protects the tendon), then complete active mobilization of the fingers in extension with the wrist extended then flexed. Electrostimulation, fluidotherapy. 3. Manipulation of light objects **Risks:** Same as in phase A, functional exclusion	**Therapeutic goals :** 1. Same as in previous phases, intensify if necessary 2. Complete functional recovery **Techniques:** 1. Specific joint mobilizations, progressive stretching of the intrinsic muscles, postures and electrostimulation (B2) 2. Functional activities adapted to the patient's professional and sporting needs **Risks:** Same as in phase A and B
ORTHOSIS	Depending on the selected option: 1. ICAM (Immediate Controlled Active Motion): wrist module + yoke 2. Static orthosis: wrist in 30° of extension, metacarpophalangeal joint between 0° and 70° (20° ++), interphalangeal joints extended	Regardless of the chosen option: 1. Yoke all the time until D35 2. After D35, the yoke is progressively taken off (night, light activities ➡ more intense activities)	Regardless of the chosen option: 1. The yoke is progressively taken off (more intense activities➡high-risk activities) 2. Orthosis to gain amplitude if necessary
	D3-D21	D21-D60	After D60

b

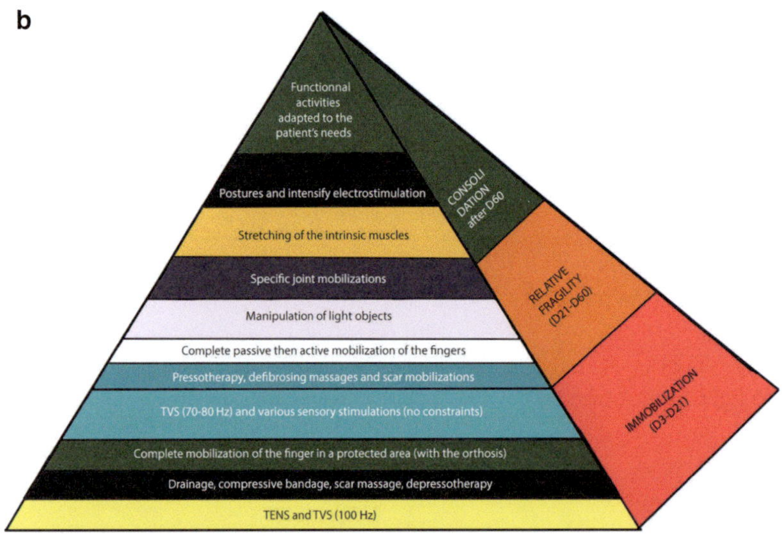

Fig. 6.35 Rehabilitation protocol (**a**) and progression pyramid (**b**) for injuries in zones 4–8

sible, but without tension and in short series (every hour, 10 repetitions for each exercise, for each joint distal to the injury).

- *Coordination and dexterity.*

Exercises for dexterity and coordination are realized at this stage, to facilitate the reintegration of the injured finger(s) into the body mapping of the hand (Fig. 6.38).

➔ After D45 (Solidity)

In this phase, the patient starts doing his sports and professional activities (aside form strength activities, only at D60). The goal is the complete functional recovery.

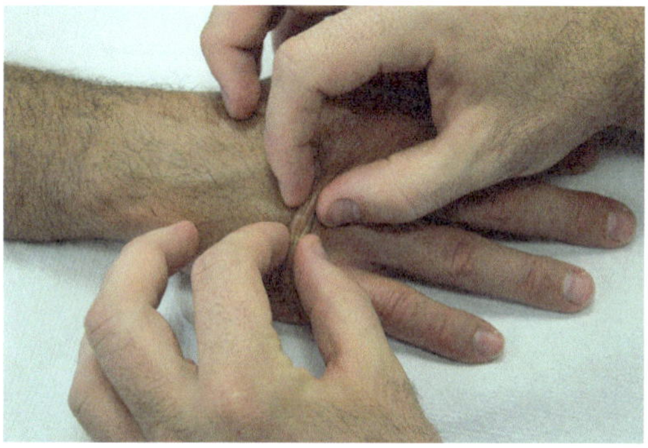

Fig. 6.36 Massages around the scar to mobilize the different gliding planes relative to each other

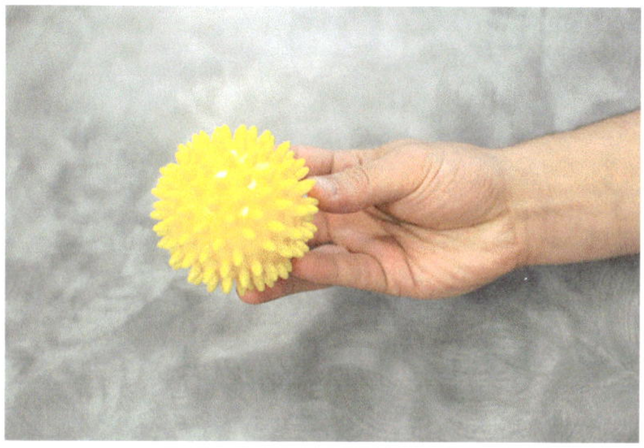

Fig. 6.38 Exercise for dexterity and prehensions

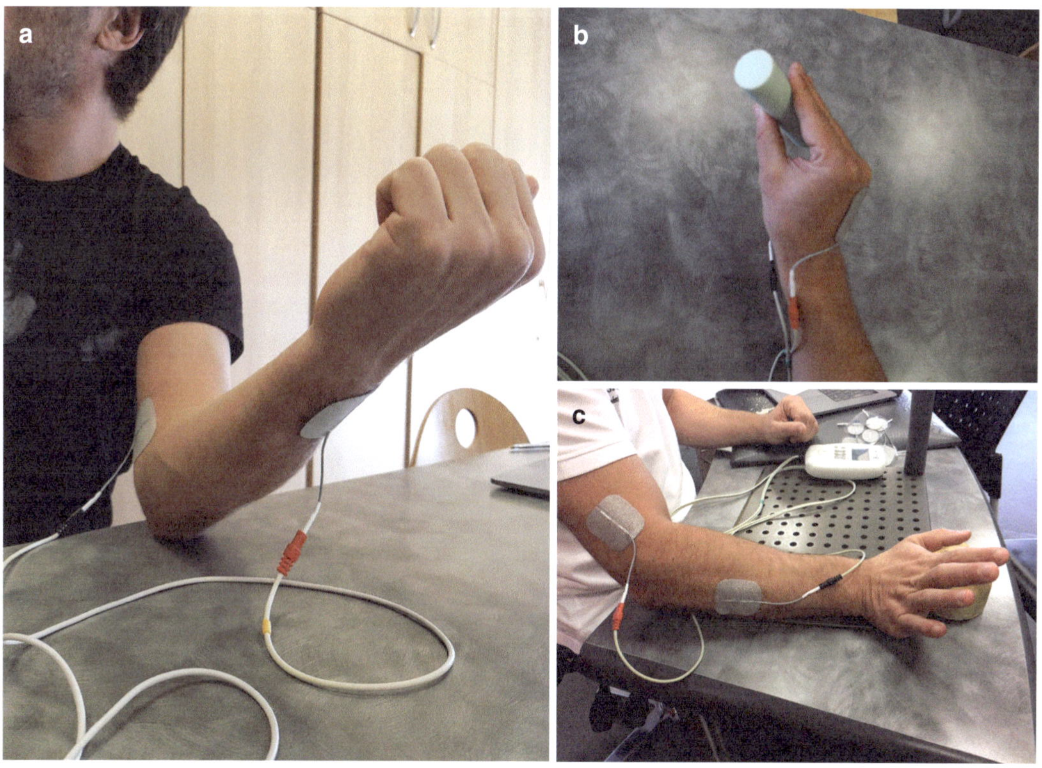

Fig. 6.37 Active electrostimulation in winding (**a**), in extension of the interphalangeal joints (**b**), or in extension of the metacarpophalangeal joint (**c**) depending on the goal

- *Total recovery of the active amplitudes.*

The techniques of the previous phase are intensified if necessary, and we add:

- Imitation exercises, by doing sequences of movements allowing an optimal gliding of the different tendinous systems of the hand (Fig. 6.39).
- Specific mobilizations of the joints with troubles in the intra-articular glidings.
- After D60, we can start stretching the intrinsic muscles: these stretches are realized if the Finochietto test is positive, which means there is a retraction of the intrinsic muscles. We stretch the interossei passively placing the hand in an "extrinsic +" position. Stretching the extrinsic musculature can be realized in

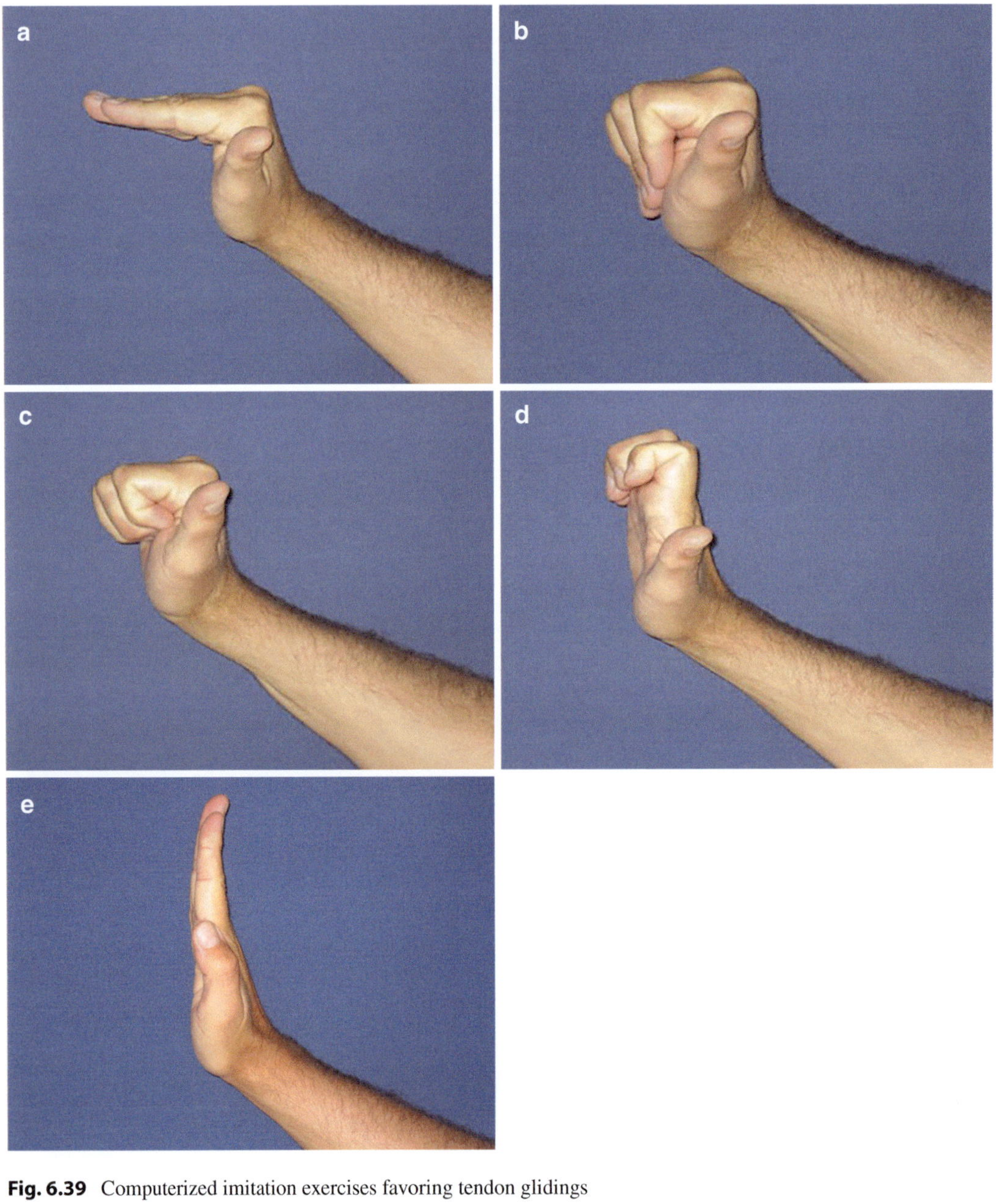

Fig. 6.39 Computerized imitation exercises favoring tendon glidings

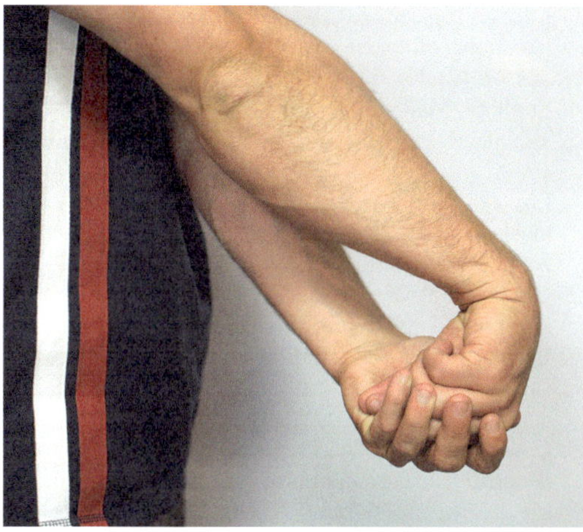

Fig. 6.40 Stretching exercises for the extrinsic muscles, realized actively or passively

the event of a retraction/disorder of the extensor gliding validated by a positive Kilgore test (Fig. 6.40).

- *Recovery of conscious and unconscious neuromuscular abilities.*

As with closed lesions, we perform dynamometric strengthening of the hand and wrist to restore the same ratio and strength characteristics as on the healthy side.

Specific exercises adapted to the patient's needs are realized to allow him/her to recover optimal function (proprioception, dexterity, coordination).

Sagittal Band Injuries (Zone 5)

The sagittal bands stabilize the extensor tendon at the level of the metacarpophalangeal joint. In the event of a radial sagittal band injury, the extensor tendon becomes unstable and may even dislocate in the ulnar intermetacarpal area of the affected finger. The injuries of the ulnar band are not symptomatic, as the axis of the extensor tendons is offset in the ulnar region in relation to the finger axis.

There are three types of sagittal band injury:

- Type 1: contusion of the sagittal band without instability.

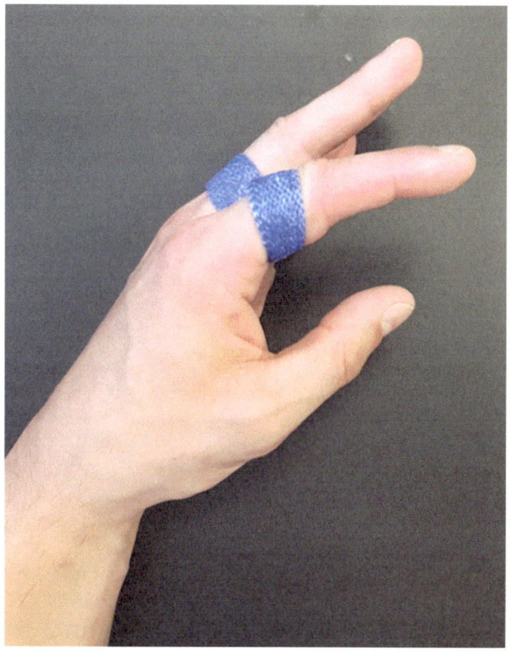

Fig. 6.41 Yoke stabilizing the extensor tendon on the back of the metacarpophalangeal joint, placing the joint in extension in relation to the adjacent fingers

- Type 2: injury of the sagittal band with instability but without complete dislocation of the tendon.
- Type 3: dislocation of the tendon in the ulnar intermetacarpal area during the flexion of the metacarpophalangeal joint.

Type 1 injuries are treated with a thermoformable plastic yoke that places the metacarpophalangeal joint in 20–30° extension relative to the adjacent finger(s). It is worn for 3 weeks.

For type 2 and 3 injuries managed within the first 3 weeks, a yoke of the same type is proposed, but it is important to check that the instability is corrected when the fingers are flexed with the yoke, and it is worn continuously for 8 weeks [13, 27] (Fig. 6.41).

Strict immobilization of these injuries does not help healing and drastically increases the risk of complications (especially stiffness and complex regional pain syndrome).

In the event of a delayed treatment (after 3 weeks), surgery is proposed, which may involve the use of the ulnar sagittal band, part of the dorsal expansion of the interossei, or a juncta to repair the damaged radial band.

After these surgeries, the same type of yoke is proposed and worn continuously for 4 to 6 weeks.

Bibliography

1. Cheung JP, Fung B, Ip WY. Review on mallet finger treatment. Hand Surg. 2012;17(3):439–47.
2. Stark HH, Boyes JH, Wilson JN. Mallet finger. J Bone Joint Surg Am. 1962;44:1061–8.
3. Wehbe MA, Schneider LH. Mallet fractures. J Bone Joint Surg Am. 1984;66(5):658–69.
4. Masméjean E, Le Bellec Y, JY. A. Lésions traumatiques des tendons extenseurs de la main. Encycl Méd Chir - appareil locomoteur. 2000;14-058-A-10:12.
5. Moradi A, Kachooei AR, Mudgal CS. Mallet fracture. J Hand Surg Am. 2014;39(10):2067–9.
6. Renfree KJ. Acute, closed tendinous mallet injuries. J Hand Surg Am. 2014;39(12):2502–5. quiz 2505
7. Leinberry C. Mallet finger injuries. J Hand Surg Am. 2009;34(9):1715–7.
8. Mesplié G, Lemoine S. Injuries of the extensor tendons, in hand and wrist rehabilitation. Springer; 2015. p. 237–74.
9. Bastien J, Rouzaud S. When should splint treatment start for a tendinous mallet finger? A retrospective review of 319 fingers. Hand Surg Rehabil. 2021;40:491.
10. Evans RB. Managing the injured tendon: current concepts. J Hand Ther. 2012;25(2):173–89. quiz 190
11. Garberman SF, Diao E, Peimer A. Mallet finger: results of early versus delayed closed treatment. J Hand Surg Am. 1994;19A n°5:850.
12. Hiwatari R, et al. Fractional fowler tenotomy for chronic mallet finger: a cadaveric biomechanical study. J Hand Surg Am. 2012;37(11):2263–8.
13. Lutz K, Pipicelli J, Grewal R. Management of complications of extensor tendon injuries. Hand Clin. 2015;31(2):301–10.
14. Smillie I. Mallet finger. Br J Surg. 1937;24:439–45.
15. Tubiana R. In: Saunders PW, editor. The hand, vol III; 1988.
16. Lin JD, Strauch RJ. Closed soft tissue extensor mechanism injuries (mallet, boutonniere, and sagittal band). J Hand Surg Am. 2014;39(5):1005–11.
17. Grau L, et al. Biomechanics of the acute boutonniere deformity. J Hand Surg Am. 2018;43(1):80 e1–6.
18. Evans RB, Thompson DE. An analysis of factors that support early active short arc motion of the repaired central slip. J Hand Ther. 1992;5(4):187–201.
19. Capon A, Watson A, England H. Therapeutic management of closed central slip injuries: outcome of a service evaluation. Hand Therapy. 2019;24(1):3–12.
20. McAuliffe JA. Early active short arc motion following central slip repair. J Hand Surg Am. 2011;36(1):143–6.
21. Wong AL, et al. The optimal orthosis and motion protocol for extensor tendon injury in zones IV–VIII: a systematic review. J Hand Ther. 2017;30:447.
22. Sharma JV, et al. Analysis of relative motion splint in the treatment of zone VI extensor tendon injuries. J Hand Surg Am. 2006;31(7):1118–22.
23. Howell JW, Merritt WH, Robinson SJ. Immediate controlled active motion following zone 4–7 extensor tendon repair. J Hand Ther. 2005;18(2):182–90.
24. Merritt WH. Relative motion splint: active motion after extensor tendon injury and repair. J Hand Surg Am. 2014;39(6):1187–94.
25. Gyovai JE, Wright Howell J. Validation of spring forces applied in dynamic outrigger splinting. J Hand Ther. 1992;5(1):8–15.
26. Vancoppenolle E. La prise en charge des cicatrices. Mémoire du diplôme inter-universitaire de rééducation et d'appareillage de la main; 2015.
27. Catalano L, et al. Closed treatment of non-rheumatoid extensor tendon dislocations at the metacarpophalangeal joint. J Hand Surg. 2006;31(2):242–5.

Injuries of the Flexor Tendons

7

Grégory Mesplié and Vincent Grelet

A huge progress has been made these last years in the surgical treatment and rehabilitation of the flexor system. However, a good knowledge of the tendon healing process and some experience in the field are required to limit the risks of tears or secondary adherences.

Classification

The Verdan and Michon classification allows us to approach their physiology according to five topographic zones (Fig. 7.1).

Fingers

Zone 1

Located below the distal insertion of the flexor digitorum superficialis, it is the area of the distal insertion of the flexor digitorum profundus. It is one of the areas where the tendon is poorly vascularized, which makes its healing longer and random in case of injury.

Zone 2

It starts at the entrance of the digital sheath and ends at the medium part of the second phalanx (lower than the two tendon strips of the flexor digitorum superficialis).

This is zone used to be called the "no man's land" by Bunnell, because it seemed impossible to repair the injuries that occurred there. The injuries in that zone are still the most complex to treat.

The two flexors share the digital canal, made up of the periosteum and the palmar ligaments of the metacarpophalangeal and proximal interphalangeal joint from behind, and the annular ligaments and cruciate pulleys in the front (Fig. 7.2).

The aim of these pulleys and annular ligaments is to maintain the flexors against the bone levers, thus permitting the complete finger winding and avoiding the "bowstring" effect.

Lastly, the flexor digitorum superficialis splits into two strips near the base of the first phalanx to let the flexor digitorum profundus pass [1, 2]. Below this chiasma, the flexor digitorum profundus becomes superficial and the flexor digitorum superficialis becomes deep. Given the complexity of this zone, Tang et al. [3] suggest dividing it into five sub-zones, zone 2C being the most complex to treat as it corresponds to the division of the flexor digitorum superficialis opposite the most powerful and thickest pulley of the synovial sheath, the A2 pulley (Fig. 7.3).

G. Mesplié (✉) · V. Grelet
Institut Sud Aquitain de la Main et du Membre Supérieur (ISAMMS), Biarritz, France
e-mail: grelet.vincent@dbmail.com

G. Mesplié (ed.), *Hand Functional Anatomy and Therapy*,
https://doi.org/10.1007/978-3-031-92505-4_7

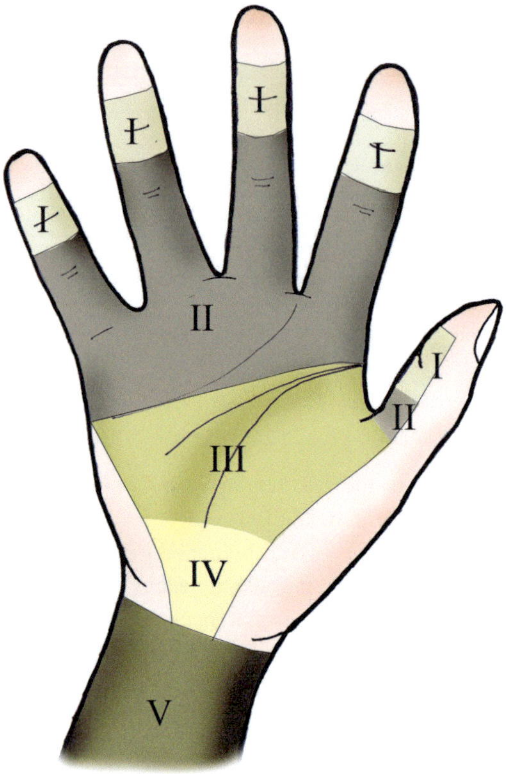

Fig. 7.1 Topographic classification of the flexor tendons according to Verdan and Michon

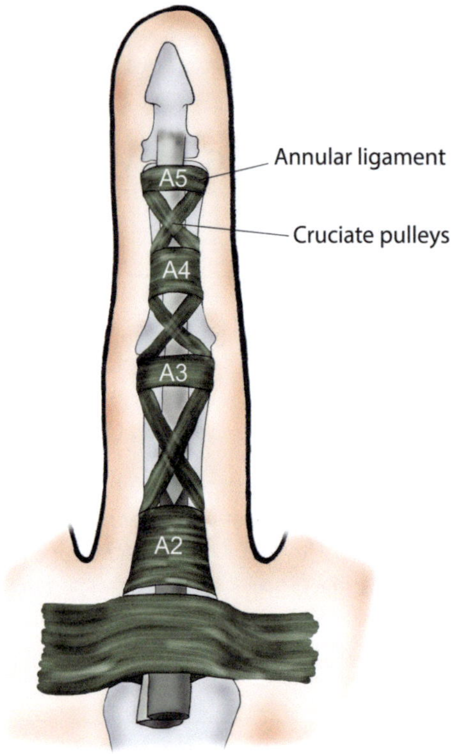

Fig. 7.2 Location of the annular ligaments and cruciate pulleys

Zone 3

Located between the distal part of the flexor retinaculum (or transverse carpal ligament) and the entrance of the digital sheath.

Zone 4

It corresponds to the carpal tunnel where the flexor retinaculum acts as the first pulley for the flexor system.

Zone 5

Located between the musculotendinous junction proximally (inferior third of the forearm) and the proximal part of the flexor retinaculum.

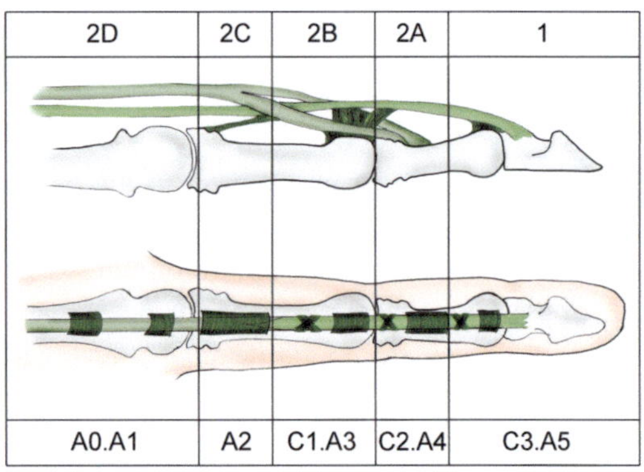

Fig. 7.3 Proposition of sub-zones for zone 2

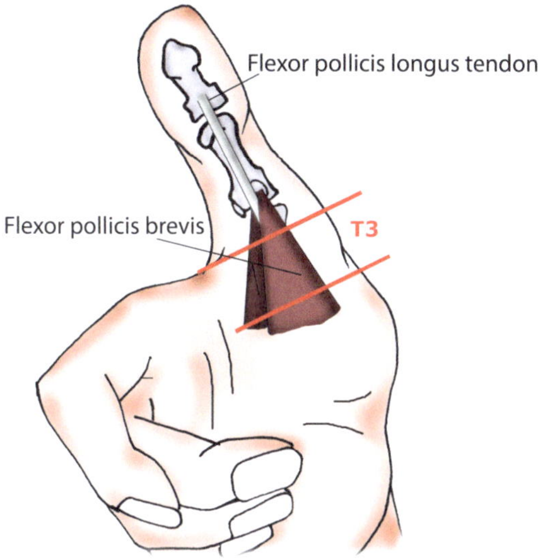

Fig. 7.4 Trajectory of the flexor pollicis longus between the two heads of the flexor pollicis brevis

Thumb

The only extrinsic muscle that makes the flexion of the thumb is the flexor pollicis longus.

The T1 zone corresponds to the ending of the flexor pollicis longus, and the T2 zone is between the A1 pulley and the proximal part of the A2 pulley. The T3 zone is located at the level of the thenar eminence (possible area of adherences with the two heads of the flexor pollicis brevis) (Fig. 7.4).

Zones 4 and 5 are the same than for the fingers.

Physiopathology

It is most frequently due to direct traumas caused by sharp objects (knife, steel plate, etc.).

However, there are three severity factors that can lower the functional prognosis:

Sharp Cut or Shredding

The surgical repair is easier in the case of sharp cut.

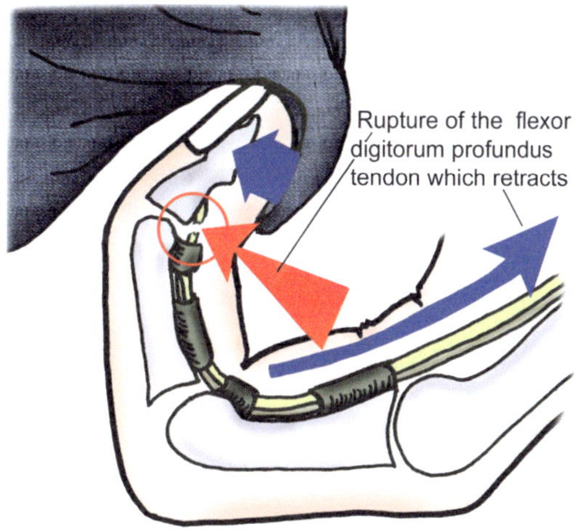

Fig. 7.5 Injury mechanism of the jersey finger

Contamination of the Injury

In case of infection, the risks of adherences and breaks are far more important.

Clamping at the Time of the Trauma

The flexors can retract higher, pulling out the vincula, which makes the repair more difficult and the healing random.

The jersey finger (or rugby finger) is the typical example of this type of injury, where the player (often a rugby player) holds back his opponent by the jersey, which leads to a rupture of the flexor digitorum profundus (often in the ring finger). The tendon can retract until the palm of the hand (Fig. 7.5).

The prognosis in this kind of injury is guarded and uncertain. It depends on the rapidity of the medical care (to limit the retraction of the tendon).

Sadly, this kind of injury is often underestimated in the field.

Healing of the Flexor Tendons

It depends on two complementary systems [4].

Vascular System

Outside the digital sheath: the flexor tendons are vascularized from their two endings (periosteum and musculotendinous junction) and by the intra-tendinous vascular system for the areas far from the extremities of the tendon.

The paratendon, surrounding the tendon, sends a structure to carry the vessels (the mesotendon) which enters the tendon, allowing its vascularization.

Inside the digital sheath, the mesotendon condenses to form vincula, supplied by anastomoses with the collateral arteries [5].

The two flexors each have two vincula, a short one near their ending and a long one higher, which infuse their dorsal part.

There still are three areas that are badly vascularized, in front of the A2 and A4 pulleys. The first one is proximal to the flexor digitorum superficialis' chiasma, and the two others are above and below the vinculum longus that approaches the flexor digitorum profundus at the level of the proximal interphalangeal joint (Fig. 7.6).

Synovial Pump

The synovial sheaths have different organizations, depending on the finger (Fig. 7.7). The flexor pollicis longus has its own sheath, from zone 4 to the T1 zone.

The index, middle, and ring fingers share a sheath with the little finger in zone 4. They each have their individual sheath in the digital canal. The little finger's sheath, shared with the other fingers, continues until the digital canal.

The synovial fluid in the sheaths plays an important role of lubrication and nutrition, by soaking the tendons in the digital canal.

It is important to note that, in the digital canal, the nutrition of the flexor digitorum superficialis is twice as important through this method as through the vascular system, and five times more important for the flexor digitorum profundus.

Thanks to these two systems, we obtain the healing of the tendon by extrinsic healing (vascular mechanism) and intrinsic healing (synovial pump).

The extrinsic healing corresponds to a fibroblastic invasion, which causes adherences. On

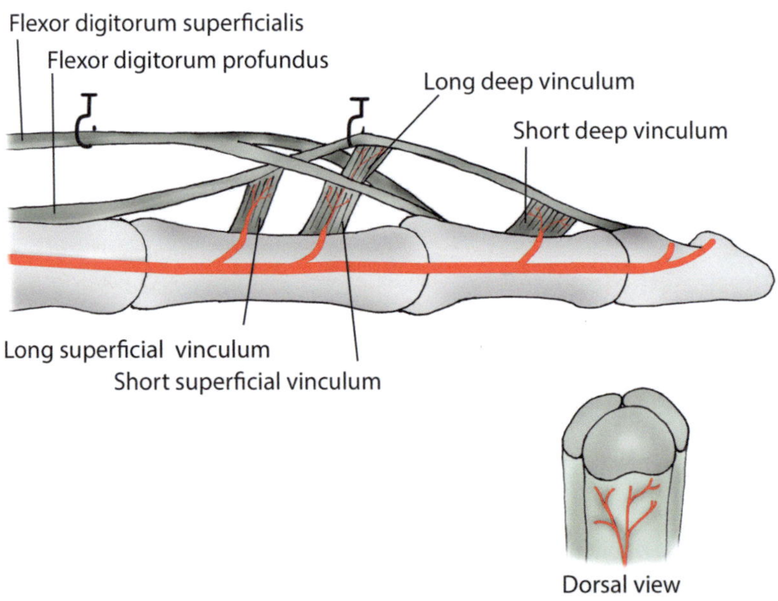

Fig. 7.6 Vincula system, participating in the vascularization of the flexor system

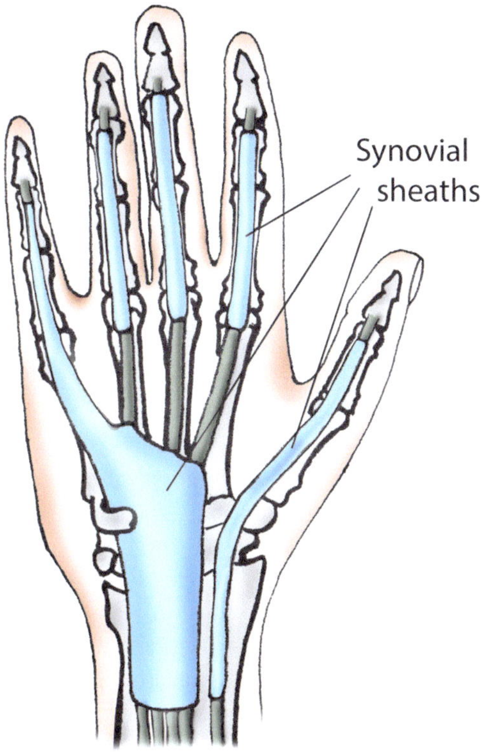

Fig. 7.7 Topography of the synovial sheaths

the other hand, the intrinsic healing is related to a phenomenon of synovial imbibition that does not create adherences.

A surgery as atraumatic as possible and an immediate active rehabilitation favor the intrinsic healing, providing a better functional recovery.

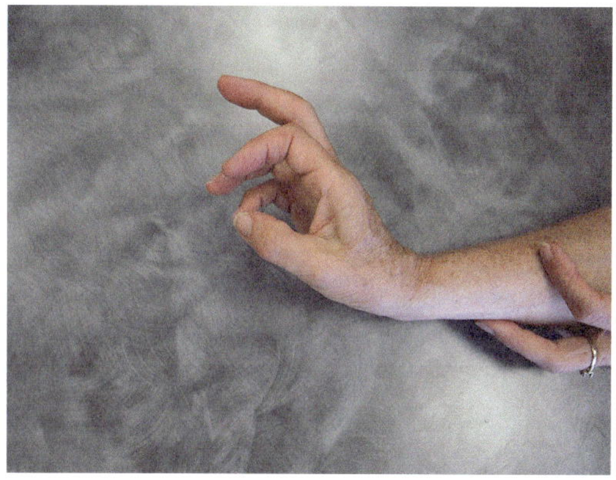

Fig. 7.8 The extension of the wrist leads to the flexion of the fingers from the index to the fifth finger if there is no tendon rupture

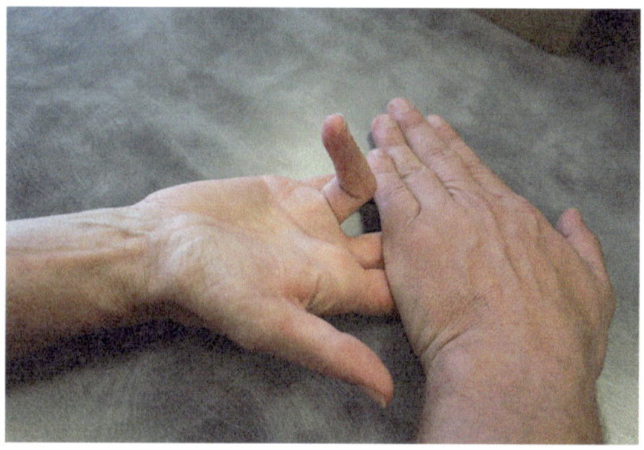

Fig. 7.9 The quadriga effect; it is impossible to flex the distal interphalangeal joint in one finger if the others are maintained in extension, because the flexor digitorum profundus is the same for all the fingers and the proper tendons of each finger become individual very distally

Clinical and Paraclinical Signs

There are various reliable tests that help reveal a sectioning of the flexor tendons:

- Tenodesis effect: as the flexor tendons are polyarticular, the mobilization of the wrist in extension leads to a progressive flexion of the fingers ("in cascade"), from the index to the little finger if there is no rupture (Fig. 7.8).
- The pressure on the muscle masses of the forearm leads to a global flexion of the fingers if there is no rupture.
- The test of the analytical active flexion of the distal interphalangeal joint, with the other fingers free, to test the flexor digitorum profundus.
- The test of the analytical active flexion of the proximal interphalangeal joint, with the other fingers extended to short-circuit the flexor digitorum profundus with the quadriga effect [6], to test the flexor digitorum superficialis (Fig. 7.9).
- The test of the analytical active flexion of the interphalangeal joint of the thumb, to test the flexor pollicis longus.

If there is any doubt, especially in case of partial injury, the exploration of the wound and even an echography if it is a closed injury (jersey finger) are essential.

Therapeutic Process and Surgical Treatment

As always in hand surgery, but even more in tendon surgery, the technique must be as precise and meticulous as possible to avoid tissue trauma, which leads to edema and adherences.

The goal of this repair is to obtain a strong primary suture, allowing an immediate controlled rehabilitation, which is the only thing that can guarantee a good functional result. The best care is ideally given by the hand emergency services.

The Lapse of Time

Ideally, the repair must be done in emergency, as the results are better than in the case of a postponed repair. In practice, it can be done during the first 48 h at the very beginning of the inflammatory phase.

The Points of Access

A meticulous trimming is always done, then enlarging incisions are made so that they are not very extensive and do not cross the flexion creases with a right angle, to avoid cutaneous cords.

Zigzag incisions (Bruner) are used, avoiding delamination and making sure to protect the neurovascular pedicles.

The Suture Techniques (Fig. 7.10)

The manipulation of the tendon's extremities must be as atraumatic as possible. If the rupture of the tendon has occurred in finger flexion, the distal extremity will have distally shifted from the wound of the synovial sheath, and it will be necessary to open the said sheath.

Treatments are adapted to the injury site, especially in zone 2 where the presence of pulleys and the decussation zone of the superficial flexors complicate the treatment [7] (Fig. 7.11).

The tendon suture must have the highest resistance possible to avoid early ruptures and allow and immediate mobilization. The tendon's anchoring must be the best possible to avoid shearing of the tendon fibers by the thread with the formation of a long callus. The suture must be as thin as possible to allow the tendon gliding, and not interfere with the healing process.

A thread with slow resorption, like a PDS with a 4/0 or 3/0 diameter, is the most used, depending on the size of the tendon, with a round needle that is less aggressive.

The classical stitch is the modified Kessler, in which a frame is made with two strands associated with a peritendinous overlock, using a 5/0 thread. By increasing the number of threads, we enhance the resistance, so the four-strand sutures are the most used nowadays, like McLarney's cruciate suture or Tsuge's two-strand looped suture (Fig. 7.12).

The peripheral overlock, combined with the suture in the middle of the tendon, ensures an optimal congruence and avoids friction at the level of the pulleys.

The repair of the flexor digitorum superficialis must always be associated with the repair of the flexor digitorum profundus, to keep the strength and independence of the finger in flexion. However, in zone 2, there is a risk of blocking of the two repaired tendons because of their volume, so the repair of only one strip of the flexor digitorum superficialis and the resection of the second one can be preferable.

Particular Cases

In Zone 1

The avulsion of the flexor digitorum profundus on the last phalanx (jersey finger), or its distal rupture, needs a trans-osseous reinsertion by the pull-out technique or an intraosseous anchor.

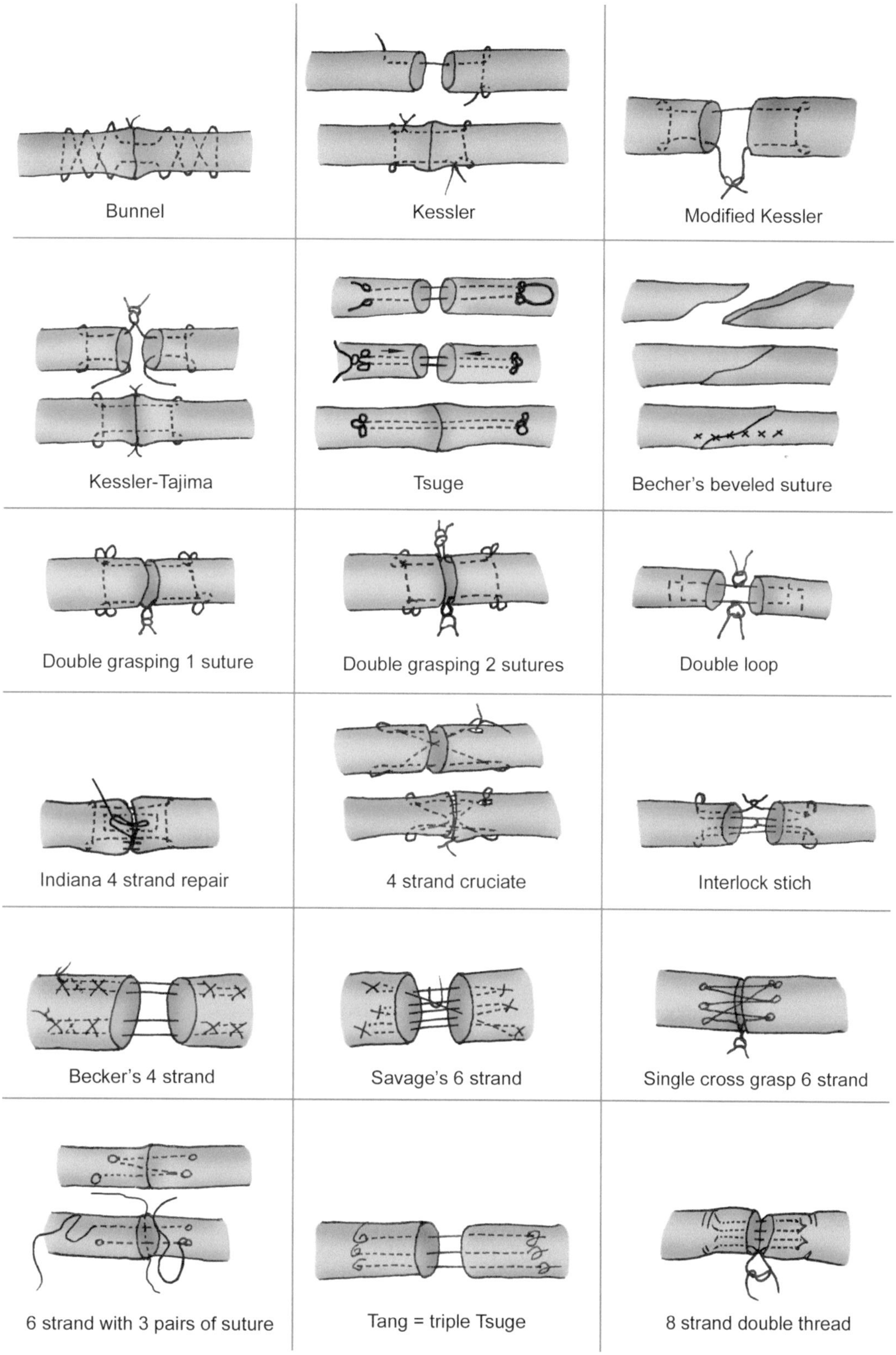

Fig. 7.10 Different types of sutures of the flexor tendons

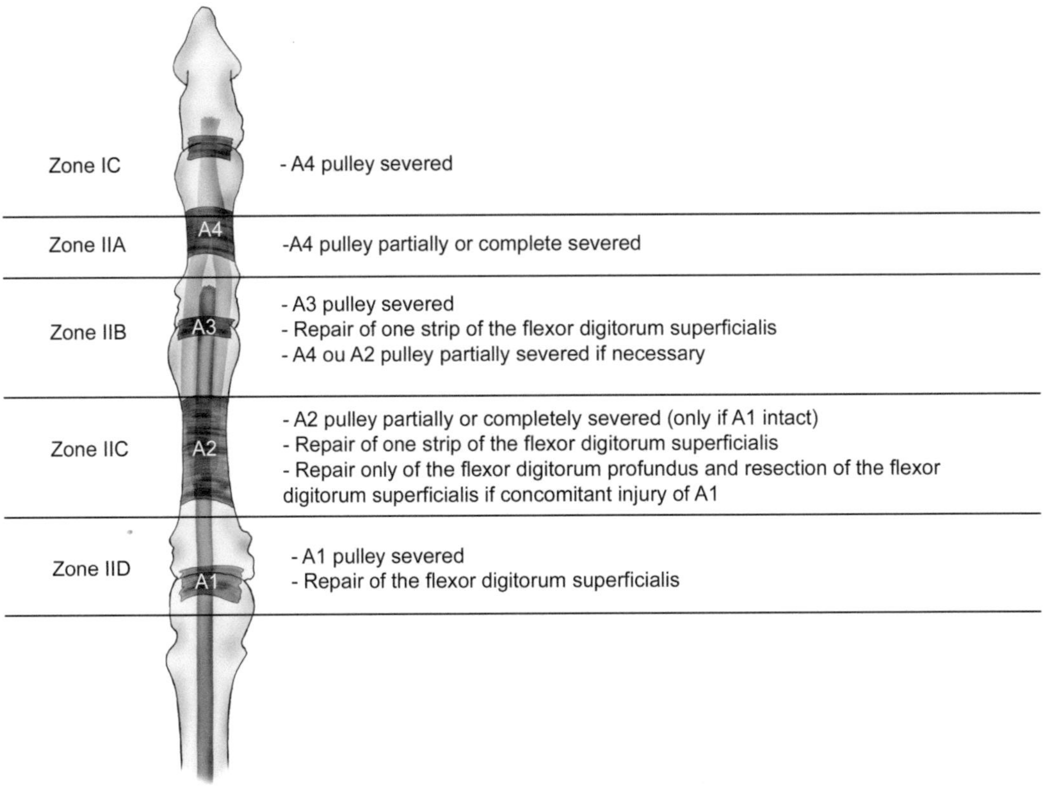

Fig. 7.11 Adaptation of the surgical treatment depending on the zone according to Giesen

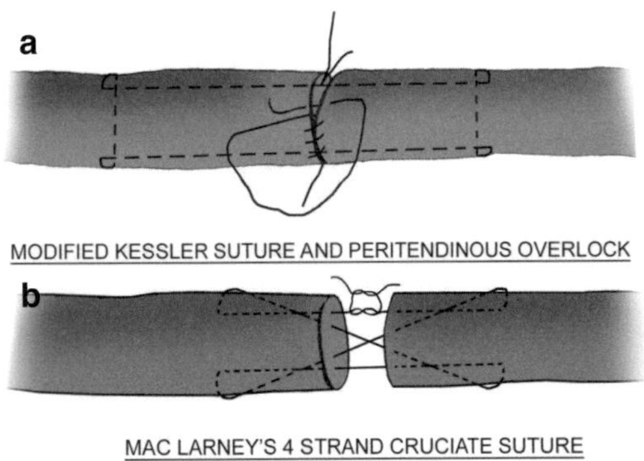

Fig. 7.12 Modified Kessler suture and peritendinous overlock (**a**), and McLarney's four-strand cruciate suture (**b**)

Partial Injury

The risks of adherences, trigger finger, or secondary rupture make us prefer a repair with a peripheral outlock if the injury is smaller than 50% of the tendon, and a suture directly in the tendon if it is bigger than that.

The Flexor Pollicis Longus

Its particularity is due to the high frequency of associated neurovascular injuries, because of the superficial location of the radial collateral pedicle. It is also due to the retraction of the proximal stump, because there is only one vinculum.

The associated multi-tissular injuries must be treated at the same time and allow an early rehabilitation.

The postoperative immobilization is carried out immediately, in a resting position for the flexor system. The early rehabilitation will be an integral part of the treatment and play an essential role in the final result.

Rehabilitation

The rehabilitation must limit the risks of adherences and avoid any rupture of the suture in priority.

A badly measured rehabilitation will lead to one of these two complications.

The immediate postoperative care (D3) [8] and early active mobilizations seem to be the two main elements of this rehabilitation, as they increase the intrinsic healing of the tendon. They also create a healing remodeling, with a longitudinal orientation of the collagen fibers and a faster maturation of the tendinous callus [8].

The mobilized tendons are therefore stronger and more mobile than the ones that are immobilized (Fig. 7.13).

Surgery and early mobilization should make it possible to reduce the "work of flexion" (WOF), i.e., the force required to actively flex the affected finger. With this in mind, the surgical procedure (Fig. 7.14) and rehabilitation should comply with certain validated principles [3, 9].

To reduce the WOF, early mobilization should consider the anatomical and physiological elements validated by science:

- The amount of gliding required to avoid adherences and promote intrinsic healing is 3 to 5 mm [10, 11]. This gliding corresponds to a "half a fist" amplitude, i.e., half the amplitude in digital winding [12].
- Resistance to tendon gliding increases exponentially with increasing digital flexion. This is especially linked to the increase in friction between the tendon and the digital pulleys [13] (Fig. 7.15).
- Friction between the tendon and the pulleys does not increase with the speed of movement [3].
- Active flexion/extension movements are the least stressful for the flexor tendons, with the

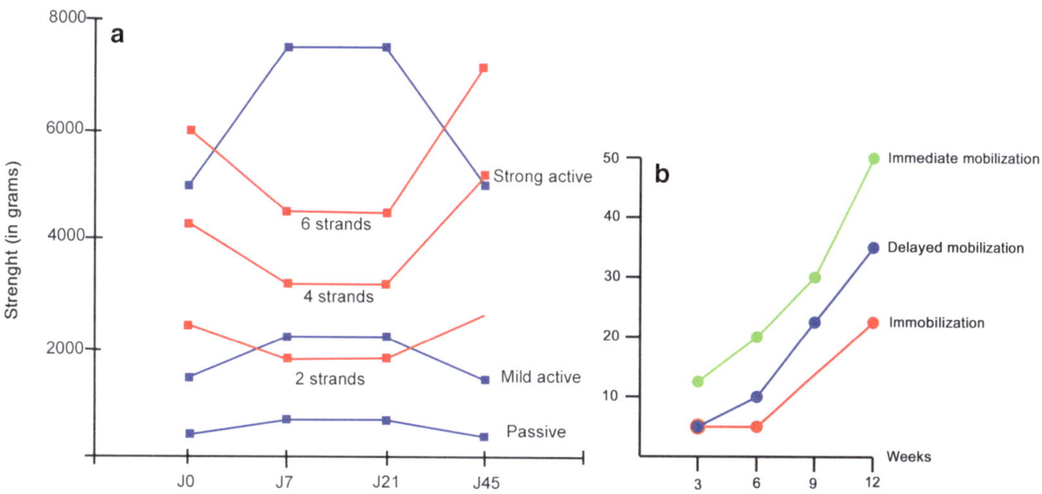

Fig. 7.13 Correlation between the type of suture mobilization and the suture strength over time (**a**) and correlation between the immobilization time and the suture strength over time (**b**)

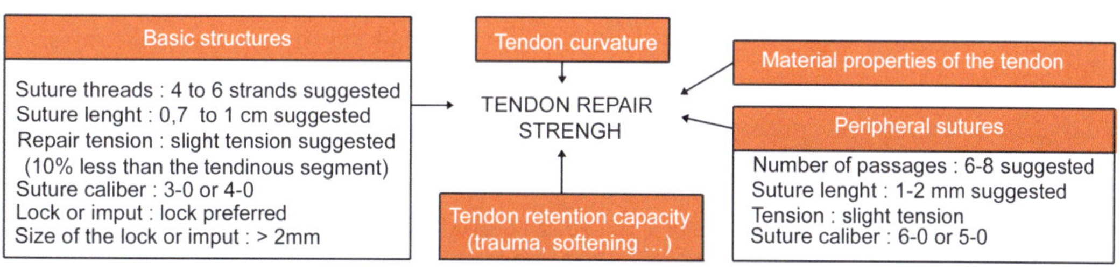

Fig. 7.14 Fundamental principles of the surgical act according to Tang

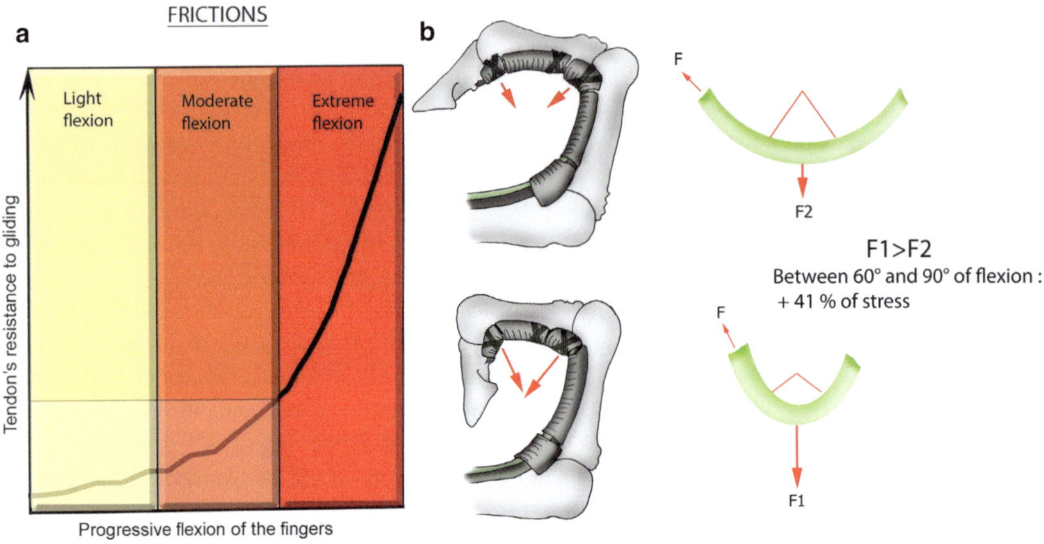

Fig. 7.15 Increase in friction depending on the winding (**a**). Moving from 60° to 90° of flexion increases the stress by 41% (**b**)

metacarpophalangeal joint at a 15° flexion and the wrist in a straight position [14, 15].

- Scientific studies have reached contradictory conclusions concerning the tensions generated by "held-placed" exercises and active flexion [14–16].
- Synergic hand work, based on the tenodesis effect, is the tendon gliding technique with the best ratio of excursion/exerted tension [15, 16].

Rehabilitation Protocols (Fig. 7.16) [17]

For the first 3 days after surgery, the patient is left to rest in an orthosis made in the operating room and in a compression bandage whenever possible. This phase limits the risk of increased inflammation and pain, which could be triggered by a mobilization carried out too early. On D3, the orthosis is made, and active mobilizations are started. The orthosis is worn for 4–6 weeks.

Postoperative Phase (D3 to D45)

From D3 to D45, the patient must keep his orthosis at all times, except during the rehabilitation session and when he does the exercises that he will have to repeat every hour at home.

This is the key phase of that kind of rehabilitation, because it is a fragility and healing phase. The physiotherapist must improve tendon gliding with as few constraints as possible to limit the risks of adherences and rupture.

During this phase, it is important to know exactly what type of injury and suture we are dealing with to use the program that best suits the fragility of the operated tendon.

The notion of a surgeon-physiotherapist team is of key importance here to obtain the best results possible!

Self-rehabilitation is essential and complements the daily sessions. The exercises must be realized every hour. They are explained to the patient and an "exercise sheet" is handed to him (Fig. 7.17).

➔ Fight Against the Edema

- Draining massage above the injury, without any "risky" maneuver for the tendon (like going to extension).
- Cryotherapy without touching the wound for the non-sterile applications. In that case, we use a cold pillow of cherry stones and apply it

a **Injuries of the flexor tendons**

	Post-operative (A)	Relative fragility (B)	Consolidation (C)
REHABILITATION	<u>Therapeutic goals</u> : 1. Fight against pain 2. Fight against trophic disorders 3. Recover passive then active mobilities 4. Prevent functional exclusion <u>Techniques:</u> 1. TENS and TVS (100 Hz) 2. Manual drainage, scar massage and depressotherapy when the scar is closed and if it is not inflammatory, ultrasounds after the scar is closed (not validated) 3. Complete passive mobilization in flexion, then active according to Groth's protocol to limit the WOF. Synergic exercises for the wrist and finger (tenodesis effect). Analytic flexion of the proximal and distal interphalangeal joints (D21). Active analytic extension until tension in a position where the flexors are shortened. 4. TVS (70-80 Hz) and various sensory stimulation (no constraint) <u>Risks:</u> ruptures and adherences if the rehabilitation techniques are maladapted to the surgery	<u>Therapeutic goals</u> : 1. Same, intensify phase 1 if necessary. 2. Recover complete active mobility (claw, analytic flexion of proximal and dorsal interphalangeal joints) 3. Improve coordination and dexterity <u>Techniques:</u> 1. Pressotherapy at defibrosing scar massages and scar mobilization 2. Stretching of the interossei (passive) then active claw, electrostimulation 3. Manipulations of light objects <u>Risks:</u> Same as in phase A, functional exclusion	<u>Therapeutic goals</u> : 1. Intensify the techniques from the two previous phases if necessary 2. Complete functional recovery <u>Techniques:</u> 1. Specific mobilizations of the joints and increase the intensities of the electrostimulation (B2). 2. Functional exercises adapted to the patient's sporting and professional needs <u>Risks:</u> Same as in phases A and B
ORTHOSIS	1. Orthosis immobilizing the wrist (0-30°), metacarpophalangeal joints (15°) and interphalangeal joints (0°) = modified Duran orthosis worn until D30-45, or Manchester orthosis worn until D45 2. Compressive bandage	Orthosis to gain amplitude after 2 months (soft tension but worn for a long period of time)	Orthosis to gain amplitude with adapted modalities if the results are not satisfactory
	D3-D45	D45-D90	After D90

b

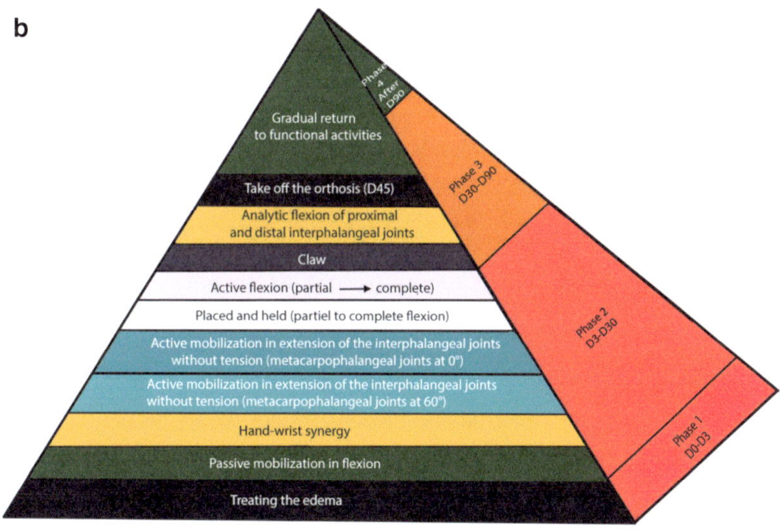

Fig. 7.16 Rehabilitation protocol (**a**) and modified progression pyramid according to Groth (**b**)

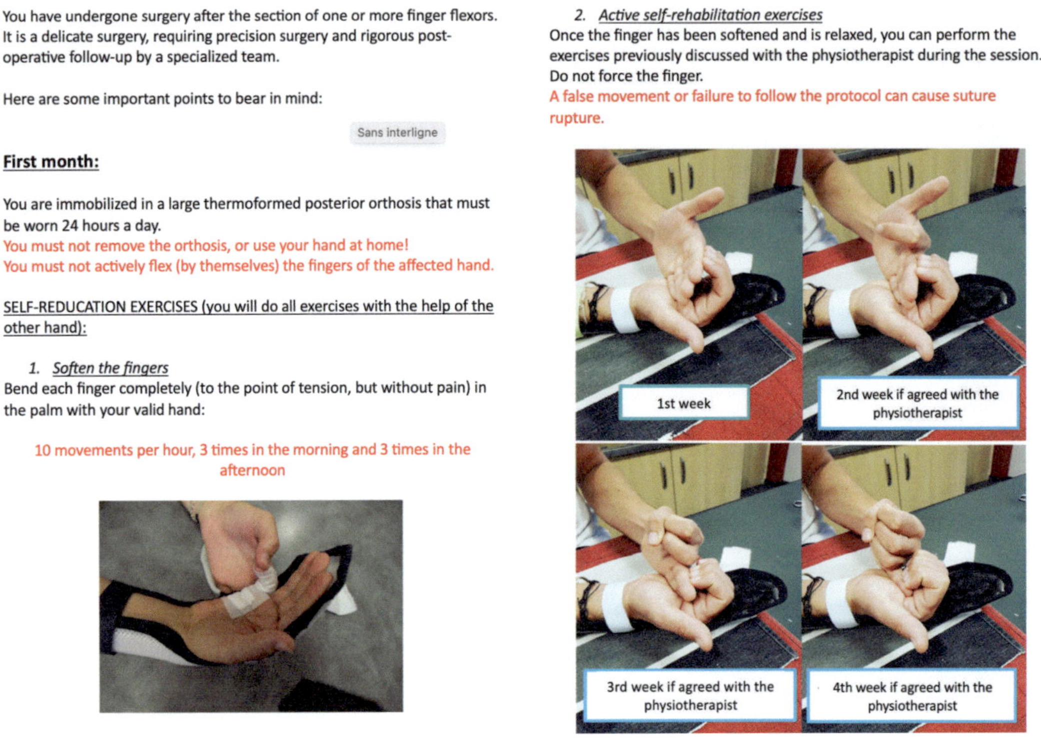

Fig. 7.17 Self-rehabilitation. The patient must make ten passive pain-free mobilizations of the affected finger every hour, without increasing the trophic disorders. An active exercise can also be done in some cases, with an ideal progression of one finger width per week

on the palm of the edematous hand during 15 to 20 min (with a bandage). The patient's hand must be maintained in a protective position during all the application. Cryotherapy also has an interesting analgesic effect.

- Compressive bandage outside the periods of self-rehabilitation if the patient knows well what the "risky" positions are for his tendon. Otherwise, he must not take the bandage off himself, which raises the issue of self-mobilizations at home, limited by this compressive system. We sometimes must give it up, as self-mobilizations at home are essential to recover mobility.
- Electrotherapy (1 Hz) is used since D21 on the edematous areas with a moderate intensity.

➔ Fight Against Pain

- Analgesic electrotherapy with a wobbled 100 Hz frequency: the active (smallest) electrode is placed near the painful area and the indifferent electrode at the level of the corresponding vertebral level. The current intensity must be set to get a "tingling" sensation, but no muscle contraction.
- Transcutaneous vibratory stimulations with a low frequency (ideally 100 Hz) and amplitude (lower than 1 mm) are applied on the painful area, moving along the trajectory of the sensitive nerve concerned by this area [18]. In case of pain when applying the device directly on the skin, we place it far from the painful area, yet always on the trajectory of the corresponding nerve. With a 70 Hz frequency, this type of mechanical vibration has a proprioceptive effect, creating an illusion of movement if we apply it along the operated tendon [19–22] (Fig. 7.18).

➔ Progressive Recovery of the Joint Amplitudes (Improving the Intrinsic Healing)

- *Passive exercises in a protected area*

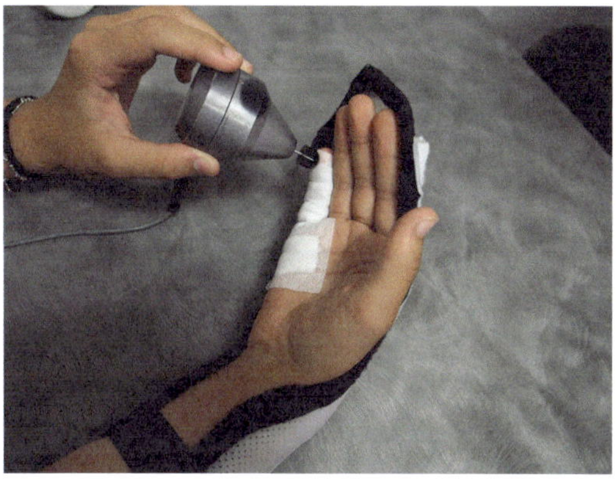

Fig. 7.18 Transcutaneous vibratory stimulations

It is the mobilization of the affected segments, in areas that do not threaten the tendon suture. The flexion is not limited, but the combined extension of various joints of the same segment is forbidden if it puts the suture in tension. The limits are different from one patient to another depending on the type of injury, the intraoperative tensioning of the suture, etc. Therefore, we must be careful and stay focus during these mobilizations and be aware of the operative report.

The passive exercises alone can be insufficient to mobilize the tendon effectively, especially in case of adherences when the "accordion effect" can be observed (Fig. 7.19). However, it is used to get the joint amplitudes back in flexion and to warm up the hand before using active techniques, which are essential in the good recuperation of the tendon gliding.

- *Active extension*

Finger winding is passive, but the patient actively returns to the extended position, still staying in protected areas. For example, we work on the interphalangeal joint extension with the metacarpophalangeal joints flexed to avoid any excessive constraint on the suture.

We use this exercise to progressively get back the amplitudes in extension, as the contraction of the extensor system is less "risky" than the passive mobilization for the suture: the patient controls the movement and stops as soon as he/she feels tension. This exercise does not avoid the

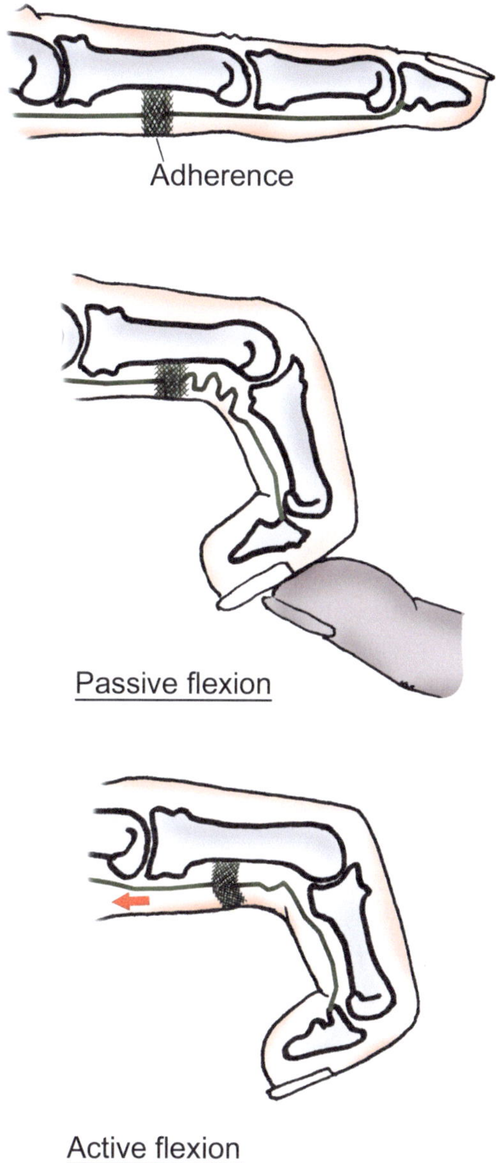

Fig. 7.19 In case of adherences, the passive mobilization alone does not allow moving the tendon suture, and an accordion effect can be observed

"accordion effect" as there is no contraction of the flexor system.

- *Placed and held*

Before this type of active work, the wrist is placed in a straight position and the metacarpophalangeal joints flexed at 15° to reduce the WOF. In the case of sutures under tension, the position is of course adapted so as not to create tension on the suture. Similarly, this work is postponed in the event of significant edema, which creates resistance to movement (increased WOF) and would be maintained by over-intensive active exercises [23]. On the other hand, the use of very light muscular contractions, without any notion of amplitude improvement, stimulates the "vis a latere" and promotes venous return through a pumping effect.

This technique can be used after warming up the hand with passive mobilizations, which limits the resistances during the contraction of the flexor tendon.

We place the finger in flexion and ask the patient to actively maintain this position. The evolution goes from an "easy" position in the intermediate race, to more difficult positions in inner or outer tendon race. In inner race, the resistance of the flexor to contraction is more important than in intermediate race because the extensor system is tensed, while it is the pretension of the flexor that increases the constraints imposed on it in outer race. Therefore, we must be very careful with the exercises in inner and outer race, which must be realized after the exercises in intermediate race.

We ask the patient to do 20 contractions, each of them lasting 3 s. He must not realize these contractions with strength, so we ask him to avoid tremors and contractions of the muscles adjacent to the one we are working with. The goal is to insist on the quality of the motor command and to get the exact contraction we are looking for. If the exercise is too difficult, we postpone it or we place the finger in a more favorable position, most of the time in intermediate tendon race. To do this, the physiotherapist can change the position of each joint of the concerned segments separately, always staying in protected areas.

- *Active exercises in a protected area*

As with "placed and held" exercises, the wrist is placed in a straight position, with the metacarpophalangeal joints flexed at 15° to reduce the WOF and the position adapted in the event of tensioned sutures.

In our experience, simple active exercises in the protected sector are preferred, as the tension generated is no greater than the resistance of a four-strand suture (Fig. 7.13), and the control of movement is often better assured than in the "placed and held" exercises. The amplitude requested at D3 (if flexible in passive) corresponds to a "half a fist" amplitude, i.e., half the amplitude of digital flexion, which is enough to limit the risk of adherences and promote intrinsic healing [12]. This amplitude is increased by one finger width per week if progress is favorable (Fig. 7.17).

We realize these exercises analytically and globally, without forcing the hand's amplitudes and always after a previous warm-up. The movements must be slow and smooth, we ask for 2 to 3 series of 10 repetitions per session. The active exercises, if they are too aggressive, can lead to a rupture or a flabbiness of the scar. Working with the four long fingers at the same time makes the realization of the movement easier and limits the constraints on the suture.

- *Cooney exercise/synergetic hand-wrist exercise*

This technique consists in going from a wrist flexion + fingers extension to a wrist extension + fingers flexion.

This exercise creates an important tendon gliding via by tenodesis effect.

However, during the first few weeks, wrist extension is limited to 45° to avoid tension on the suture. As tendon excursion is greater in the wrist (6.5 cm) than in the fingers (2.5 cm) [4] (Fig. 7.20), a wrist extension greater than 45° creates noticeable tension on the tendon, even with the fingers fully flexed [24].

➔ Flexibility of the Scar (As Soon As It Is Closed)

- *Massage of the scar*

When the vitro-pressure test is greater than 2 s, we can begin scar massage and mobilization

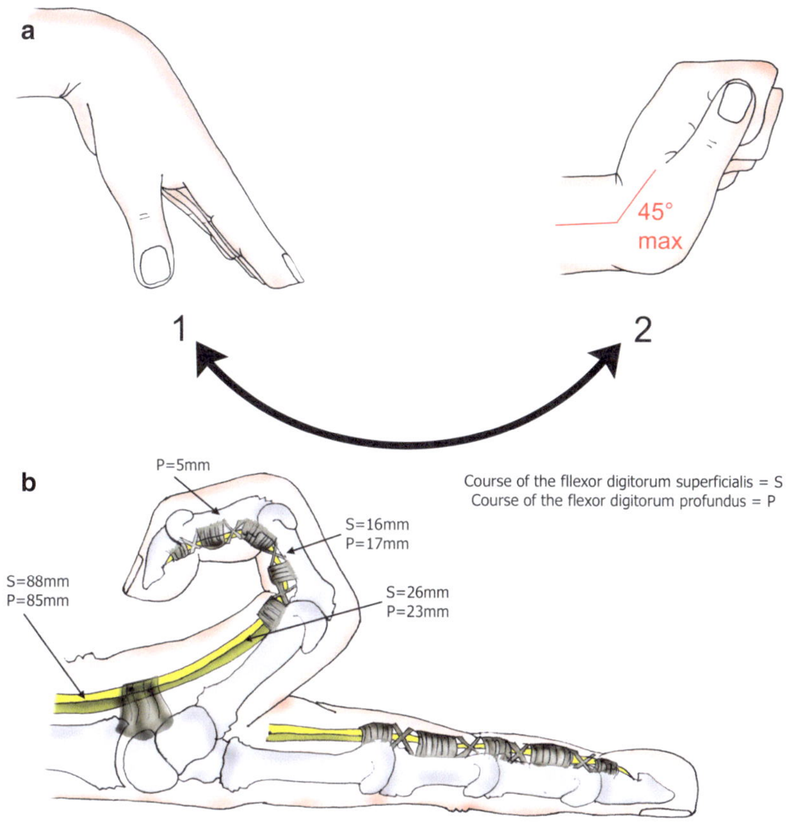

Fig. 7.20 Because of the tenodesis effect, the extension of the wrist leads to the flexion of the fingers (**a**). The wrist extension must not be greater than 45° during the first weeks in order not to put tension on the sutured flexor tendon (**b**)

techniques. Without any distraction of the scar, we mobilize it to try to free the different gliding planes and soften the scar. We use sanding techniques, sliding pressures, and palpating and rolling massage in the areas where it can be done.

- *Depressotherapy*

We use this device with the usual procedures for the treatment of scars, but with the orthosis to limit the risks of dangerous maneuvers for the tendon.

Relative Fragility Phase (D45 to D90)

During this phase, we keep doing the previous techniques, intensifying their application. The orthosis is removed for all the daily activities but kept during "risky" activities.

The importance of the different techniques depends on the healing of the patient.

If the patient has an intrinsic healing, there are less adherences, and the active mobility can be satisfactory. There is less risk of stiffness than of rupture (which is still unusual in this phase).

If the patient has an extrinsic healing (big finger, hypertrophic scar), the finger is not very mobile, and there still are trophic disorders. The risk of stiffness is important.

Of course, ideally, at D45 the patients should all have developed an intrinsic healing, but we note that it is not always the case, even for the patients followed by a specialized team (genetic factor, associated injuries, waiting before medical care).

Some new techniques are used in this phase:

➔ Fight Against Trophic Disorders

Pressotherapy techniques with compression from distal to proximal can be used to fight trophic disorders that can still remain in this phase of the rehabilitation.

➔ Recover Mobility

- *Electrostimulation.*

In this phase, we can use striomotor currents to accompany the patient's active contraction. It helps improve the tendon glidings and therefore fighting against possible adherences.

They are especially useful when the patient has a deficit of motor control, because the current efficiently stimulates the targeted muscle even if the motor command is not optimal.

The placement of the electrodes depends on the muscle we want to stimulate (see chapter "Physical Agents" in Volume 1).

- *Intrinsic muscle stretching.*

The interossei and lumbrical muscles should be differentiated, as their stretching modalities are different.

The interossei can be stretched by the extrinsic + position of the hand, regardless of the wrist position.

The lumbrical muscles are stretched only if this position is realized with the wrist in extension, as the lumbrical muscles do not have a proximal bone insertion: the insertion is on the flexor digitorum profundus that moves from distal to proximal when placing the wrist in extension (Fig. 7.21).

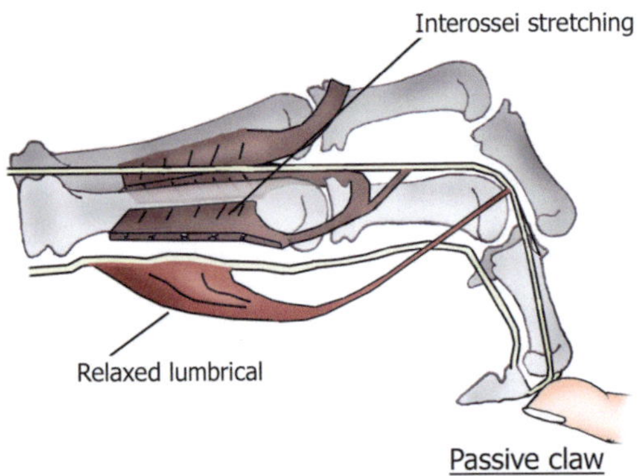

Fig. 7.21 The passive placement in the extrinsic + position does not stretch the lumbrical muscles, but the active placement does

- *Computerized imitation exercises.*

It consists in imitating the pictures on the screen during all the time they are on display.

The positions have been defined by Wehbé [25] and allow obtaining a complete tendon gliding for the flexor digitorum superficialis and the flexor digitorum profundus, and a maximal differential gliding between the two of them (Fig. 7.22).

- *Improving the coordination and dexterity.*

The patient is asked to perform manipulations of increasing difficulty and intensity to improve coordination and dexterity.

Solidity Phase (After D90)

This phase corresponds with the patient getting back to work and doing sports.

We keep doing the previous techniques and intensify them to get closer to the patient's daily needs and the flexor tendons' function (Fig. 7.23).

Orthotic Treatment

Immobilization Phase

Several types of orthoses have been proposed for the postoperative phase, but in the current state of knowledge, two options should be preferred:

➔ Modified Duran

In this orthosis, the wrist is positioned between 0 and 30° flexion, the metacarpophalangeal joints between 15° and 30° of flexion, and the interphalangeal joints in a straight position, if this is actively possible (Fig. 7.24).

If this is not the case, the suture may have been realized under tension, and the orthosis is made in the patient's position of maximum active extension, then remolded according to the progress made in active extension. The finger must never be brought into passive extension; otherwise the surgical repair will break!

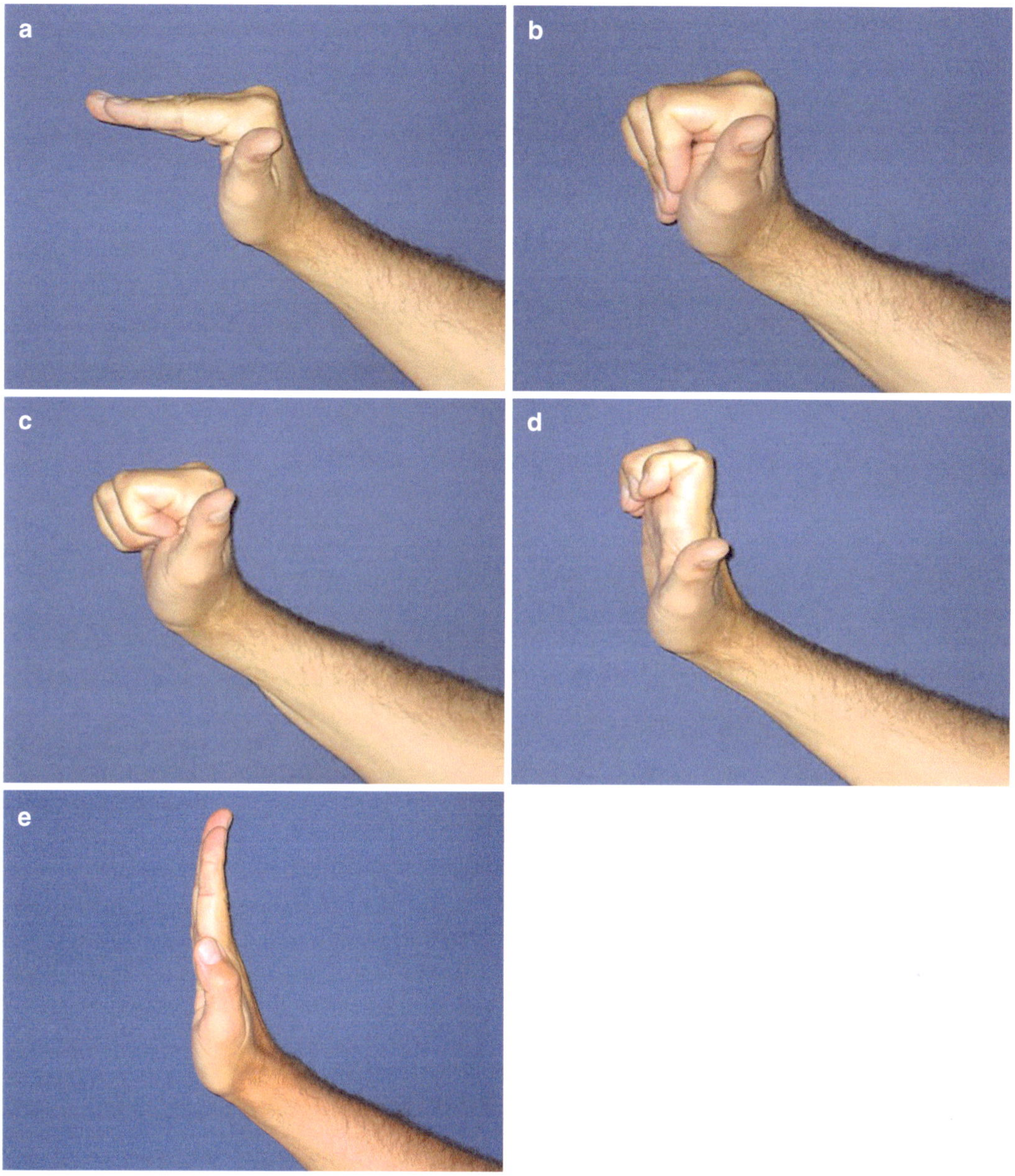

Fig. 7.22 Slide show for imitations of the positions defined by Wehbé, which allow a maximal differential gliding between the flexor digitorum profundus and the flexor digitorum superficialis

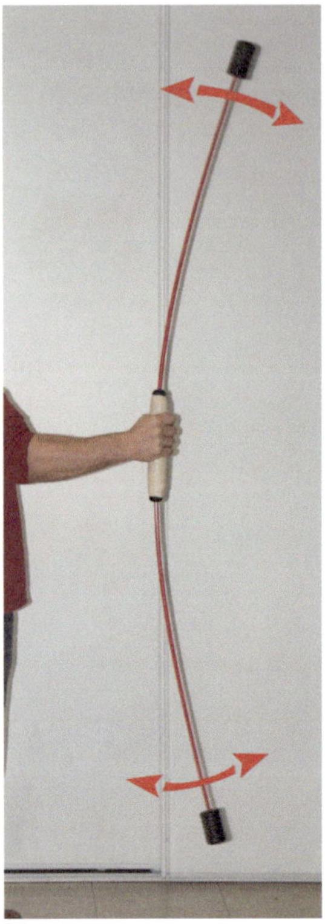

Fig. 7.23 Functional exercises according to the patient's functional needs

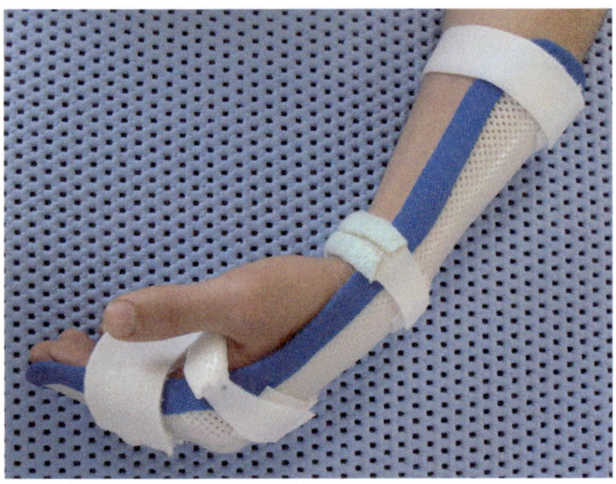

Fig. 7.24 Modified Duran orthosis

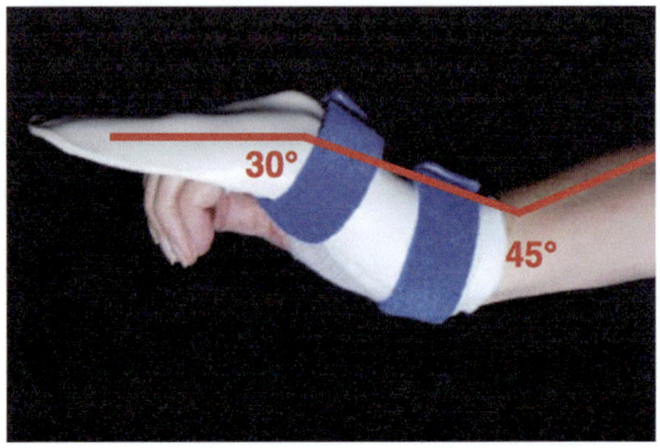

Fig. 7.25 Manchester orthosis (according to Peck)

After D21, the orthosis can be reshaped by moving the wrist further into extension or even by letting the wrist free, especially if the flexed wrist position is poorly tolerated. The orthosis is worn for 45 days.

➔ Manchester Orthosis

The purpose of this orthosis is to allow the synergetic hand/wrist work throughout the day. The metacarpophalangeal joints are placed at 30° of flexion, with the interphalangeal joints free and the wrist extension limited to 45° to avoid creating tension on the tendon at the end of its amplitude [24] (Fig. 7.25).

The results obtained with this method appear to be significantly superior, despite a rupture rate 10% higher than the control group immobilized with a modified Duran orthosis [24].

After D60

In case of flessum of the interphalangeal or metacarpophalangeal joints, we realize a postural orthosis (see chapter "Common Hand and Wrist Orthoses" in Volume 1) (Fig. 7.26).

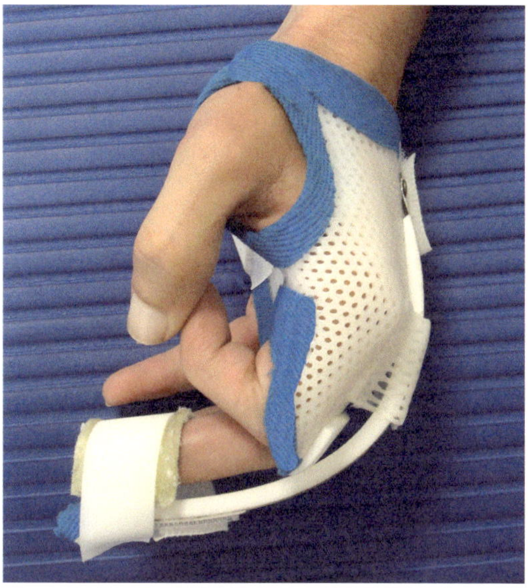

Fig. 7.26 Dynamic extension orthosis in case of flexum

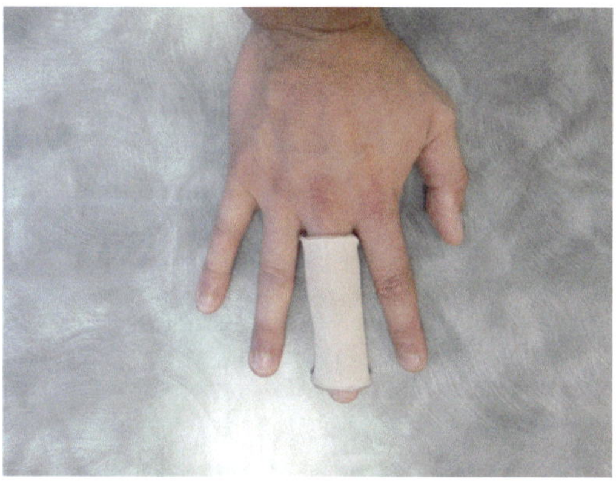

Fig. 7.27 Silicone muff for an anti-edematous effect and healing improvement

The use of a silicone tube can also be very beneficial, as it combines an anti-edematous effect (by compression) and an anti-flessum effect and improves the healing state (Fig. 7.27). The posture, maintained by the silicone tube, is not very intense, so we can use them since D45 if the trophic and healing disorders persist.

Particular Cases

Injuries of the Flexor Pollicis Longus

The rehabilitation protocol follows the same principles as in the rehabilitation of the fingers, adjusting to the physiological and architectural particularities of the flexor pollicis longus.

There are a few things to keep in mind:

- The orthosis places the wrist in 30° of flexion, significantly reducing the tension on the flexor pollicis longus [26].
- The flexor pollicis longus is a very powerful muscle, so the patient must control its contraction during the first phase to avoid any risk of rupture.
- In the T2 zone, its tendon can stick to the two heads of the flexor pollicis brevis, which can limit its gliding.

Jersey Finger (or Rugby Finger)

It is an injury of the flexor digitorum profundus in the ring finger, caused by a tear that occurs in a closed chain.

Their classification allows us to know their gravity and surgical treatment.

The application of the rehabilitation protocol is more or less careful, depending on the vascular state of the tendon (tear of its short distal vincula).

Bibliography

1. Mesplié G, Grelet V. Injuries of the flexor tendons, in hand and wrist rehabilitation. Springer; 2015. p. 275–306.
2. Kapandji, I.A., Physiologie articulaire tome 1—Membre supérieur. 2005: Maloine.

3. Tang BT, et al. Tendon surgery of the hand. Elsevier Saunders; 2012.
4. Strickland JW. The scientific basis for advances in flexor tendon surgery. J Hand Ther. 2005;18(2):94–110.
5. Tang JB. Clinical outcomes associated with flexor tendon repair. Hand Clin. 2005;21(2):199–210.
6. Schreuders TA. The quadriga phenomenon: a review and clinical relevance. J Hand Surg Eur. 2012;37(6):513–22.
7. Giesen T, Calcagni M, Elliot D. Primary flexor tendon repair with early active motion: experience in Europe. Hand Clin. 2017;33(3):465–72.
8. Bigorre N, et al. Primary flexor tendons repair in zone 2: current trends with GEMMSOR survey results. Hand Surg Rehabil. 2018;37(5):281–8.
9. Savage R. The search for the ideal tendon repair in zone 2: strand number, anchor points and suture thickness. J Hand Surg Eur. 2014;39(1):20–9.
10. Strickland JW. Flexor Tendon Repair. Hand Clin. 1985 Feb;1(1):55–68.
11. Duran R, Houser R. Controlled passive motion following flexor tendon repair in zones II and III. In: The American Academy of Orthopaedic surgeons: symposium on tendon surgery in the hand. Mosby St Louis; 1975.
12. Meals C, Lalonde D, Candelier G. Repaired flexor tendon excursion with half a fist of true active movement versus full fist place and hold in the awake patient, vol. 7. Plast Reconstr Surg Glob Open; 2019. p. e2074.
13. Wu YF, Tang JB. Tendon healing, edema, and resistance to flexor tendon gliding: clinical implications. Hand Clin. 2013;29(2):167–78.
14. Kursa K, et al. In vivo flexor tendon forces increase with finger and wrist flexion during active finger flexion and extension. J Orthop Res. 2006;24(4):763–9.
15. Edsfeldt S, et al. In vivo flexor tendon forces generated during different rehabilitation exercises. J Hand Surg Eur. 2015;40(7):705–10.
16. Sapienza A, et al. Flexor tendon excursion and load during passive and active simulated motion: a cadaver study. J Hand Surg Eur. 2013;38(9):964–71.
17. Groth GN. Pyramid of progressive force exercises to the injured flexor tendon. J Hand Ther. 2004;17(1):31–42.
18. Roll JP. Stimulation vibratoire transcutanée et douleur. Douleurs Éval – Diagn – Trait. 2019;20(5):226–31.
19. Thyrion C, Roll JP. Perceptual integration of illusory and imagined kinesthetic images. J Neurosci. 2009;29(26):8483–92.
20. Roll JP, et al. Inducing any virtual two-dimensional movement in humans by applying muscle tendon vibration. J Neurophysiol. 2009;101(2):816–23.
21. Roll R, et al. Illusory movements prevent cortical disruption caused by immobilization. NeuroImage. 2012;62(1):510–9.
22. Gerlac, D., Mobiliser « sans mobiliser » Utilisation des vibrations comme moyen de récupération des amplitudes articulaires. Les feuillets du GEMMSOR.
23. Wu YF, Zhou YL, Tang JB. Relative contribution of tissue oedema and the presence of an A2 pulley to resistance to flexor tendon movement: an in vitro and in vivo study. J Hand Surg Eur. 2012;37(4):310–5.
24. Peck FH, et al. The Manchester short splint: a change to splinting practice in the rehabilitation of zone II flexor tendon repairs. Hand Ther. 2014;19(2):47–53.
25. Wehbe MA, Hunter JM. Flexor tendon gliding in the hand. Part I. In vivo excursions. J Hand Surg Am. 1985;10(4):570–4.
26. Rappaport PO, et al. Effect of wrist and interphalangeal thumb movement on zone T2 flexor pollicis longus tendon tension in a human cadaver model. J Hand Ther. 2015;28:347.

Part IV

Finger Amputations

8 Traumatic Amputations

Amélie-Anne Vienne

Introduction

Amputation of one or more fingers has functional, aesthetic, and psychological consequences.

This type of injury involves functional after-effects that impact on the patient's participation and quality of life.

There are many surgical techniques available, depending on the initial trauma.

Their goal is to ensure the function of the injured limb, manage the aesthetic aspect, and limit sensory after-effects.

Rehabilitation and orthopedic devices are essential and complementary to surgical treatment to optimize a return to function and promote occupational activities. As they are indissociable from the surgery, collaboration between the medical and paramedical teams is essential.

A.-A. Vienne (✉)
Service Ergothérapie Appareillage, CHU Sud Réunion, Saint-Pierre, France

General Information

Epidemiology and Prevalence [10, 11, 36]

The prevalence of amputations mainly affects active men between 40 and 60 years old. The literature does not describe a right/left prevalence, dominant or non-dominant side.

The fingers most affected are the index and middle fingers, and 51% are distal amputations (third phalanx).

The vast majority (85%) involves one single finger.

Etiology and Context of the Injury [11, 36]

Finger amputations are 90% traumatic in origin. They can also be caused by complications of trauma to the tendons or bones, severe burns, infections or congenital malformations, etc.

During surgical and paramedical management, the cause and circumstances of the trauma are important elements to determine. They give decisive indications for the treatments implemented in follow-up care.

The most frequent etiology involves domestic accidents (DIY) and accidents at work (manual jobs).

G. Mesplié (ed.), *Hand Functional Anatomy and Therapy*,
https://doi.org/10.1007/978-3-031-92505-4_8

The most common mechanism of injury is saw and tool blade cuts. These represent a cost of $2000 billion per year worldwide.

Amputations are also often caused by crushing, avulsions, clipper wounds, and pressure injections.

Treatment Time [10, 11, 14]

An amputation is a "complex" wound, combining tissue, bone, nerve, and vascular lesions, sometimes at multiple sites, so there are many criteria that determine the functional outcome and duration of overall treatment.

We can distinguish three classes of factors:

- Pre-injury factors: the patient and his/her initial state of health, age, psychological state, medical history, etc.
- Injury factors: the injury mechanism, the quality and integrity of the mutilated structures, the management of immediate care, the conservation of the injured structures, etc.
- Post-injury factors: surgical gesture(s) and treatment, postoperative care, rehabilitation and orthosis, motivation, grief management, after-effects, etc.

It has been reported that 50% of people affected by this type of injury must stop working for more than 2 months, with an average absence of 6 months.

The duration of treatment and time off work is reported to be longer in the case of digital reimplantation and in cases where secondary surgery is envisaged.

This is explained by the need to keep the concerned area immobilized to respect tissue, vascular and nerve healing, and bone consolidation times.

It should be noted that in the case of skin and flap grafting, functional recovery is even later, with the majority of after-effect being permanent.

Surgical Treatment

The surgical tools for amputations are many, with three types and stages of surgery:

- Primary post-traumatic surgery, which aims to act immediately after the trauma
- Secondary reconstructive surgery, which aims to restore and optimize the function of the mutilated limb and which may be considered in the short to medium term
- Revision surgery, which aims to provide solutions to the after-effects and which is discussed in the medium to long term

22% of traumatic amputations require revision surgery and/or secondary surgery.

Each surgical procedure is carefully considered in its own timeframe, with the aim of achieving the best possible functional outcome, preventing complications as far as possible and minimizing after-effects.

In addition to the injury and structural-technical criteria, the patient's profile (age, activities, needs) helps to determine the most appropriate treatment.

Primary Surgery

The management of a single or multiple digital amputation injury is an absolute emergency. The patient is most likely to require treatment within a few hours after the accident.

The injured finger(s), trophic and vascular status, type of wound, site of injury, future functional benefits and risks, and the patient's profile are all criteria that will determine the medical team's choice of emergency procedure.

There are two possibilities for surgical treatment:

- Revision amputation, which consists in shortening, improving, covering, and regularizing the traumatic stump(s).

- Reimplantation of the amputated part(s) may be envisaged when the conditions are right.

We will see the indications, particularities, and principles of these two surgical techniques.

Regularization Amputation

➔ Generalities [10]

Regularization amputation is indicated in cases where the amputated part does not meet the conditions necessary for reimplantation. It can also be a secondary procedure in the event of a reimplantation failure, in the case of major after-effects (functional discomfort, pain, neuromas, infections, etc.), or in the case of certain pathologies such as ischemia, tumors, etc.

In Western countries, the initial management of traumatic amputations by regularization accounts for 83% of surgical procedures. In some countries, such as Asia, amputation of one or more fingers has a negative aesthetic or social stigma attached to it. Known as "Yubitsume" in Japan, amputation of the ring or little finger is a strong sign of dereliction of duty. It also carries the cultural stigma of banditry. As a result, regularizations are kept to a minimum, accounting for only 25% of surgical procedures.

➔ Surgical Principles [7]

Two main considerations are considered during the surgical procedure:

- Sufficient coverage of the stump with soft tissue remains an absolute priority over preservation of segment length.
- Prevention of symptomatic neuroma is also a major concern. It is essential to treat the nerve during the first stage of surgery.

Neglect of the nerve leads to a symptomatic neuroma in 36% of cases. End-to-end suturing of the two palmar nerves, burial in the bone, and thermo-coagulation all help to avoid this type of complication.

The after-effects are less severe in the case of primary suturing of the stump and directed healing in younger patients. A higher prevalence of grafts and transplants is reported in people with morbidities.

➔ Postoperative Management

The after-effects of regularization procedures are fairly rapid, with an average of 2 months off work.

Healing of the stump is the most important postoperative requirement.

Mobility remains the priority and should not be hindered by an orthosis or even a contention bandage.

It is rare for the patient to benefit from orthoses and hand rehabilitation, given that most injuries involve the distal phalanges of a single finger. However, functional after-effects and discomfort are frequent.

The goal of rehabilitation is to reduce the risk of vascular, sensory, and functional complications, as well as problems with the motor pattern, stiffness, and deformity, and to avoid pejorative compensations. Details are given in the rehabilitation section.

It also aims to remind the patient of instructions and inform him/her of how to behave during the healing period (stop smoking, skin monitoring, declive, daily gestures to be limited or encouraged).

➔ After-Effects and Complications [1, 10, 11, 14, 18]

78% of patients report long-term (2–4 years) symptomatic complications that have a significant impact on their daily participation and quality of life.

Sensory after-effects are major and predominant.

45% of patients reported incapacitating paresthesia, 34% recurrent and troublesome algohallucinoses and phantom pain, and 61% expressed intolerance to cold at the level of the scar.

For 60% of patients, sensory disorders are due to insufficient coverage, neuroma, and inguinal disorders (very frequent given the proportion of distal amputations).

Aesthetic damage is also an issue that has a considerable impact on the quality of life.

Digital Reimplantations

➔ Generalities [9, 17]

The circumstances of the trauma, the mutilated finger(s), the grade of avulsion, the patient's age, state of health, motivation, and access to follow-up care are decisive criteria in the surgical choice of reimplantation of one or more fingers.

According to Chung and Alderman, the absolute contraindications are:

- Life-threatening injury, making prolonged anesthesia impossible.
- Incapacity for rehabilitation and aftercare.
- Acute psychiatric illness.
- Non-functioning limb.
- Medical history increasing morbidity.
- Significant contamination of the amputated area.
- Prolonged ischemia: the acceptable warm ischemia time is 6–8 h for a limb and 10–12 h for a finger. It can be extended to 24 h with correct handling (cooling). The shorter the time to revascularization, the better the return to sensitivity.

➔ Preoperative Principles [5, 29, 33]

The preoperative protocol and management of the amputated finger can significantly limit iatrogenic soft-tissue damage.

The preoperative protocols for preservation and storage of the amputated part can reduce the risk of complications and after-effects by 20–60%.

The aim is to allow the quickest possible cooling in a dry or humid environment, ideally at 10°. The direct cooling of the tissue is detrimental to the tissue.

➔ Postoperative Care

It should be noted that this type of surgery always requires a global postoperative care, including hand therapy.

Referral to a specialized center is often indicated. Lack of access to specialized follow-up care may be a contraindication to this surgical technique.

Vascular survival is the priority. Once guaranteed, the time required for bone consolidation, the nerve sutures, the presence of surgical arthrorise material, and the healing are all criteria that will determine the start of rehabilitation and the chosen resources.

Regarding the postoperative orthopedic devices:

- The orthosis enables protective positioning and immobilization of the injured structures while respecting the principles of damage prevention.
- The surgeon will determine which structures are to be preserved, protected, or immobilized, based on the surgical procedure(s) performed.
- An orthosis, usually articular, may be prescribed.
- The whole limb (wrist, hand, and finger(s)) or part of it (hand + finger(s) or finger(s)) may be concerned by the orthosis.
- The therapist in charge of making the orthosis must respect the medical indications of the prescribing surgeon.
- In this case, the person in charge of making the orthosis must respect the general principles of orthoses concerning the tensions put on the tissues, nerves, and vascular structures.
- Unless contraindicated, the reference position is: wrist straight, metacarpophalangeal joint at 40° flexion, and proximal and distal interphalangeal joints in extension.
- To prevent functional complications, the patient should be rapidly referred to a rehabilitation specialist.
- Early rehabilitation should follow the general principles of traumatology, with the aim of preventing the effects of prolonged immobilization and its consequences.

➔ After-Effects and Complications [4, 10]

The major complication is vascular. The reimplanted part may not survive. In this case, regularization or secondary surgery may be indicated.

Major after-effects are common to traumatic injuries of the hand (stiffness, deformity, sensory disorders, limb perception disorders, etc.).

The patients' function and quality of life are described as better after reimplantation than after regularization.

Patients are more satisfied when these gestures concern the thumb or the distal parts of several fingers, but also and above all when the patient's care pathway includes specific follow-up care and adapted rehabilitation.

Secondary Surgery (Fig. 8.1)

Generalities [11]

In 22% of amputations, secondary surgery is required.

A distinction will be made between surgical procedures for the revision of after-effects and reconstructive techniques.

After-Effects Surgery

These are the usual techniques used in planned orthopedic surgery of the hand. Their goal is to improve functional outcome.

They take place more or less at a distance from the primary surgery.

They depend on certain symptomatic problems and persistent clinical signs that do not or no longer respond to rehabilitation.

Techniques such as tendon transfer, tenolysis, arthrolysis, nerve surgery, arthrodesis, grafting, prosthesis, etc. can be applied surgically.

Reconstructive Surgery [13, 22, 40]

Today's therapeutic tools are much more effective and advanced, thanks to objective analysis of functional and aesthetic results and the advent of reconstructive microsurgery and plastic surgery.

It is important to keep things in perspective, viewing secondary surgery as the possibility of a significant gain in function, comfort, and improvement of the situation.

The therapeutic goal is to improve the function of the hand with a clamp between the thumb and fingers that is thin, stable, sensitive, strong, mobile, and, if possible, aesthetically pleasing.

This type of surgery should be considered soon after the initial trauma, before the mourning process has been completed. Once this period has passed, the risk of increased perceptual disturbance and psychological damage increases considerably.

Interdisciplinary support and collaboration (surgeon, rehabilitator, psychologist) is essential to ensure coherent and optimal care.

Particular care must be taken to discuss the planned techniques with the patient.

Beforehand, the situation must be analyzed in depth, considering the patient's needs and establishing in detail the benefits and disadvantages.

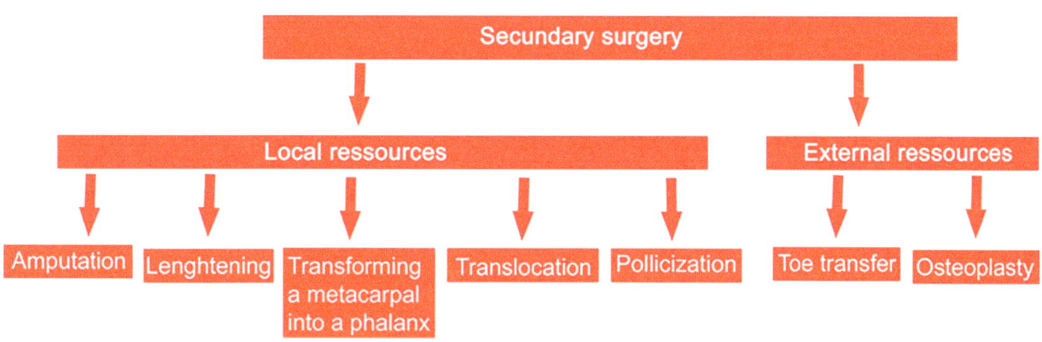

Fig. 8.1 Secondary surgery. (Picture by Amélie-Anne Vienne)

Two categories are distinguished:

- Techniques using local resources: the goal is to reorganize the digital capital and harmonize the structures with the hand's own resources.
- Techniques using resources external to the injured limb.

➔ Techniques Using Local Resources

- *Proximal Amputations* [22, 27, 34]
  Indicated when the amputated finger or even the whole limb is functionally impaired (lack of strength, stiffness) or more often for aesthetic reasons.
  It is unavoidable when the reimplantation fails and can sometimes be associated with a digital translocation: this technique consists of removing the digital stump proximally.
  When the digital segment is removed entirely, it is a digital translocation.
  In the case of translocations, certain consequences need to be considered, such as a reduced range of motion and a significant loss of grip strength, which may hinder a return to professional activity, for example.
  The aesthetic benefits are significant, with the removal of the stump or an unattractive interdigital space.
- *Transforming a Metacarpal into a Phalanx* [23]
  This is the oldest reconstructive technique, described by Hugier in 1874. The goal is to create an intermetacarpal commissure and mobility in the thumb or fifth finger, to create an opposition of a finger and a functional pinch.
  This technique can be used for multi-digital injuries.
- *Matev's Metacarpal Lengthening* [31]
  This method is indicated when the skin coverage is excellent.
  The lengthening of the metacarpal and soft tissues is achieved by an osteotomy and distraction wires, with a gain in length of up to 3 cm.
  Spontaneous consolidation as described by Matev's technique requires a long treatment period (4–5 months).
  Kessler proposes to reduce this period to 1 month by adding a systematic bone grafting and an accelerated lengthening.
  Functional results are reliable and well-recognized.
  Most often used on the first metacarpal, it tends to limit the commissural opening, requiring certain surgical precautions and adequate positioning during treatment.
- *Digital Redistribution or Pollicization* [12, 16]
  This type of procedure is most often applied to the thumb and in cases of complex multi-finger amputation.
  Innervated and vascularized tissues from a healthy or mutilated finger are harvested to reconstruct a damaged finger.
  The benefits are functional gain through thumb lengthening, good healing, and improved sensory quality. These results are proportional to the quality of the harvested tissues.

➔ Techniques Using External Grafts

- *Toe transfer* [15, 28, 43]
  Since the first successful toe transfers 1966, the foot has emerged as an essential tissue resource. Methods have evolved to balance the ratio of functional and aesthetic consequences of the donor foot to those of the recipient hand.
  It imposes certain conditions, such as the operator's mastery of microsurgical techniques, an age limit for the patients (under 45), and exemplary motivation and compliance with rehabilitation.
  The total transfer of the second or third toe is now widely indicated and offers highly satisfactory results, both functionally and aesthetically.
- *Osteoplasty* [2, 20, 22, 32]
  This technique combines the harvesting of a flap and a bone graft to lengthen the amputated finger.
- A great deal of studies has been carried out to limit the observed after-effects:

- At the recipient site: bone resorption, delayed consolidation, sensory and trophic disorders
- At the donor site: aesthetic damage, secondary fractures, pain
- At the general level: several operative steps, prolonged immobilization

In most cases, it is the last resort when toe transfer cannot be done on an elderly subject or on a non-dominant limb.

- *Indications depending on the injured finger* [44] (Fig. 8.2)
  - *Thumb*

    The more proximal the amputation, the more limited the impact on daily participation. Reconstructive techniques are envisaged to lengthen the finger and optimize its action or even replace it.

    Several factors must be considered, such as the tissue condition of the mutilated thumb (trophicity, tissue elasticity), the patient's age, sex, lifestyle, state of health, needs, and the consequences of the technique used on the harvesting site, depending on the method employed.
  - *Injuries of a single finger*

    In the case of amputations through the first phalanx, the sometimes very short stump may be of limited functional interest. Proximal amputation or digital translocation techniques are considered if the patient expresses symptoms (functional discomfort, disabling pain, or significant aesthetic damage) that interfere with the daily use of the limb.

    For amputations through the second phalanx, a toe-transfer reconstruction can provide perfectly satisfactory functional results when the patient is young and according to certain criteria.
  - *Complex injuries involving amputations of several fingers or even both hands*

    The priority is to restore a functional and efficient pinch function.

    The technique(s) employed depend on the integrity of the thumb and the quality of the remaining tissue. Surgery can be performed in several stages.

Treatment and Rehabilitation

The follow-up care and rehabilitation depend on the severity of the amputation, its location, and the surgery realized.

As we have seen, complications and aftereffects are frequent.

After surgery, rehabilitation can be carried out in a multi-professional or specialized center (hand SOS, hand clinic, functional rehabilitation center) or in private practice, depending on the

Concerned finger	Injury site	Major impact	Indicated technique
Thumb	Proximal to the interphalangeal joint	Prehension Pinch Functional ++	Lenghtening Pollicization Osteoplasty Toe transfert
Finger	Through the second phalanx	Sensory Aesthetic	Toe transfert
	Through the first phalanx	Functional Aesthetic Stifness Pain	Proximal amputation Digital translocation Aesthetic protheses
Several fingers	All techniques = priority to the thumb and functional pinch Phalangization Myoelectric prostheses Aesthetic prostheses		

Fig. 8.2 Summary of indications according to the affected finger(s). (Picture by Amélie-Anne Vienne)

availability of care, the medical indications, and the patient's choice.

Communication between therapists is essential to coordinate practices and ensure a real coherence in the patient's care.

The primary goal is to restore limb function.

Therapists must consider the patient's profile and needs to reestablish an effective level of occupation (Fig. 8.3).

Rehabilitation is indicated in three phases:

- Primary care: short term, following initial surgery (regularization or reimplantation), with several degrees of precociousness, to prevent after-effects.
- Secondary care: medium term, to maintain and restore mobility to affected areas. It can also prepare a secondary surgery.
- Palliative management of after-effects and stiffness: in the medium to long term, this involves treating the after-effects of the injured limb.

Rehabilitation goals and methods concern the prevention and treatment of trophic status, stiffness and mobility, prehension, segmental exclusion, sensory disorders and phantom pain, the patient's psychological state and quality of life, and planning or making the limb's device.

Trophicity

Trophic assessment is an important part of any amputation procedure. Special precautions must be taken during rehabilitation and after-care.

Vascularization

The vascular survival of the reimplanted and amputated segment is a priority.

Nursing care must be regular and attentive to the skin's condition.

The dressing must be light, so as not to disturb the mobility of the wrist, healthy fingers, and injured finger. The smallest possible dressing rule should be applied (Fig. 8.4).

If the patient is a smoker, preventive information on the vascular consequences of smoking should be provided, and the patient may be referred to specific support (associations, prevention networks).

During treatment, the rehabilitator must monitor and report in the clinical assessment the pres-

	Third phalanx		Second phalanx		Proximal finger	
Indicator	Risk	Prevention	Risk	Prevention	Risk	Prevention
Motricity	Stiffness in the distal interphalangeal joint or even in the proximal interphalangeal joint, deformation of the finger(s), swan-neck, flessum, mallet finger	Maintain mobility while respecting the healing process	Stiffness of the proximal interphalangeal joint, flessum of the metacarpophalangeal and proximal interphalangeal joints, boutonnière deformity, swan-neck	Maintain mobility while respecting the healing process	Stiffness of the metacarpophalangeal joint, disruption of hand architecture	Maintain mobility while respecting the healing process
Prehension	Reorganization of the grips between the thumb and the fingers	Stimulation of the grips	Complete reorganization of the grips between the thumb and the fingers	Stimulation of the grips	Finger not functional for prehension, possible opposition of the fifth finger	Reorganization of the prehension
Exclusion	Stiffness of the finger(s), body mapping disorder	Integration of the finger(s), graded motor imagery	Stiffness of the finger(s), body mapping disorder	Integration of the finger(s), graded motor imagery	Exclusion of the injured finger	Integration of the finger(s), graded motor imagery
Sensitivity	Pain at the tip of the stump, nail disorders, sensory disorders	Sensory rehabilitation and orthoses (function and discharge), dermatological care to the nail	Pain at the tip of the stump, sensory disorders	Sensory rehabilitation and orthoses (function and discharge)	Pain at the tip of the stump, functional discomfort with the adjacent fingers (friction)	Sensory rehabilitation and orthoses (function and discharge)

Fig. 8.3 Functional consequences depending on the finger and the level of the amputation. (Picture by Amélie-Anne Vienne)

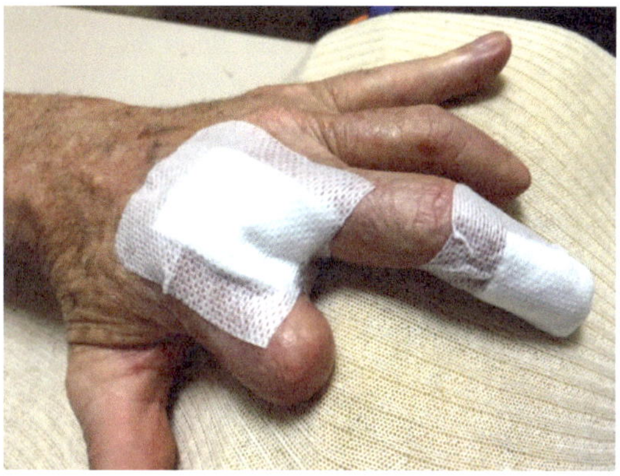

Fig. 8.4 Simple dressing on a hand. (Picture by Amélie-Anne Vienne)

ence of objective vasomotor signs (difference in coloring, difference in temperature, etc.).

Scar

The rehabilitator is vigilant to the evolution of the scar throughout the cicatricial maturation period (18 months).

To optimize healing, standard silicone tubes and silicone-coated dressings or interfaces can be suggested (Figs. 8.5, 8.6, and 8.7).

Silicone tips and dressings may be used during the day, but must comply with two requirements:

- Their length must allow the full mobility of the finger.
- The inhibition of the finger's pulp must not impair its function.

Devices for mobilization and cicatricial compression can be proposed to the patients (Figs. 8.8 and 8.9).

Phaneras

When the nail is preserved, the possibility of inguinal complications must be considered. A brittle, irregular, and fragile nail has a long and uncertain evolution. This has an impact on many daily activities, such as dressing up, personal care, intimacy, etc.

The repercussions on function are major, and this type of injury is essential to treat. Dermatological referral may be indicated (Fig. 8.10).

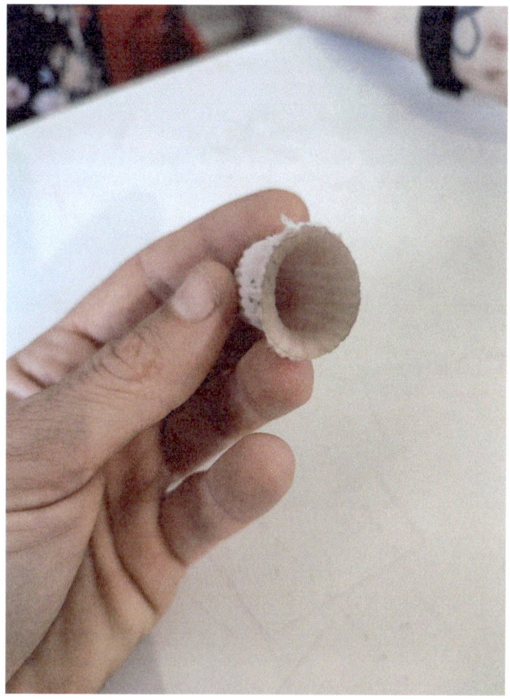

Fig. 8.5 Commercial silicone fingertip. (Picture by Amélie-Anne Vienne)

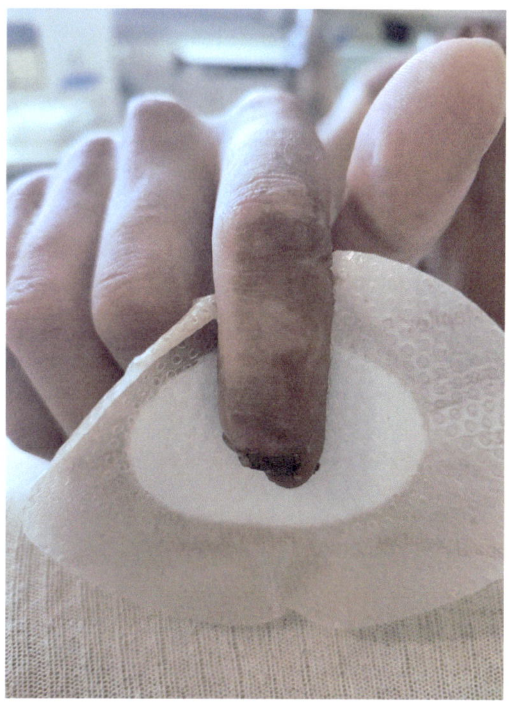

Fig. 8.6 Silicone dressing. (Picture by Amélie-Anne Vienne)

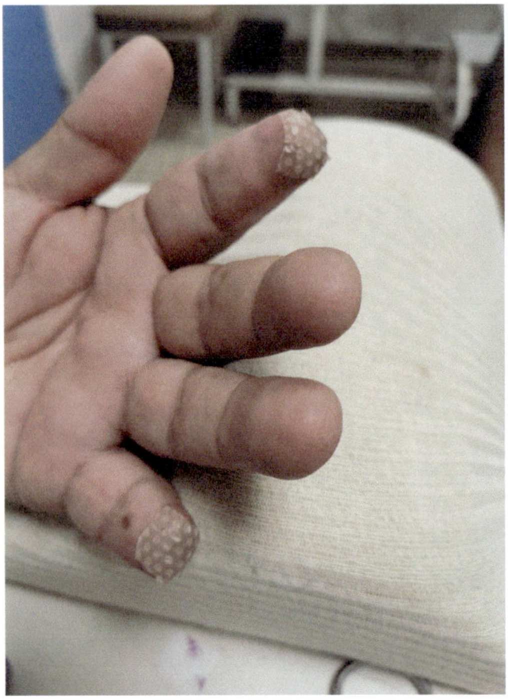

Fig. 8.7 Silicone interface. (Picture by Amélie-Anne Vienne)

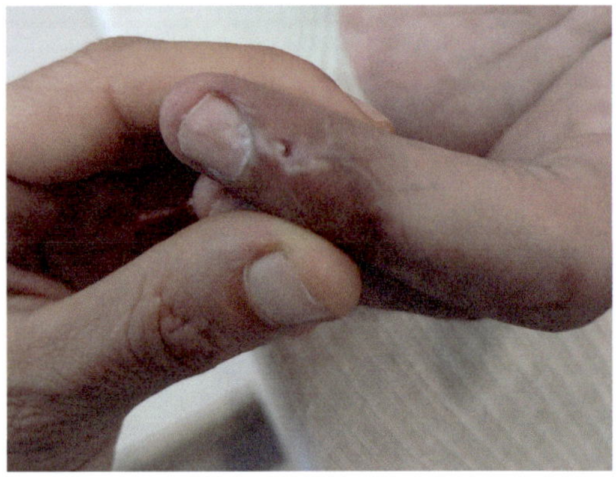

Fig. 8.8 Bud on scar after 9 months of evolution. (Picture by Amélie-Anne Vienne)

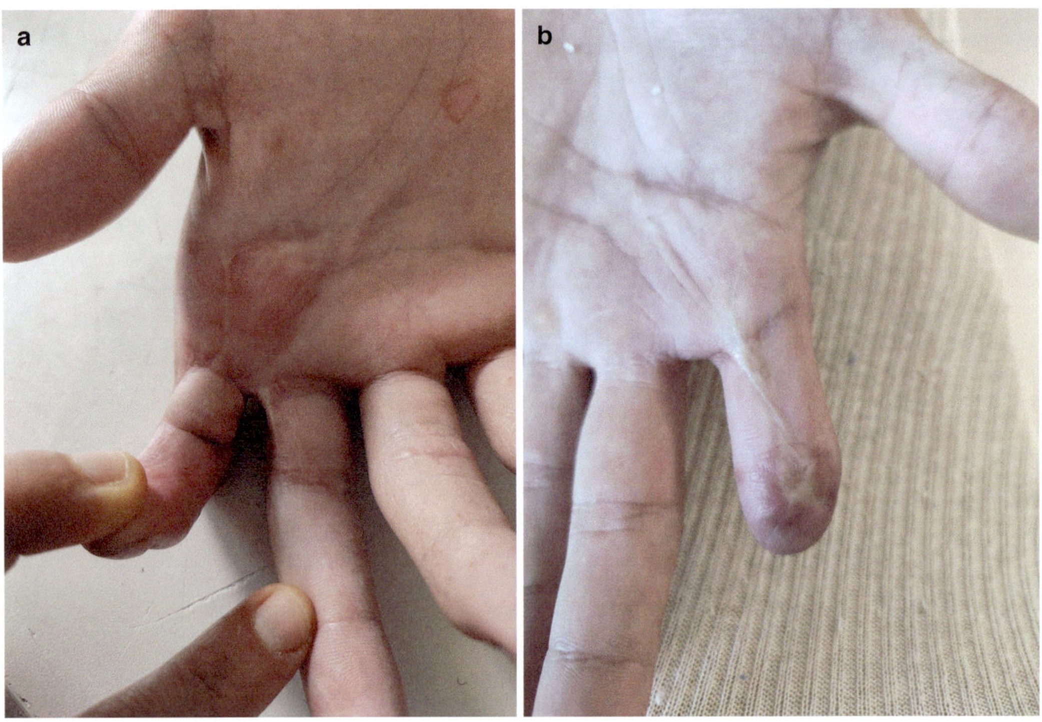

Fig. 8.9 Interdigital hypertrophic linear cords on an injury after 6 months. (Picture by Amélie-Anne Vienne)

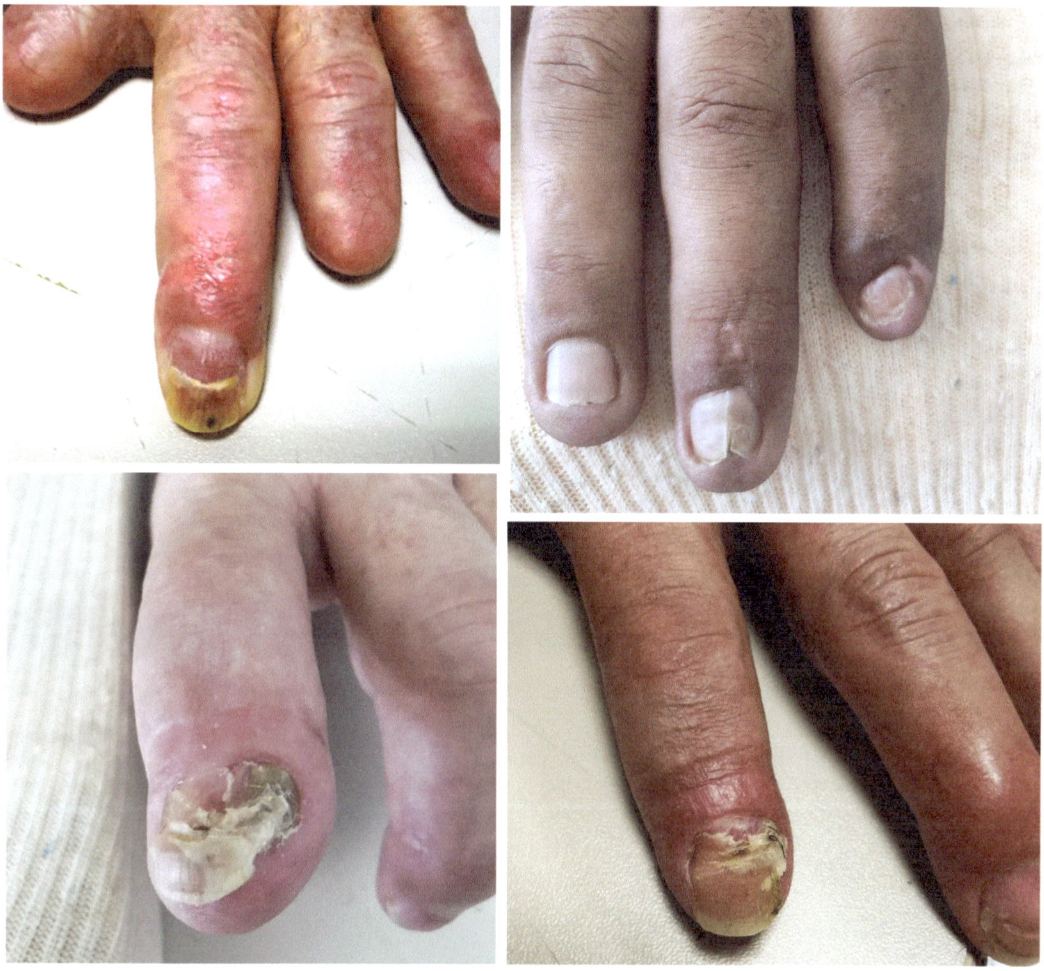

Fig. 8.10 Skin appendages alterations in distal finger amputations and reimplantations. (Picture by Amélie-Anne Vienne)

As with scarring complications, the rehabilitator can suggest custom-made orthoses to protect the concerned area, or siliconized materials, which can primarily help preserve the use of the finger (Figs. 8.11, 8.12, and 8.13).

Covering the Stump

The rehabilitator may observe a bony protrusion at the end of the stump. Cutaneous tension and the predominance of an irregular tip may indicate a lack of overlap (Fig. 8.14).

A further radiological assessment may reveal a bony displacement or the failure of the graft, for example.

The rehabilitator may suggest an orthotic protection or a tip to protect the fingertip and preserve the cutaneous integrity. Surgical advice may also be indicated.

Stiffness

Stiffness is a common complication of traumatic injuries of the hand and can have a variety of ori-

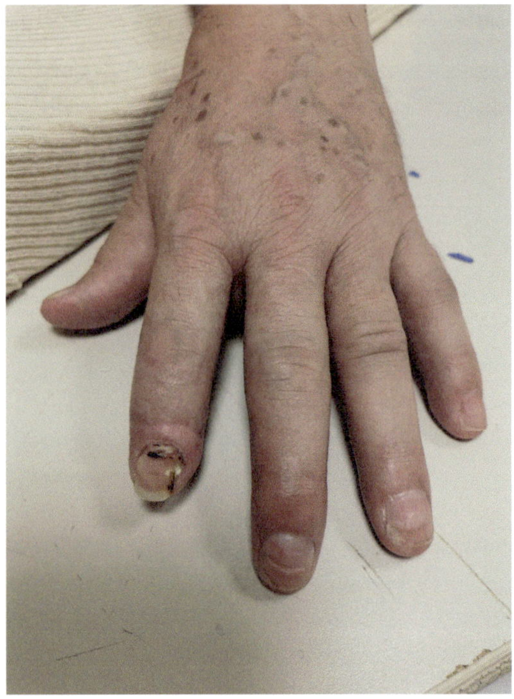

Fig. 8.12 State of the nail. (Picture by Amélie-Anne Vienne)

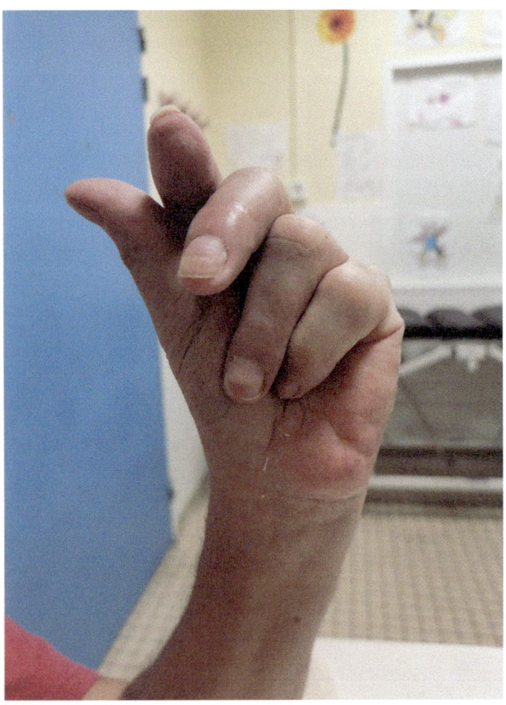

Fig. 8.11 Exclusion in extension of the index due to discomfort and pain. (Picture by Amélie-Anne Vienne)

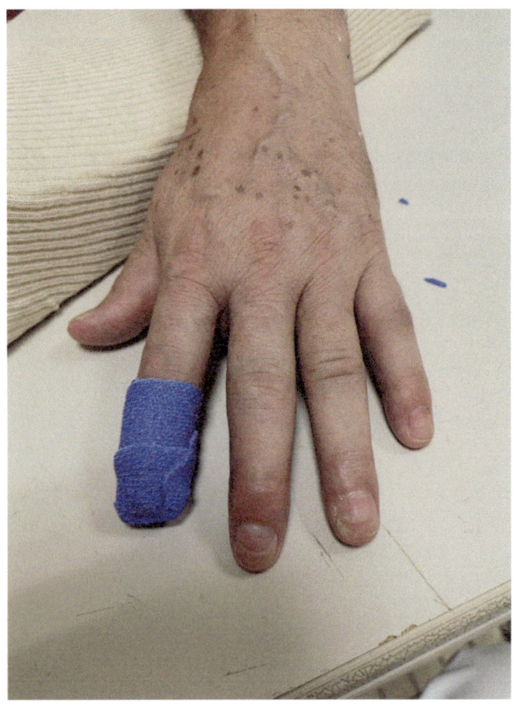

Fig. 8.13 Inguinal protection with thermo-woven fingertip orthosis. (Picture by Amélie-Anne Vienne)

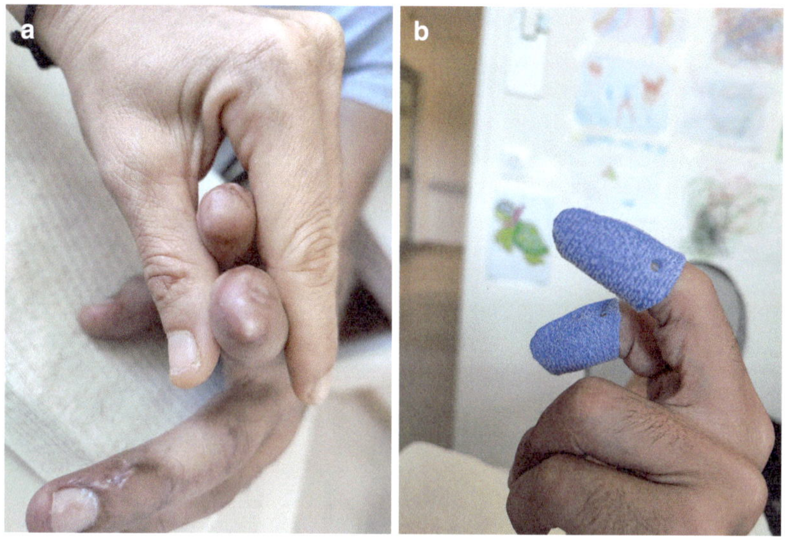

Fig. 8.14 Stump tip of the second phalanx of the third finger (**a**). Protection with a discharge tip (**b**). (Picture by Amélie-Anne Vienne)

gins, which need to be determined during a detailed clinical assessment.

The principles of rehabilitation are identical to those for complex traumatic injuries to the hand.

From the beginning, the goal is to fight against edema, ensure correct positioning of the structures, and promote the mobility of the healthy or injured segments while respecting the indications and limits imposed by the time required for recovery and consolidation of the bone, nerve, vascular and tissue structures, etc.

The literature indicates that rehabilitation is rarely indicated in the case of regularization.

However, stiffness is a frequent complication, and early rehabilitation is essential to prevent the consequences of a prolonged immobilization.

The goal is to maintain the mobility of the structures and avoid the consequences of a prolonged immobilization.

The more proximal the amputation, the greater the risk of stiffness.

Stiffness is more frequent with proximal injuries, for several reasons:

- The segments are small, and this disturbs the synergic balance of the finger's flexion at the bone level.
- The proximal interphalangeal joint is a joint that rapidly and durably stiffens.
- The damage to systems (tissue, fibrous, capsuloligamentous, etc.) essential to the biomechanical balance of the finger.

Stiffness will be assessed and managed using appropriate techniques, depending on its origin(s) (Figs. 8.15, 8.16, and 8.17).

Prehension

By observing the patient's gestures, the rehabilitator must identify the functional impact of the

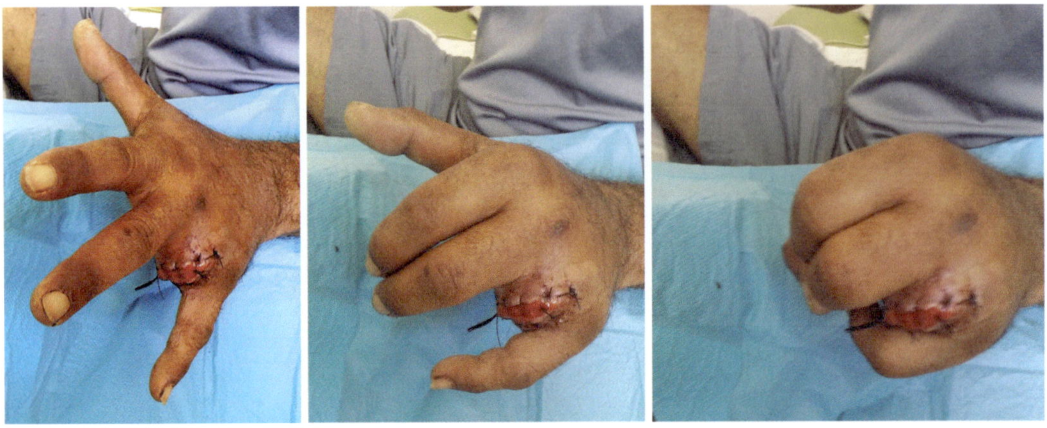

Fig. 8.15 Immediate postoperative surgery after a regularization amputation of the fourth finger. (Picture by Amélie-Anne Vienne)

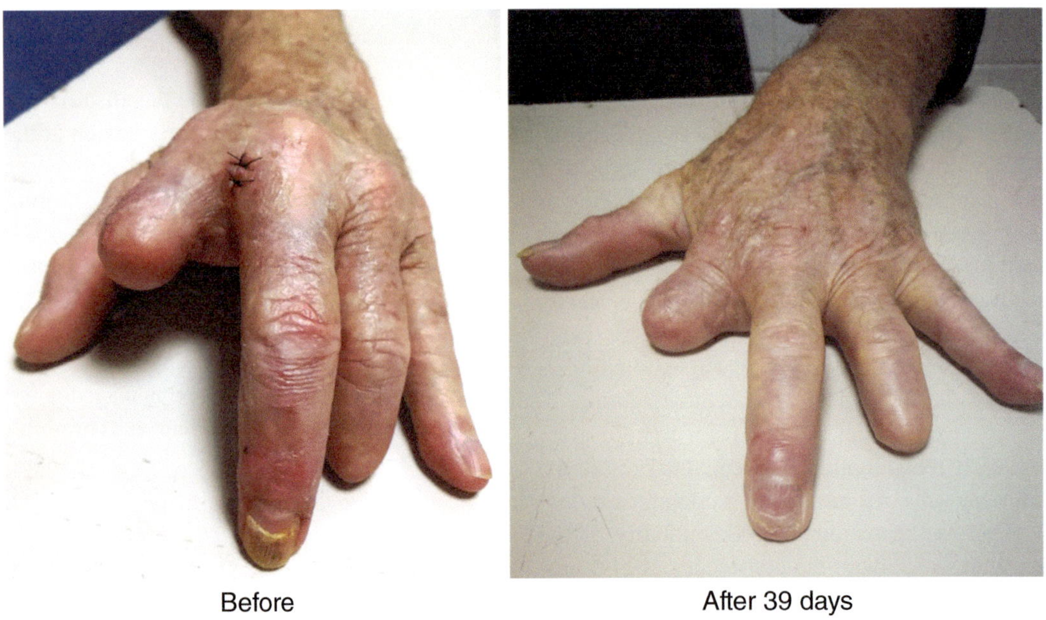

Fig. 8.16 Recovery of full hand extension in 39 days with rehabilitation and mobilization devices for flexion and extension. (Picture by Amélie-Anne Vienne)

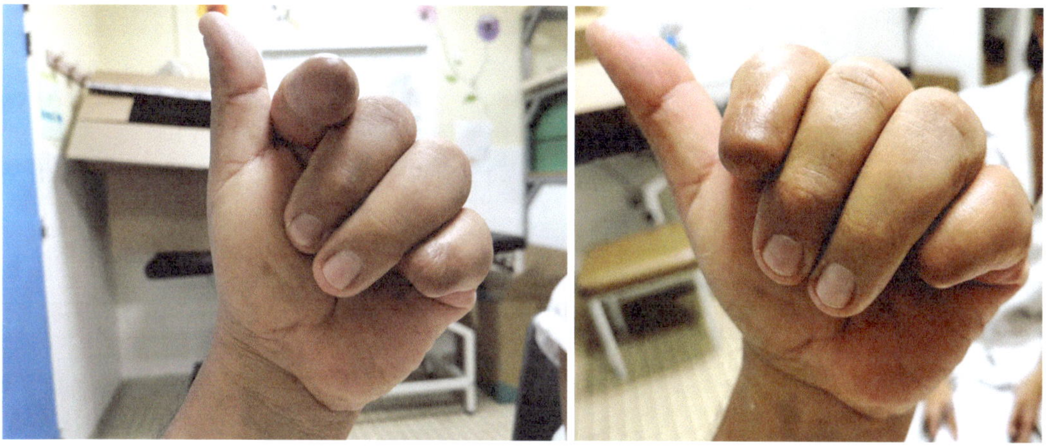

After 14 days

Fig. 8.17 Recovery of flexion in 14 days with rehabilitation and mobilization devices for the flexion of the proximal interphalangeal joints of the second and fifth fingers. (Picture by Amélie-Anne Vienne)

injury and anticipate strategies for compensating and reorganizing the prehension.

Fine Pinching

A shortened thumb or a lesion of the second and third fingers implies the limitation or prevention of bi- and tri-digital fine pinching.

In most cases, the patient will avoid the contact between the thumb's pulp and the first two fingers' pulps.

Two situations must be differentiated:

- In the case of a loss of thumb length, the patient will compensate with a safe and effective pinch, most often using the key pinch. In this case, the rehabilitator focuses on strengthening the thumb's pronator muscles, including the first dorsal interosseous muscle, to maintain the muscular balance (Fig. 8.18).
- The patient avoids contact with the tip of a finger: pinching is possible but not performed. This may be because of pain, stiffness, or segmental exclusion, which needs to be defined and treated accordingly (Figs. 8.19, 8.20, 8.21, and 8.22). The assessment can be done using specific fine dexterity tools such as the Nine-Hole Peg Test 1985 for qualitative measurement, and the Key Pinch dynamometer for quantitative measurement.

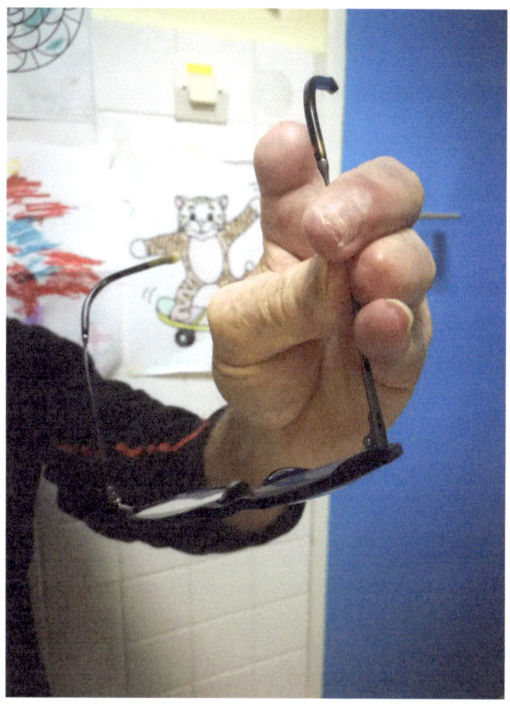

Fig. 8.18 Fine pinch compensated by the third and fourth fingers because of the lack of length in the index. (Picture by Amélie-Anne Vienne)

Rehabilitation exercises for fine prehension are varied, and the rehabilitator must encourage the use of objects related to the patient's daily activities.

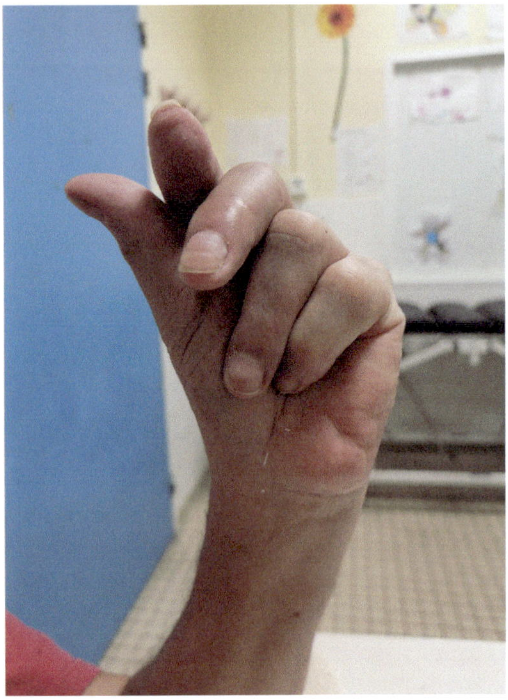

Fig. 8.19 Disorganization of the prehension because of stiffness and exclusion of the index. (Picture by Amélie-Anne Vienne)

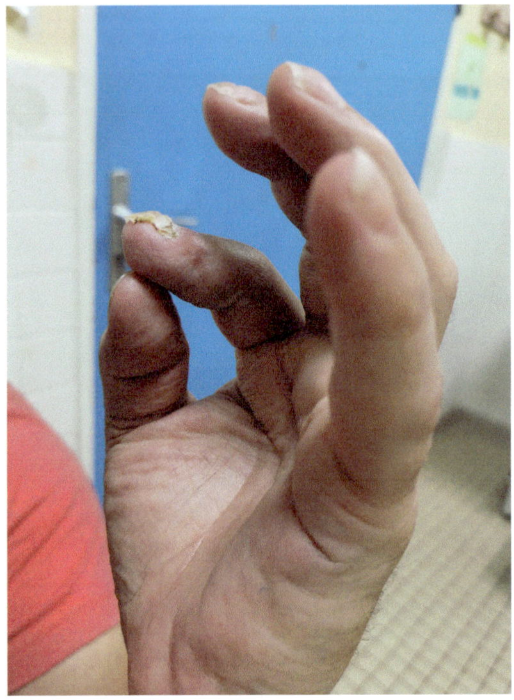

Fig. 8.21 Stimulation of the opposition between the pulps of the thumb and the index. (Picture by Amélie-Anne Vienne)

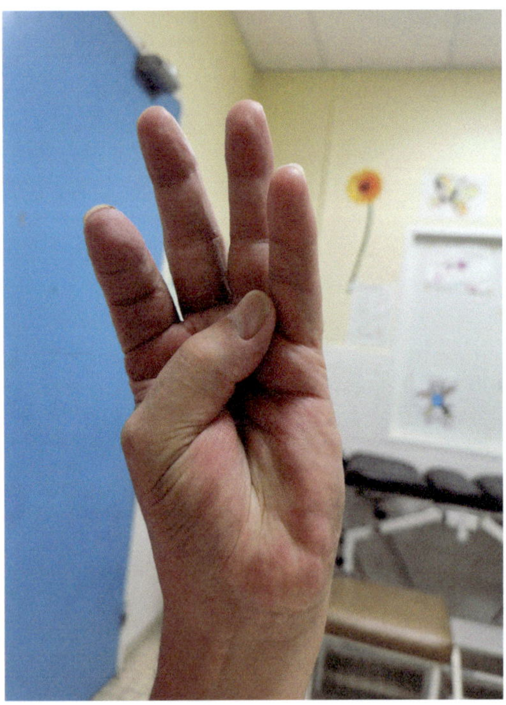

Fig. 8.20 Opposition with no opening of the commissure. (Picture by Amélie-Anne Vienne)

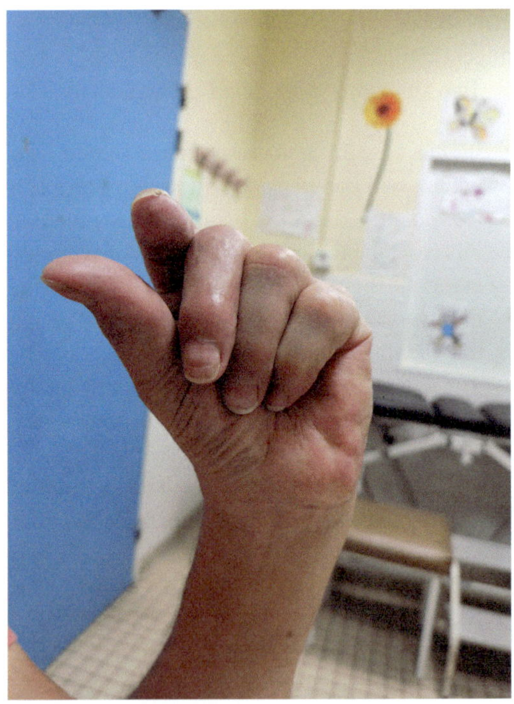

Fig. 8.22 Improvement of winding after 20 days of rehabilitation and orthoses. (Picture by Amélie-Anne Vienne)

Force Grips

Gesture reorganization may also concern the force grips. As with fine pinching, stiffness is the main cause of reorganization.

In Chase amputations, a lack of strength persists over time, due to the removal of a finger and (part of) its metacarpal and its muscular and architectural consequences (Figs. 8.23, 8.24, and 8.25).

Strength is assessed by dynamometric quantitative measurements (Grasp Test Jamar, digital strength measurement tools) and qualitative measurements of the grip on common objects.

Rehabilitation aims to highlight compensations and reestablish a safe, functional grip.

Segment Exclusion

The disruption of the cortical pattern is very common, due to the lack of one or more fingers, prolonged immobilization, stiffness, or pain.

Early mobilizations with active exercises and preventive motor imagery prevent the onset of segmental exclusion (Figs. 8.26, 8.27, 8.28, 8.29, and 8.30).

When it is persistent, the rehabilitator will undertake a step-by-step motor imagery and proprioceptive rehabilitation.

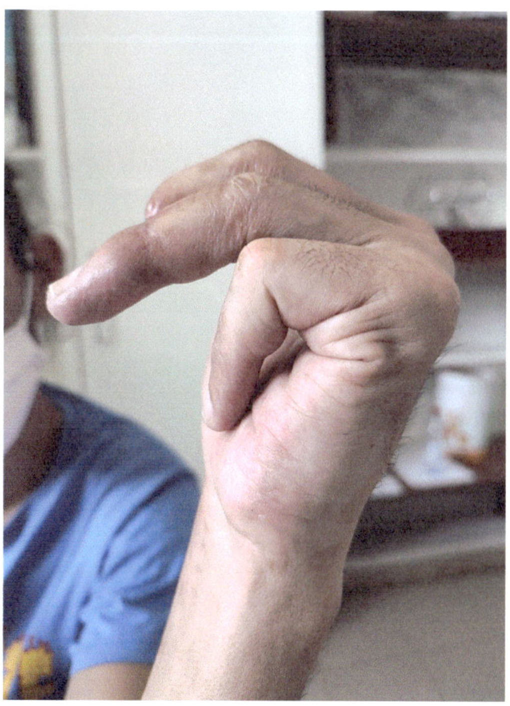

Fig. 8.23 Loss of mobility in flexion of the proximal interphalangeal joint of the third and fourth fingers, making the strength grips impossible. (Picture by Amélie-Anne Vienne)

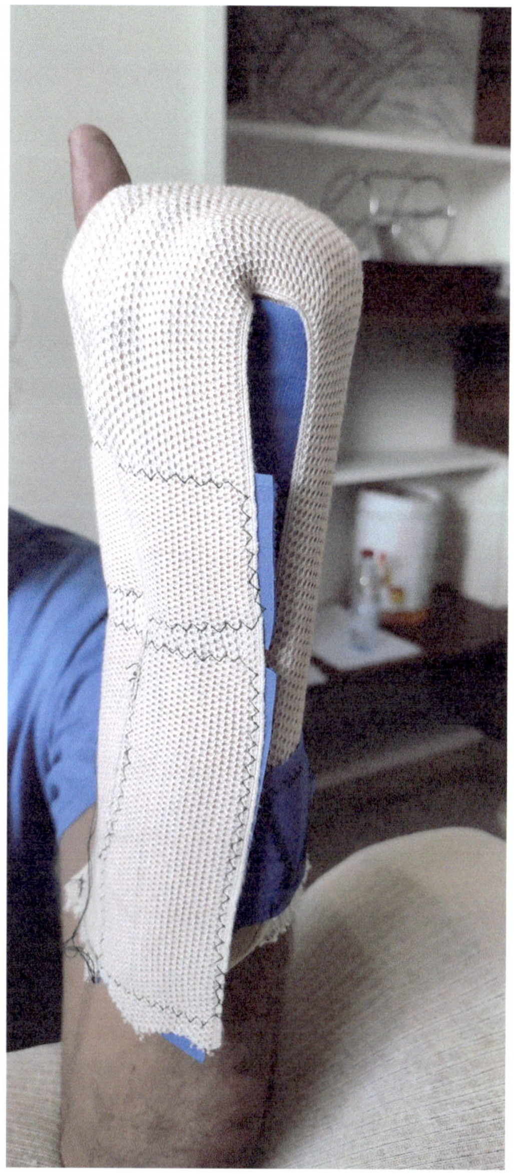

Fig. 8.24 Device for dynamic mobilization in flexion of the metacarpophalangeal and proximal interphalangeal joints (three times a day, 15 min maximum). (Picture by Amélie-Anne Vienne)

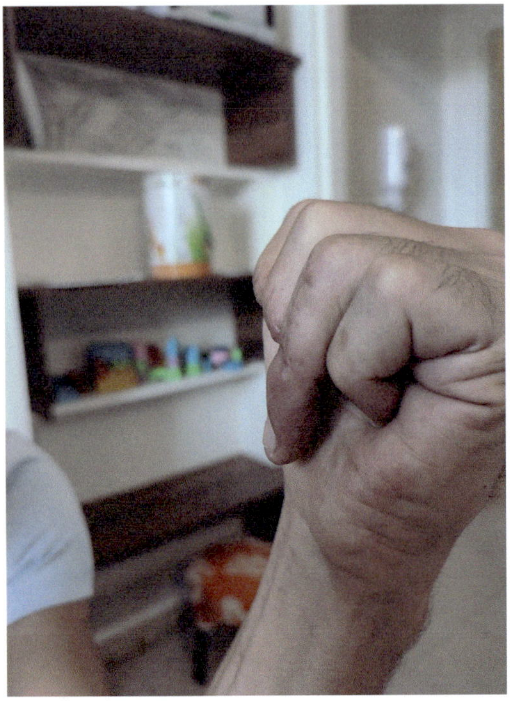

Fig. 8.25 Improvement of winding at D49 with rehabilitation, mobilization devices, and devices for the fingertip. (Picture by Amélie-Anne Vienne)

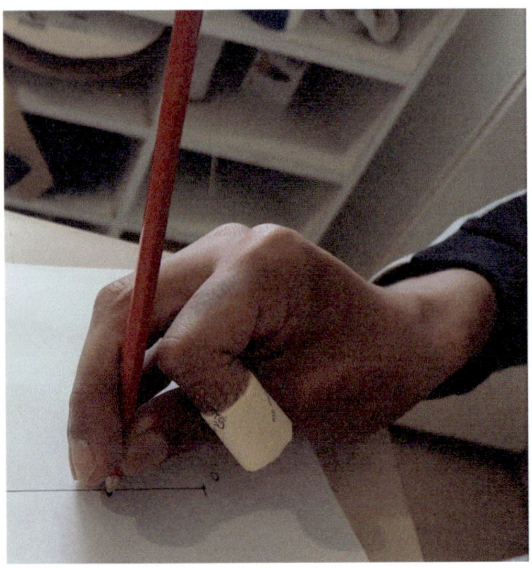

Fig. 8.26 Segmentary exclusion of the index. (Picture by Amélie-Anne Vienne)

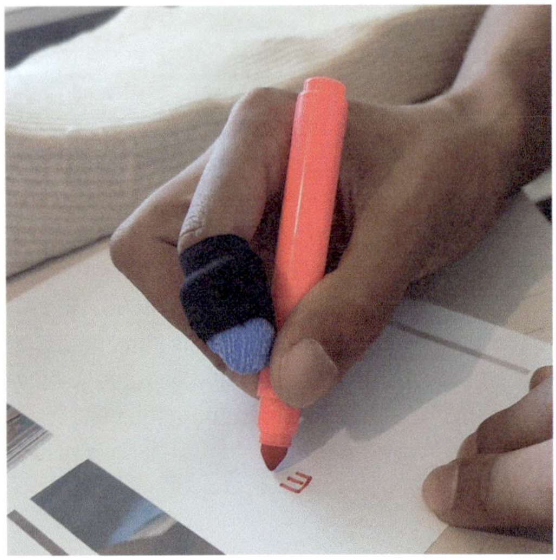

Fig. 8.27 Immediate motor inclusion with a protection cap and rehabilitation. (Picture by Amélie-Anne Vienne)

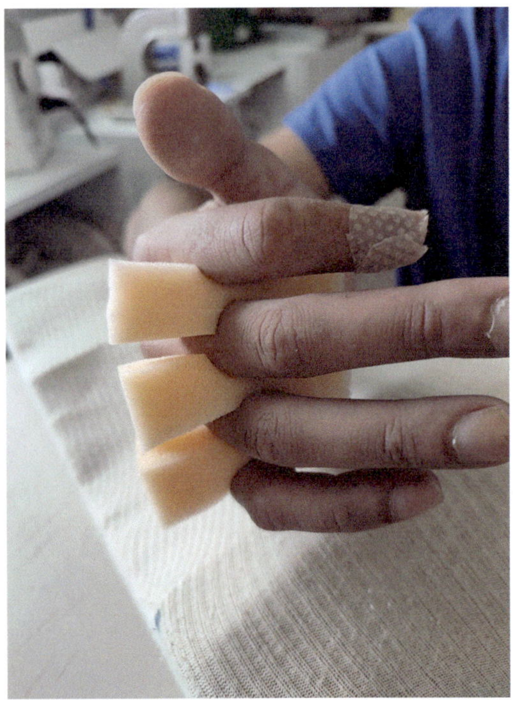

Fig. 8.28 Self-rehabilitation tools: Taylor Wedges. (Picture by Amélie-Anne Vienne)

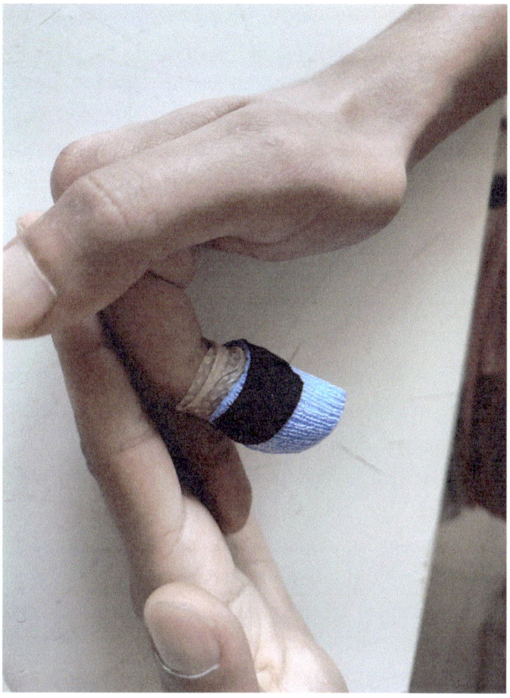

Fig. 8.29 Self-rehabilitation for the active extension of the proximal interphalangeal joint with tip. (Picture by Amélie-Anne Vienne)

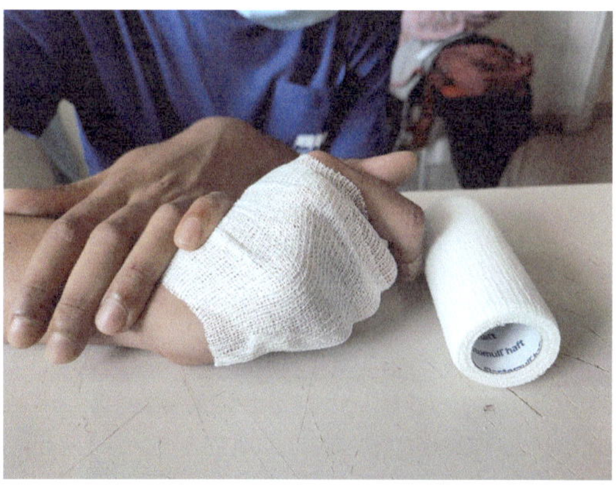

Fig. 8.30 "Constraint therapy" exercise. Inhibition of adjacent fingers and stimulation of the index finger extension (combined with motor imagery using laterality recognition and explicit internal and external motor imagery). (Picture by Amélie-Anne Vienne)

As with prehension rehabilitation, the mental images and exercises used should be as close as possible to the patient's usual daily gestures (tools, daily activities, driving, etc.).

Sensory Disorder and Phantom Limb

An amputation inevitably involves nerve damage to the sensory branches of the concerned limb.

Sensory disturbances and stump pain are frequent and disabling.

The patients may express pain, discomfort, abnormal sensations, etc.

During the assessment, the therapist must identify pain due to an excessive nociception, sensory disorders, and the expression of the phantom limb.

Sensory Disorders

The sensory clinical assessment allows the functional signs to be objectified and the type(s) of sensory disorders described by the patient to be determined.

These symptoms are present in the area proximal to the injury and are more or less extensive.

They may be painless, such as paresthesia, hypoesthesia, or anesthesia, or painful, such as dysesthesia, allodynia, or hyperalgesia.

The therapist then establishes the conclusions of the qualitative and quantitative sensory assessment and applies the appropriate rehabilitation techniques.

Phantom Limb [3, 8, 25, 38, 39]

The phantom limb is a sign found in 80% of upper limb amputations.

However, it is not specific to these injuries and can be found following peripheral or central nerve injuries.

Symptoms tend to decrease over time but are long-lasting in 30% of amputees.

Phantom limb is expressed by sensations or pain in the part of the limb that is amputated, which is distant from the injury and therefore no longer physically present.

Cortical reorganization is one of the most frequently cited reasons for this phenomenon.

The mechanism involves a reduction of the area of the somato-sensory cortex corresponding to the amputated part, while adjacent areas expand until they take over the place of the affected part.

The neurons are still present and now respond to stimuli from neighboring areas (Fig. 8.31): the hand area lies between the area of the face and the area of the forearm. When the hand is amputated, a stimulation of the upper face or forearm can, for example, create the perception of the absent limb.

There are two forms of phantom limb expression:

➔ Phantom Sensations

These are non-painful symptoms experienced in the missing limb, in the form of strange sensations and/or paresthesia.

The patient describes strange sensations such as itching, movement, position in space, volume and shape, contact, and temperature.

The patient describes paresthesia such as tingling, electricity, needles, and tingling.

These functional signs tend to decrease with activity and over time.

Their impact on occupation and daily life is reported to be low.

➔ Phantom Pain [6, 42]

The patient describes pain in the amputated part.

He may express:

- Nociceptive pain: it is often identical to the one perceived at the time of or just after the trauma. 50% of these signs appear during the first postoperative week and are proportional to the preoperative pain.
- Dysesthesia such as burning, electric shocks, and painful cold.
- Paralysis or cramps of the amputated limb.

Phantom pain can appear up to a year and a half after amputation and is largely favored by the presence of a persistent stump pain.

Palliative drug treatments are limited and unsatisfactory in the long term. However, as the direct link between post-traumatic pain and phantom pain has been established, preventive analgesia is considered and recommended.

The therapist can use the following techniques [26, 30, 41]:

- Electrotherapy: use of TENS with medullary or cortical stimulation to desensitize and help manage the pain.
- Physical activity: helps to relax the muscles and reduce the symptoms during activity.
- Massage: optimizes muscle relaxation and helps to manage the edema.
- Application of heat: activates the blood flow and reduces symptoms.
- Visual afference therapy: mirror therapy and virtual reality therapy have helped some people to manage pain more effectively.
- Alternative therapies such as acupuncture, hypnosis and hypno-analgesia, and magnetotherapy are sometimes mentioned in the treatment of these disorders.
- Orthotic devices: off-loading and functional and fingertip protection orthoses to limit the fingertip pain and stimulate nearby cortical areas.
- Prosthetic devices: functional or social prostheses to reduce and prevent phantom pain.

Psychological Impact and Grief

When an amputation trauma occurs, mourning is an unavoidable psychological process for the patient.

Three main stages make up normal mourning:

- The shock phase: often short, the patient is stunned by the trauma, the information is too brutal, and he/she may express denial or even anger.

- The reactionary depression phase. The patient becomes aware of the trauma and may experience symptoms such as sadness, guilt, feelings of mutilation, loss of desire and motivation, and social isolation.
- The termination phase: acceptance of the situation. It is then possible to rebuild one's life and more actively consider social, professional, and sporting rehabilitation.

The normal course of grief is around 6 months.

Abnormal Grief

Abnormal grief can be pathological or complicated [19, 35]:

- Pathological grief: the grief process triggers a psychiatric illness. The signs are major, and the diagnosis is made by competent medical staff.
- Complicated grief: the person is unable to reach the end of his/her grief. This type of complication is identified in 39% of upper limb amputations (according to the study by Pomares Coudane).

Risk factors are [37]:

- The absence of any attempt at reimplantation.
- The level of the amputation: isolated thumb amputations, multi-digital amputations, and macro-amputations.
- The traumatic circumstances of the accident: assault victims, road accidents with concomitant death, work accidents in an already dysfunctional context, etc.

The Rehabilitator and Grief

Throughout the process, the rehabilitator observes changes in the patient's mood and listens to his/her symptoms and needs.

The therapist may identify certain signs that indicate the risk of complicated grief or a need for specific support, such as:

- The risk of delayed mourning: the therapist observes a significant gap between the extent of the trauma and the patient's reaction. The patient is doing very well, even too well, despite a major injury. The patient is unaware of the injury since it occurred. He/she ignores reality and expresses plans that are not consistent with the therapeutic indications.
- The risk of inhibited mourning: a gap may be perceived between the clinical signs objectivized during the assessment and the symptoms. The symptoms are generalized, diffuse, and expressed as very important, whereas the objective clinical signs collected by the therapist do not allow them to be objectified. The patient shows no feelings and focuses only on the somatic.
- The risk of chronic grief: the most frequently found in cases of amputation. The therapist will observe a state of depression that lasts over time (more than 6 months). The patient is unable to move forward with his/her plans and cannot envisage his/her readaptation. There is a deep sense of mutilation, and aesthetic discomfort is felt to be long-lasting. This makes it impossible to return to professional, sporting, or social activities.
- The risk of transfer of skills: patients may confide in their physiotherapist about their feelings, interpreting rehabilitation as a privileged place of expression. They may seek to be listened to by their rehabilitator, who may go beyond their skills. His/her attitude and needs can interfere with and compromise the rehabilitation.

In all cases, the role of the rehabilitator is to invite the patient to seek psychological support or even to refer him/her to the local team to pursue his/her approach and refocus the objectives of the treatment.

Devices

There are two types of devices: small devices (orthoses) and large devices (prostheses).

Orthoses

The indications for orthotic devices are:

- Consolidation and healing of structures, with joint immobilization orthoses

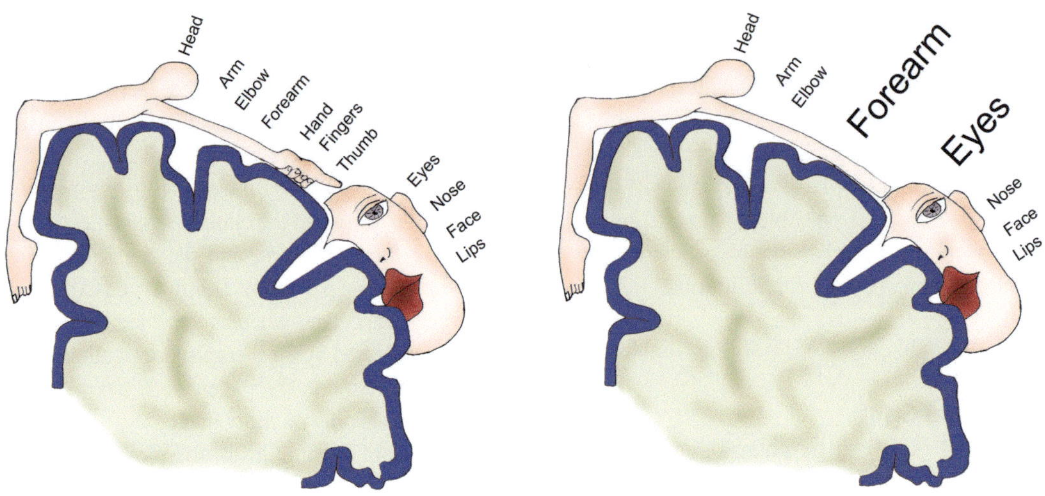

Fig. 8.31 Diagram of a healthy somato-sensory cortex VS a damaged somato-sensory cortex reproduced from Benjamin Cummings' illustration of the homunculus. (Picture by Amélie-Anne Vienne)

- Recovery of mobility, with mobilization and dynamic orthoses
- Function and protection, with discharge and fingertip orthoses

➔ Functional and Protective Orthoses

The main goal is to make the finger functional and enable the injured finger to be included in the prehension process.

These devices have one or more of the following roles:

- To relieve a painful contact zone
- To protect the skin and the stump scar for certain activities
- To alleviate inguinal disorders
- To reassure the patient in his/her daily professional and sporting activities

➔ Stump-Tip Orthoses

These are small devices ideally made from lightweight thermo-woven materials. More rigid or plastic materials should be avoided because of the sound they can produce when contacting with objects.

Principles:

- The mobility of the finger joints must be free and comfortable.
- The convergence of the fingers must be respected when winding them.

These orthoses can be simple or benefit from the addition of an off-loading device for one area of the finger.

They are used daily for certain activities. The tips are secured with a non-compressive adhesive strip.

A trial period with a prototype lasting a week or two may be recommended. The patient can then suggest adjustments, and the therapist can make several spare models or adapt the orthoses as required (Figs. 8.32, 8.33, 8.34, and 8.35).

Discharge can be made with an elastomer paste. Molding is done on the finger with the discharge cut out. Thermoformable textile material is molded on top, creating a vacuum in the area of painful contact (Figs. 8.36, 8.37, 8.38, 8.39, 8.40, 8.41, and 8.42).

➔ Functional Orthoses

Tailor-made devices can also be made to protect small stumps during daily activities (Fig. 8.43).

Prostheses [24] (Fig. 8.44)

Prosthetic devices are part of the amputee's therapeutic tools and are almost systematically used on the lower limb, but are less common on the upper limb.

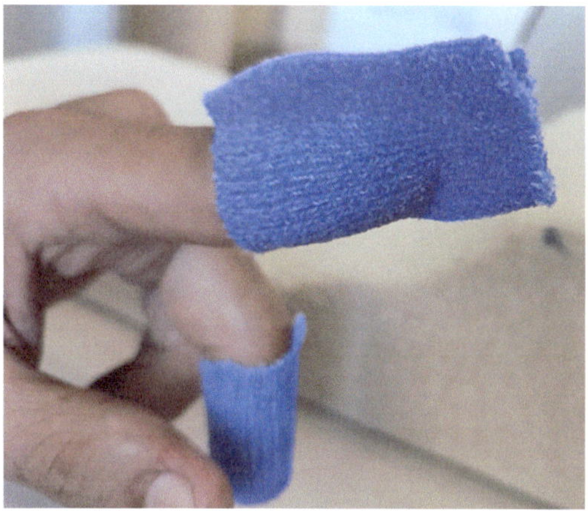

Fig. 8.32 Molding of a textile thermoformable tip. (Picture by Amélie-Anne Vienne)

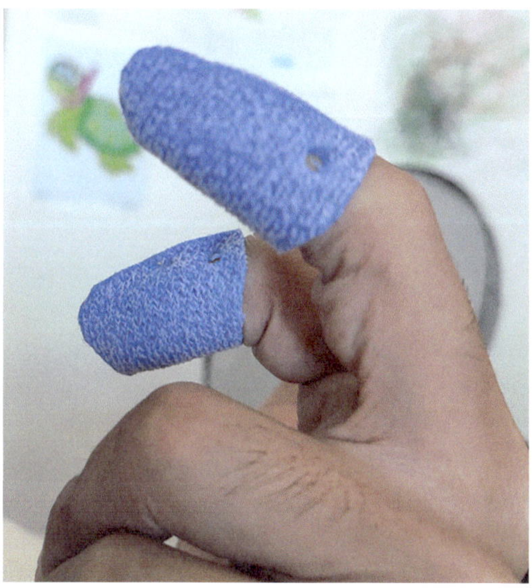

Fig. 8.33 Verification of the fingers' mobility with the tip. (Picture by Amélie-Anne Vienne)

Developments in technology and techniques now make it possible to offer more effective systems that can be adapted to the specific needs of amputee patients.

This is often a multidisciplinary project in line with the patient's needs.

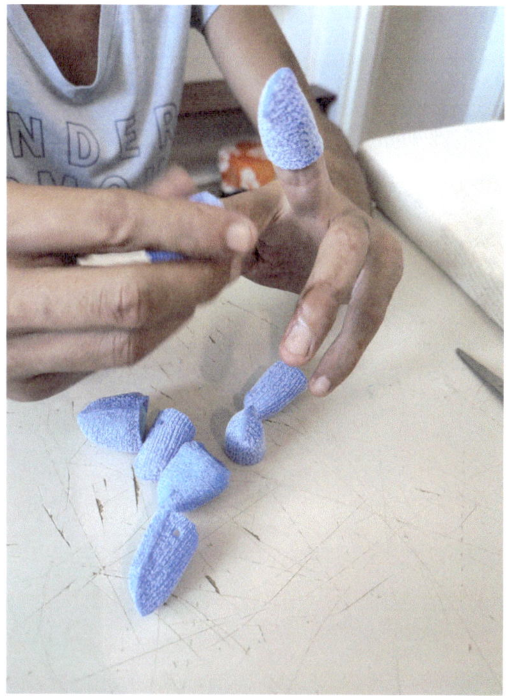

Fig. 8.34 The patient sets the tips. (Picture by Amélie-Anne Vienne)

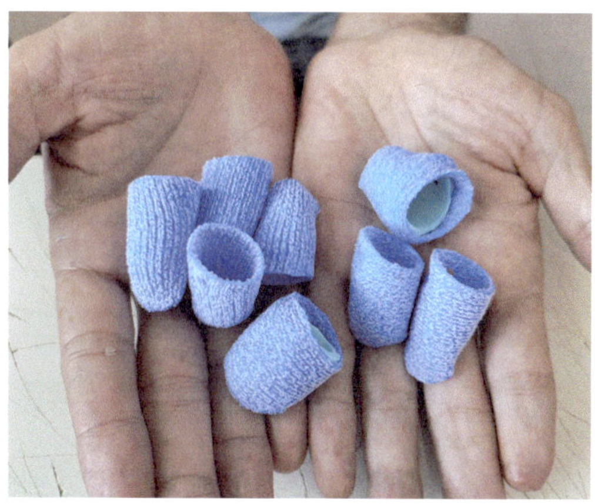

Fig. 8.35 Tailor-made supply of tips with discharge for sports and without discharge for everyday use. (Picture by Amélie-Anne Vienne)

A rigorous preparation is essential to propose the most appropriate system(s) for the situation.

There are three different prosthetic systems.

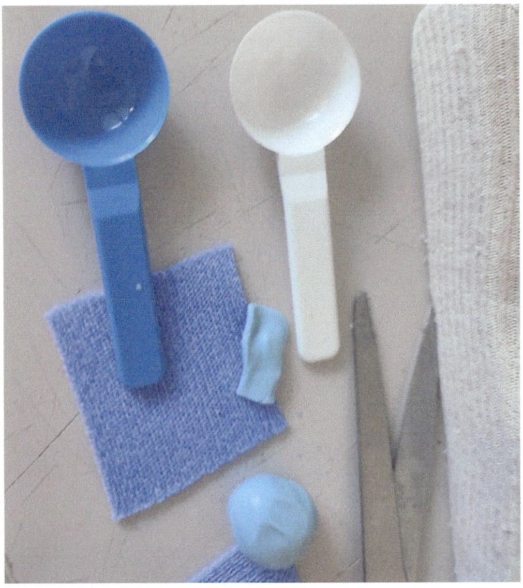

Fig. 8.36 Material: mixed elastomer paste. (Picture by Amélie-Anne Vienne)

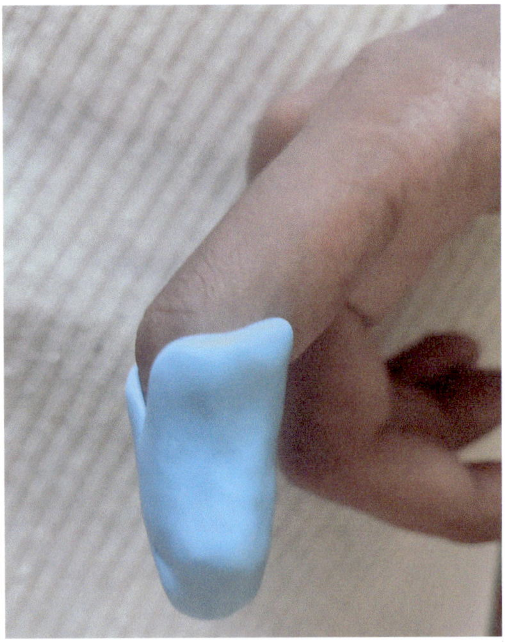

Fig. 8.37 Delicate molding of the paste in the fingertip. (Picture by Amélie-Anne Vienne)

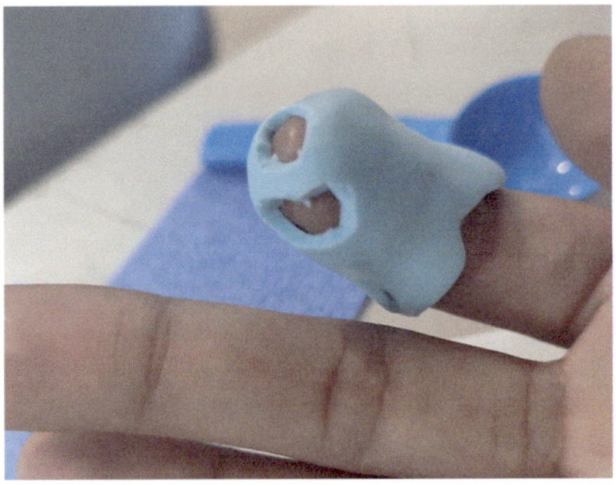

Fig. 8.38 Discharge of the painful zones and tailor-made adjustments. (Picture by Amélie-Anne Vienne)

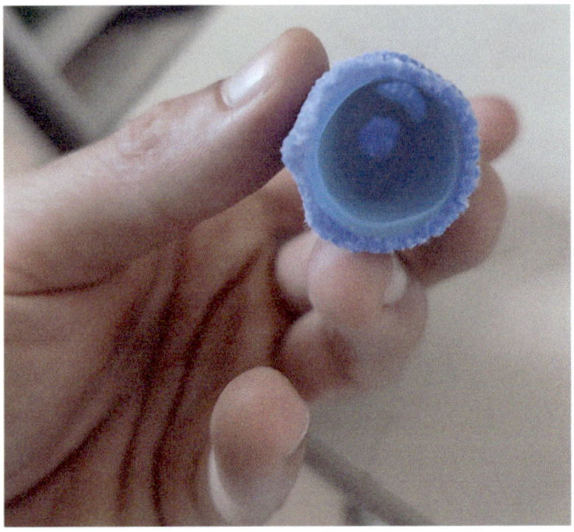

Fig. 8.39 Molding of the thermoformable textile on the hardened elastomer paste. (Picture by Amélie-Anne Vienne)

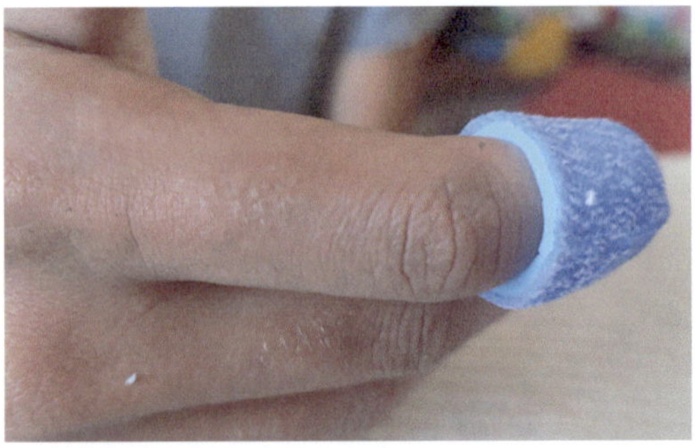

Fig. 8.40 Installation on the finger. (Picture by Amélie-Anne Vienne)

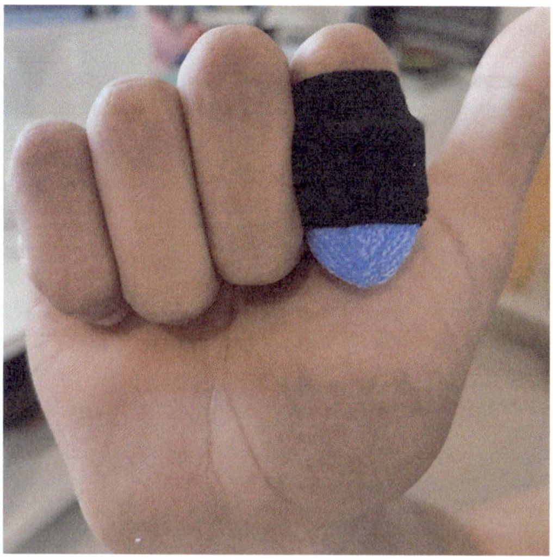

Fig. 8.41 Fixation on the finger with a simple adhesive. (Picture by Amélie-Anne Vienne)

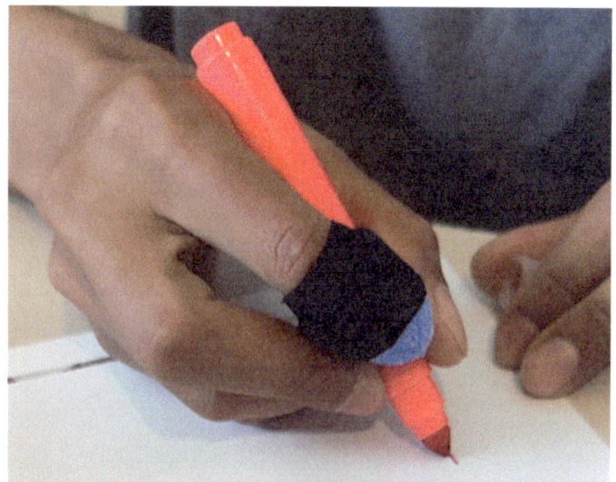

Fig. 8.42 Function with the tip. (Picture by Amélie-Anne Vienne)

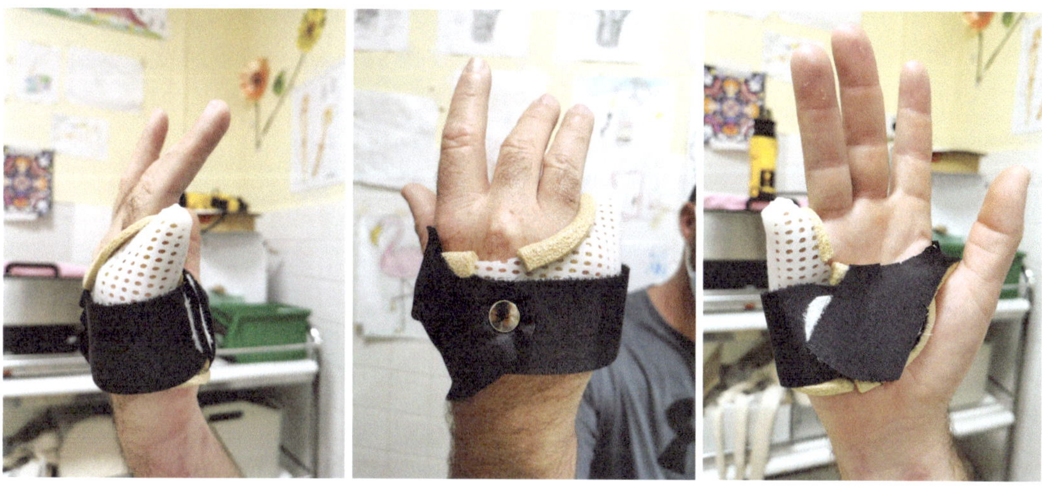

Fig. 8.43 Metacarpophalangeal functional gauntlet: protection of the stump of the fifth finger with discharge for professional activity. (Picture by Amélie-Anne Vienne)

➔ Aesthetic Prostheses

Known as "social life" prostheses, they are made of silicone or PVC, and they reproduce the amputee's limb as closely as possible to reality.

These prostheses can be fitted to any level of amputation, even the most distal.

They provide a significant aesthetic benefit, and even if this is not their primary objective, they can help the hand to function by lengthening it and enabling it to be used in certain activities (tapping, touching, holding). The visual illusion of a "complete limb" can also help to re-establish the patient's cortical pattern.

➔ Mechanical Prostheses

These are functional and have a socket and an articulated endpiece, enabling the fixed grip or the addition of a technical aid or tool specific to a daily, professional, or sporting activity.

They are indicated for complete hand amputations or trans-metacarpal amputations at the most distal level.

	Need	Goal (s)	Inclusion criteria	Counterindications
Aesthetic protheses	Aesthetic Functional very limited	Visual aesthetics Cortical pattern Sensory Protection of the stump	Any age Any amputation level No cognitive limitation	Functional need Altered cutaneous state or medical counterindication
Mechanical protheses	Functional in strength: moderate to important Sports activities Adding technical aids	Pinch or static grip Prehension with strength Resuming social and professional activities	Any age Level proximal to the metacarpophalangeal joints Sufficient cognitive level to learn the mechanism	Aesthetic need Bilateral amputation Insufficient grip for stability Weight
Myoelectric protheses	Functional in strength: little Aesthetic	Functional for daily activities Visual and cortical simulation	Adults and teenagers Specialized center Quality proximal myoelectric stimulus Patient's motivation	Limited cognitive abilities Need for grips with strength Prosthesis weight

Fig. 8.44 Summary of prosthesis types. (Picture by Amélie-Anne Vienne)

They can be covered by an aesthetic glove, but this is not their primary purpose.

➔ Myoelectric Prostheses

Technological advances now make it possible to offer articulated electric prostheses with a range of functions.

They work with voluntary muscle stimulations and programmed movements.

Research has led to the development of elaborate, high-performance systems.

The installation of this type of equipment requires a follow-up with a multi-professional team trained in this type of product, comprising a PMR, an ortho-prosthetist, a physiotherapist, and an occupational therapist. The approach involves a preliminary assessment and a trial and learning period and requires specific equipment.

Bibliography

1. Abi-Chahla ML, Choughri H, Gay A, Pelissier P, Sawaya E, Sommier B. Evaluation à long terme de la reconstruction digitale après amputation distale. Revue d'une série de 181 cas. Chir Main. 2013;32(6):433.
2. Allieu Y, Gomis R, Bahri H. Lambeau inguinal compose cutanéo-osseux prédiculé à la main en urgence. Discussion à propos d'un cas de reconstruction du pouce. Ann Chir Plast. 1981;26:159–62.
3. Attal N, Bouhassira D. Dossier: les douleurs neuropathiques. Paris: Institut UPSA de la Douleur; 2000.
4. Barbary S. Plaies complexes: replantations. In: La traumatologie des parties molles de la main. Approches pratiques en orthopedie traumatologie. Paris: Springer; 2011. p. 269–91.
5. Barbato B, Salsac AV. Finger and thumb replantation: from biomechanics to surgical applications. Hand Surg Rehabil. 2020;39(2):77–91.
6. Bosmans JC, Geertzen JH, Post WJ, van der Schans CP, Dijkstra PU. Factors associated with phantom limb pain: a 3 years prospective study. Clin Rehabil. 2010;24(5):444–53.
7. Bouteille C, Saade F, El Rifai S, Obert L, Pluvy I, Loisel F. Techniques to prevent symptomatic neuroma in digital amputation. Hand Surg Rehabil. 2022;41(2):234–9.
8. Chen R, Cohen LG, Hallett M. Réorganisation du système nerveux à la suite d'une blessure. Neurosciences. 2002;111(4):761–73.
9. Chung KC, Alderman AK. Replantation of the upper extremity: indication and outcomes. J Am Soc Surg Hand. 2002;2(2):78–93.
10. Chung KC, Yoon AP, Malay S, Shauver MJ, Wang L, Kaur S. Patient-reported and functional outcomes after revision amputation and replantation of digit amputations the FRANCHISE multicenter international retrospective cohort study. JAMA Surg. 2019;154(7):637–46. https://doi.org/10.1001/jamasurg.209.0418.
11. Conolly WB, Goulston E. Problems of digital amputation: a clinical review of 260 patients and 301 amputation. Aust N Z J Surg. 1973;43(2):118–23.

12. Dautel G. Le doigt banque. In: Merle M, Dautel G, editors. La main traumatique, l'urgence. 2nd ed. Paris: Masson; 1997. p. 331.
13. Del Pinal F. Severe mutilating injuries to the hand: guidelines for organizing the chaos. J Plast Reconstr Aesthet Surg. 2007;60(7):819–27.
14. Detammaecker R, Strugarek C, Pomares G, De Almeida YK, Dap F, Dautel G. Acceptation, reprise du travail et résultats fonctionnel des amputations basimetacarpiennes des doigts longs: série rétrospective de 41 patients. Hand Surg. 2016;35(6):437.
15. Foucher G, Merle M, Maneaud M, Michon J. Microsurgical free partial toe transfer in hand reconstruction: a report of 12 cases. Plast Reconstr Surg. 1980;65:616–27.
16. Foucher G, Braun F, Merle M, Michon J. Le doigt banque en traumatologie de la main. Ann Chir. 1980;34:693–8.
17. Gold AH, Lee GW. La réimplantation des members supérieurs: concepts actuels et sélection des patients. J Trauma. 1981;21:551–7.
18. Haddad B, Maes-Clavier C, David E, Rotari V, Najjari H. Résultats des régularisations après amputation distales des doigts longs emportant la 3e phalange – à propos de 69 cas. Hand Surg. 2018;37(7):400.
19. Hôpitaux Universitaires de Genève (HUG). Vivre avec une amputation: informations destinées au patients. 2010. http://hug-ge.ch/_library/pdf/actualite_sante/Amputation.pdf.
20. Hu W, Martin D, Foucher G. Baudet J Thumb reconstruction by the anterior interosseous osteocutaneaous island flap. Eur J Plast Surg. 1994;17:10–6.
21. Hu W, Le Nen D, Dubrana F, et al. Le réseau anastomotique dorsal du poignet. conception nouvelle de la base anatomique commune de trois lambeaux en îlot à flux rétrograde de l'avant bras. Ann Orthop Ouest. 1998;30:105–16.
22. Hu W, Le Nen D, Kerfant N, Henry AS, Trimaille A, Monneire C, Claudic Y, Ta P. Secondary digit reconstruction of mutilated hand. Ann Chir Plast Esthet. 2019;64(5–6):694–708.
23. Huguier PC. On replacing the thumb with its metacarpal, by enlarging the first interosseous space. Arch Gen Med. 1874;1:78.
24. Jacques J, Verbraeken E, Vanmarsenille J-M. L'appareillage de l'amputé du membre supérieur, médecine physique et réadaptation. Louv Med. 2019;138(4):193–8.
25. Jensen TS, Krebs B, Nielsen J, Rasmussen P. Immediate and long-term phantom limb pain in amputees: incidence, clinical characteristics and relationship to pre-amputation limb pain. Pain. 1985;21(3):267–78.
26. Kooijman CM, Dijkstra PU, Geertzen JHB, Elzinga A, Van der Schans CP. Phantom pain and phantom sensations in upper limb amputees: an epidemiological study. Pain. 2000;87(1):33–41.
27. Le Viet D. La translocation de l'auriculaire par osteotomie intracarpienne. Ann Chir. 1980;40:145–23.
28. Leung PC. Thumb reconstruction using second-toe transfer. Hand Clin. 1985;1(2):285–95.
29. Lloyd MS, Teo TC, Pickford MA, Arnstein PM. Preoperative management of the amputated limb. Emerg Med J. 2005;22:478–80.
30. Lotze M, Birbaumer N, Erb M, Huse E, Flor H. Does use of a myoelectric prothesis prevent cortical reorganization and phantom limb pain? Nat Neurosci. 1999;2(6):501–2.
31. Matev I. The distraction method in reconstructive surgery of the thumb and fingers. Handchirurgie. 1979;11(3–4):153–6.
32. Nicoladoni C. Daumenplastik. Wien Klin Wochenschr. 1897;10:633–70.
33. Oomman A, Tickunas T, Javed M, Yarrow J, Azzopardi E, Azzopardi EA, Whitaker IS. Changes in perceptions regarding correct preoperative storage and transfer of amputated digits: a 5 year follow up. Microsurgery. 2014;34(1):76–7.
34. Peze W, Iselin F. Cosmetic amputations of the long finger with carpal osteotomy. Ann Chir Main Memb Super. 1984;3:232–6.
35. Philippin Y. Deuil normal, deuil pathologique et prévention en milieu clinique. InfoKara. 2006;21(4):163–6.
36. Pomares G, Detammaecker R, Montoya-Faivre D, Dap F, Dautel G. Amputations du membre supérieur, 10 ans d'expérience d'un SOS main. Hand Surg. 2016;35(6):435.
37. Pomares G, Coudane H, Dap F, Dautel G. Impact psychologique des amputations traumatiques du membre supérieur. Hand Surg Rehabil. 2019;38(6):415.
38. Roullet S, Nouette-Gaulain K, Brochet B, Sztark F. Douleur du membre fantôme: de la physiopathologie à la prévention. Ann Fr Anesth Reanim. 2009;28(5):460–72.
39. Shukla GD, Sahu SC, Tripathi RP, Gupta DK. Phantom limb: a phenomenological study. Br J Psychiatry. 1982;141(1):54–8.
40. Tubiana R. Mutilations complexes-mutilation touchant à la fois le pouce et les doigts. In: Tubiana R, editor. Traité de chirurgie de la main, vol. 3. Paris: Masson; 1993. p. 968–76.
41. Wartan SW, Hamann W, Wedley JR, McColl I. Phantom pain and sensation among British veteran amputees. Br J Anesth. 1997;78:652–9.
42. Weeks SR, Anderson-Barnes VC, Tsao JW. Phantom limb pain: theories and therapies. Neurologist. 2010;16(5):277–86.
43. Yu ZJ. Reconstruction of a digitless hand. J Hand Surg Am. 1987;12(5):722–6.
44. Yu ZJ, Ho HG, Chen TC. Microsurgical reconstruction of the amputated hand? J Reconstr Microsurg. 1984;1(2):161–5.

Part V

Entrapment Syndromes

9 Physiopathology of Entrapment Syndromes

Grégory Mesplié and Olivier Léger

The evolution of entrapment syndromes is histologically and symptomatically well known, but the speed of progression depends on personal factors such as smoking, alcohol consumption, obesity, hypothyroidism, and diabetes.

Physiological Evolution

The severity of the injury depends not only on the intensity of the compression but also on its duration. Even a low-intensity compression (20–30 mmHg), prolonged over time, can cause severe nerve damage [1].

Histopathologically, the first symptom is an increase in intraneural pressure, leading to an endoneurial edema, which in turn causes an increase in intraneural pressure. At this stage, the nerve function is preserved, and the axonal flow is normal.

After a while, these disturbances lead to a thickening of the connective tissue, which may result in a loss of nerve gliding.

Without an effective treatment, the progression is towards a localized then diffuse demyelination of the nerve fibers, culminating in axonal degeneration [2] (Fig. 9.1).

G. Mesplié (✉) · O. Léger
Institut Sud Aquitain de la Main et du Membre Supérieur (ISAMMS), Biarritz, France

G. Mesplié (ed.), *Hand Functional Anatomy and Therapy*,
https://doi.org/10.1007/978-3-031-92505-4_9

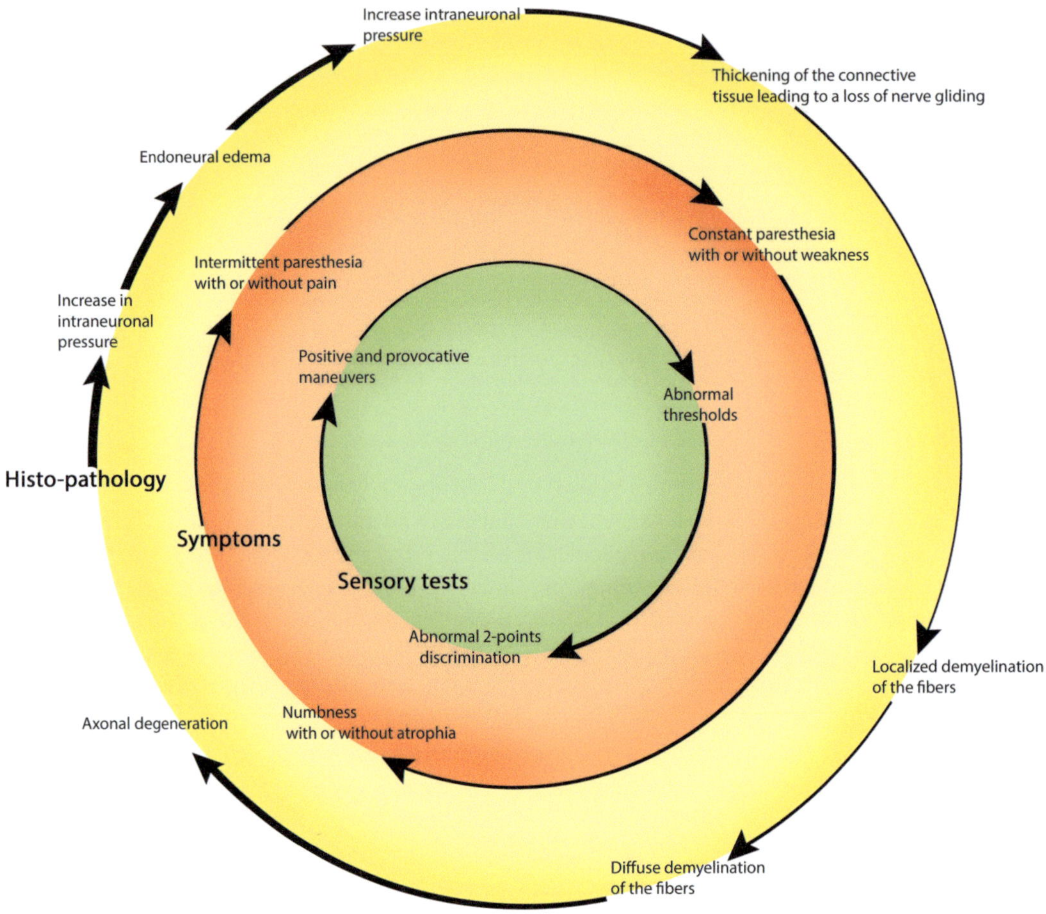

Fig. 9.1 Correlation between histopathology, symptoms, and sensory tests in entrapment syndromes

Symptomatological Evolution

The symptomatologic progression is not proportional to the histological progression, and the onset of a "moderate" symptomatology is associated with significant anatomical lesions (Fig. 9.1).

The use of provocative maneuvers is essential to highlight a nerve damage before it becomes too extensive.

Neurogenic Pain or Mechano-Sensitivity

Neurogenic pain is nociceptive nerve pain. The nociceptive fibers of a nerve itself, or nervi nervorum, signal an aggression or injury to the nerve without axonal damage.

The NP4 test (see chapter "Clinical Examination of the Wrist and Hand" in Volume 1) is negative but not nonexistent.

Pain is usually intermittent and may be triggered by pseudo-Tinel tests, tensioning, and provocative movements. Cutaneous movements modify the symptoms.

Neuropathic Pain

Neuropathic pain corresponds to a nerve damage with axonal lesion.

The NP4 test is positive; pain can be permanent and is always associated with cutaneous sensory disorders. It involves damage to the vibrotactile system.

The pain is referred to as Aß pain, since it is not related to damage to the small-diameter fibers (C fibers) carrying the nociceptive afferences, but to damage to the afferent fibers carrying the vibrotactile sensitivity (Aß fibers).

Bibliography

1. Rydevik B, Lundborg G, Bagge U. Effects of graded compression on intraneural blood blow. An in vivo study on rabbit tibial nerve. J Hand Surg Am. 1981;6:3–12.
2. Ellis R, et al. Is there a relationship between impaired median nerve excursion and carpal tunnel syndrome? A systematic review. J Hand Ther. 2017;30(1):3–12.

10 Entrapment Syndromes of the Median Nerve

Grégory Mesplié and Olivier Léger

Like the ulnar and radial nerves, the median nerve originates from the brachial plexus and travels along the upper limb, ending with sensory fibers at the digital level. It can therefore be compressed along its entire course, including at the level of its roots or the thoracic outlet. In this chapter, we will only deal with compression sites distal to the elbow.

Carpal Tunnel Syndrome

The carpal tunnel syndrome is a set of clinical signs meaning there is an entrapment of the median nerve at the level of the carpal tunnel.

It is the most frequent pathology of the hand and mostly occurs bilaterally in 50-year-old women.

Physiopathology

There is a dual physiopathology in this syndrome:

First, the ischemia of the median nerve, which explains the increase of symptoms during the night and the alleviating maneuvers described by the patients.

Second, intracanal hyper-pressure (from 3 to 30 mmHg), causing the apparition of symptoms. It can be related to several causes:

- Fractures of the inferior extremity of the radius.
- Tenosynovitis of the flexors, inflammatory rheumatism, hormonal changes (pregnancy, myxedema), diabetes. Aside from obvious metabolic contexts, tenosynovitis is present only in 4% of the cases, making the synovectomy useless.
- Intracanal tumors, muscular anomalies (hypertrophic lumbricals, palmaris longus or flexor digitorum superficialis with a distal or digastric muscle belly, Frohse palmaris profundus from the anterior side of the radius to the deep side of the superficial palmar aponeurosis).
- Repeated flexion-extension movements, often related to a professional or sports activity.

Despite the large number of possible causes, it is most often idiopathic.

The two mechanisms are probably intricately linked [1]. The preponderance of one or the other can explain the different electro-clinical observed forms. In fact, the median nerve at the level of the wrist is composed of 50% big fibers, which are the only ones explorable by EMG and sensitive to pressure. The small fibers (C fibers and fibers of

G. Mesplié (✉) · O. Léger
Institut Sud Aquitain de la Main et du Membre Supérieur (ISAMMS), Biarritz, France

G. Mesplié (ed.), *Hand Functional Anatomy and Therapy*,
https://doi.org/10.1007/978-3-031-92505-4_10

the sympathetic system) are more sensitive to ischemia.

Clinical and Paraclinical Signs

The presence of digital acro-paresthesia, sometimes felt like pain, and mostly during the night seems to be the most characteristic sign. The fifth finger is usually not damaged.

The Phalen test can be used to demonstrate a median nerve injury in the carpal tunnel. Its validity is interesting, especially if associated with a compression at the level of the carpal tunnel [2]. Tinel pseudo-test can be used along the median nerve proximal to the carpal tunnel (sensitivity 70%, specificity 98%) [3].

The Scratch Collapse Test can be used in addition to the other elements of the clinical and paraclinical assessment, although its validity remains highly debated [4–6].

A hypoesthesia in the territory of the median nerve and an atrophy of the external thenar muscles make the diagnosis obvious, but are, fortunately, very rare as they mean we are dealing with a severe deficit form of the syndrome.

Other than the following neurologic injuries, the Raynaud syndrome is the key element of the differential diagnosis.

The EMG is essential as it studies the distal motor latency and the speed of the sensorial conduction and allows:

- Confirming the diagnosis.
- Assessing the severity.
- Looking for an associated neurologic injury realizing a double crush syndrome: compression of the ulnar nerve in the elbow, radicular compression or thoracic outlet syndrome; diabetic neuropathy, for example. In the case of double crush syndrome, it is hard to tell which pathology causes which symptoms. The carpal tunnel treatment is simple (contrary to the previous pathologies) and should therefore be proposed first.

There are 10% false negatives. They are starting forms with damage of the small fibers that are explored on the assessment or a transitory damage of a small number of big fibers. In these cases, a test infiltration is essential.

Ultrasound can also be used to assess the condition of the median nerve at the carpal tunnel [7].

Medical and Surgical Treatment

A conservative treatment (orthosis, gestures, corticoid infiltration) is possible, with 30–75% of improvement depending on the authors. It is therefore difficult to know if this improvement is due to a lull in the pathology or if it is a therapeutic effect [8].

Without treatment, 23% of patients have a worsened symptomatology, 29% remain stable, and 48% have a significant recovery [9].

Infiltration often betters the speed of the nervous conduction after 1 month but does not change the spontaneous evolution after 1 year, unlike the surgery that we realize after a loss of 2.7 m/s.

The surgical treatment is essential in three cases:

- If there is a sensorial or motor deficit. When there is deficit there usually is little pain, with a major axonal loss. It occurs more often in old patients and may be a particular form of the pathology, the evolution from painful subjective forms to forms with deficit being poorly known. Surgery clearly improves the symptoms.
- In the case of a neurogenic path of the abductor pollicis brevis, the other parameters only reflect the importance of the conduction block.
- If the symptoms persist after 1 year.

Surgery is very efficient, with an almost immediate relief. Aside from all the secondary effects that can happen in every hand surgery, some specific secondary effects are frequent and can persist until 6 months post-surgery in 25% of the cases, justifying the cessation of work because of loss of strength and pillar pain. They are related to hypertrophic healing of the retinaculum or slight modifications in the architecture of the carpal bones.

Some publications demonstrate that complex surgeries of the root canal like synovectomy or endo-neurolysis are useless, and that an incision in the axis of the fourth finger is safe. Therefore, several authors have suggested the endoscopic section of the retinaculum and have presented their results in the early 1990s.

The endoscopic technique allows a better postoperative comfort and an earlier use of the hand, as well as a shorter leave from work. However, the results 6 months after surgery are the same, except maybe for the strength recovery [10].

Endoscopy is reliable, with a relapse rate comparable to the conventional technique and a close failure rate (0.05%).

The complications are more frequent than with the conventional technique but are resolving most of the time. In 2/3 of the cases, the complication is the contusion of the nerve or the branch of the third space occurring when preparing the ligament or introducing the endoscope. Their frequency remains low but there is an unavoidable learning curve.

The technique with one opening seems to have better results than the one with two openings, and it is logical to reduce the scar as much as possible, especially in a contact area.

Contrary to the conventional technique, the endoscopic liberation allows conserving the inter-thenar fascia and the superficial palmar aponeurosis.

To avoid any neuroma in the palmar cutaneous branch of the median nerve, the cutaneous incision must stay medial to the palmaris longus. However, similar branches intended to innervate the skin of the hypothenar eminence arise from the ulnar nerve (cutaneous palmar branch of the ulnar nerve and nerve of Henlé), and only a small incision (endoscopic) decreases the risk of neuroma.

Rehabilitation and Orthotic Treatment

Without Surgery or Preoperative

When the nerve damage is moderate, rehabilitation and wearing a resting orthosis can delay or even avoid surgery. This treatment is only efficient in some cases, most of the time when the inflammation has mechanical causes.

➔ Rehabilitation

It is about fighting against inflammatory phenomena and, depending on the indications, mobilizing the median nerve.

- **Fight against trophic disorders and pain**

This is based on the association of cryotherapy, pressotherapy, analgesic vibrotherapy, and draining massages that can help reduce the intra-canal edema, therefore participating in the decompression of the median nerve in the carpal tunnel.

In the case of neurogenic pain (mechanosensitivity) and neuropathic pain (without allodynia), fasciatherapy techniques combined with taping can have very interesting effects. The therapist moves the skin in different directions and, if an improvement in symptoms is observed, applies a tape reproducing the maneuver performed.

Scottish baths (or contrast baths) have not been shown to be effective, either before or after surgery [11].

- **Longitudinal massages**

These massages are applied on the accessible area of the nerve that is the closest to the painful area.

It consists in realizing a longitudinal pressure along the nerve along 3–4 cm to improve vascularization and enable axonal flows [12].

The ideal pressure recreates the distal symptomatology without creating pain. It is maintained a few minutes, until we obtain a variation of the initial response.

The preferential area is proximal to the flexors' retinaculum, where the nerve is not reachable.

In this area, the nerve is located on the ulnar side of the flexor pollicis longus and the flexor carpi radialis, and on the radial side of the palmaris longus.

The patient is placed in decubitus, with a 30° flexion of the elbow. After finding the median nerve, longitudinal maneuvers are realized along it.

Another way to apply this technique consists in pressing the median nerve and slowly mobilizing the wrist in flexion/extension. It is not the finger but the nerve that moves, which can be better tolerated by the patient.

- **Fight against perineural adherences**

These exercises improve glidings between the median nerve and the adjacent tissues, which limits the compressive constraints and improves vascularization.

These techniques are particularly effective in neurogenic pain, without axonal injuries. In more severe stages, their indication seems less obvious.

- ***Nerve mobilizations***

The goal of the nerve mobilizations is to mobilize the median nerve respective to the adjacent tissues to limit the risks of compression and ischemia [13, 14].

We avoid the Upper Limb Tension Tests, described by Butler in 1991. These maneuvers are diagnostic, not therapeutic.

In fact, nerves do not tolerate stretching well: an 8% stretching causes venous obstruction, a 15% stretching causes ischemia, and a 20% stretching causes nerve rupture [15].

We therefore prefer gliding maneuvers, which allow twice more excursion than tension maneuvers, with 8.5 times less tension [16] (Fig. 10.1) (see chapter "Neurodynamic Mobilizations" in Volume 1).

Nerve mobilizations can also be achieved by imitating animated images using a slide show [17] (Fig. 10.2).

- ***Mobilizations of the tissues adjacent to the nerve***

Alternating contraction-relaxation-stretching of the adjacent muscles allows a perineural pumping that improves local trophicity and maintains the inter-tissue glidings.

This mobilization of the tissues around the nerve can be realized alternating movements in the wrist and fingers, allowing a dissociative contraction of the muscles adjacent to the median nerve.

- ***Massages against fibrosis***

They are realized along the median nerve, on the anterior part of the forearm, at the level of the flexors' retinaculum and the thenar muscles.

We use dot-shaped massages, glided pressures, and kneading that improve local trophicity, fight against perineural fibrosis, and relax the muscles adjacent to the nerve.

- ***Self-rehabilitation***

Self-rehabilitation exercises include mobilizations, longitudinal self-massages, and cryotherapy.

The mobilizations are realized several times a day in all the amplitudes of the wrist and elbow to improve the neural gliding.

The longitudinal massages are realized three times a day for 1–2 min (until there is a modification of the perception) at the level of the median nerve.

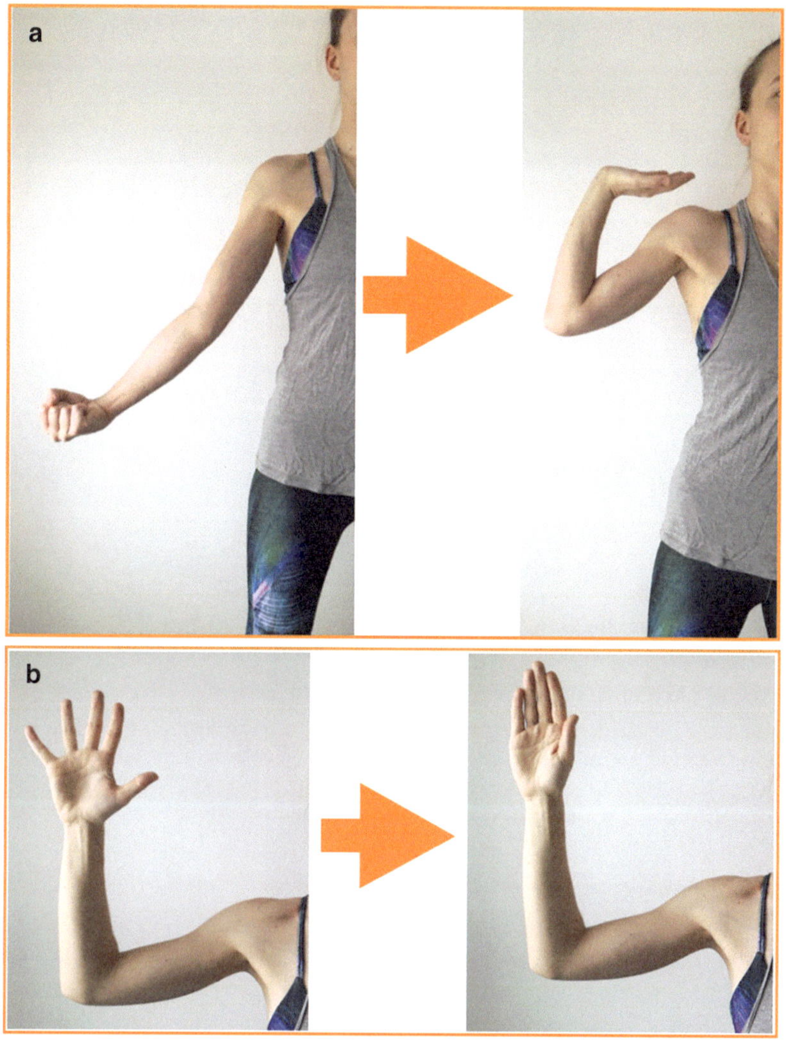

Fig. 10.1 (**a**) Tension-free gliding of the median nerve: extension of the elbow in supination, wrist and finger flexion/flexion of the elbow in pronation, wrist and finger extension. (**b**) Mobilization of the median nerve in the carpal tunnel according to Meng et al.: shoulder abduction, 90° elbow flexion, neutral wrist position, finger abduction/adduction. (Picture by Josette Mesplié)

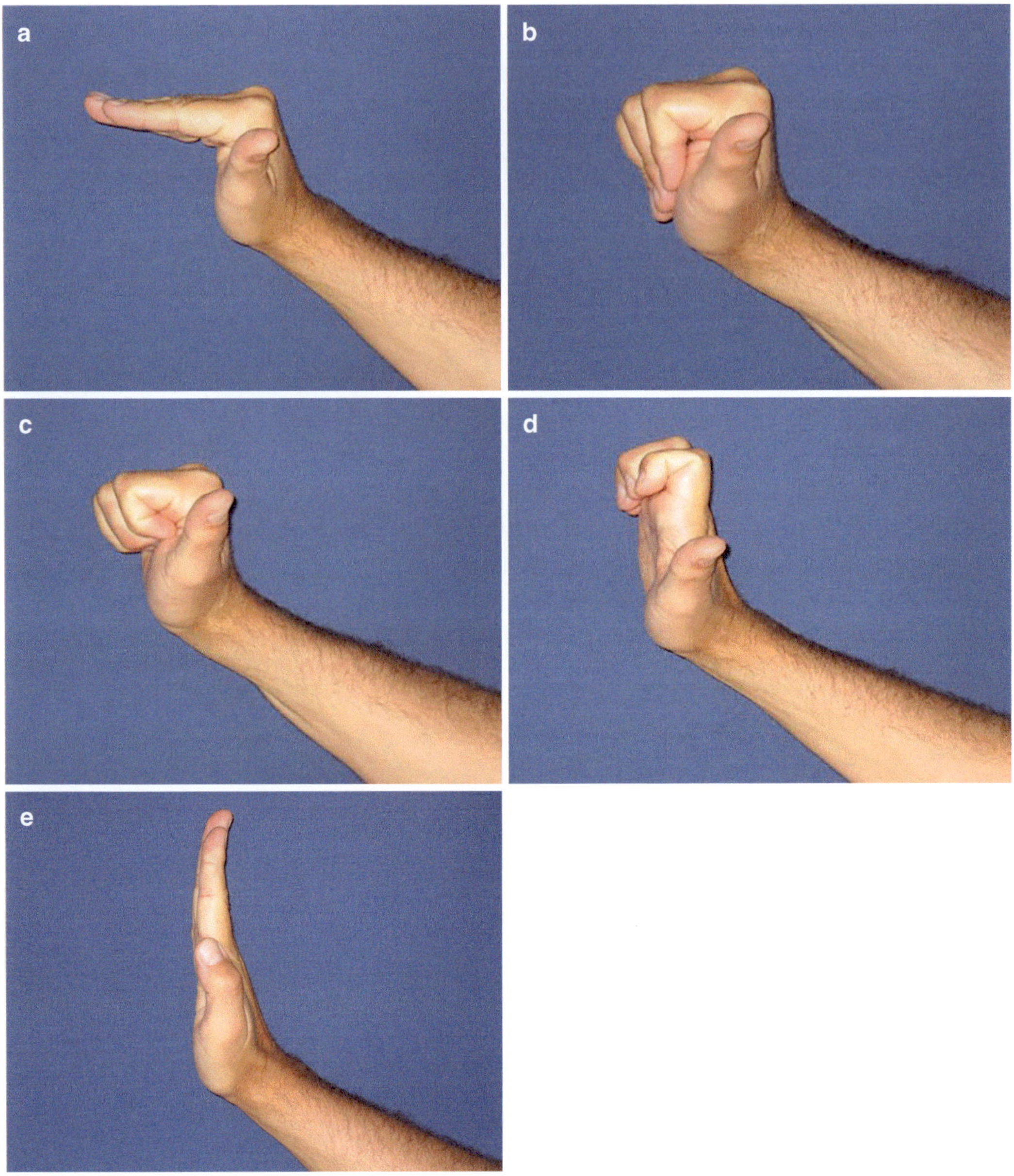

Fig. 10.2 Imitation exercise to mobilize the median nerve. (Picture by Coline Geoffroy)

- **Strength recovery**

At this level of compression, the injuries are not beyond the stage of neurapraxia or stage 1 of Sunderland. The motor assessment of Daniels and Worthingham is most often 4.

The muscles concerned by the compression of the median nerve in the carpal tunnel are the pollicis abductor brevis, the opponens pollicis, the short fascicle of the flexor pollicis brevis, and the two radial lumbrical muscles.

Therefore, we propose several exercises reinforcing these anatomical elements.

- ***External thenar muscles***

We ask the patient to realize an anteflexion of the thumb against a resistance placed on the radial side of the first phalanx to stimulate the external sesamoid muscles, and on the radial side of the first metacarpal for the opponens pollicis (Fig. 10.3).

The strengthening evolves depending on the progression, until 2 months, when the flexor retinaculum is healed.

We add electrotherapy to the voluntary contraction of the patient, with currents of wide amplitude (150–200 μs) and a frequency of 20–30 Hz to stimulate type 1 muscle fibers (Fig. 10.4).

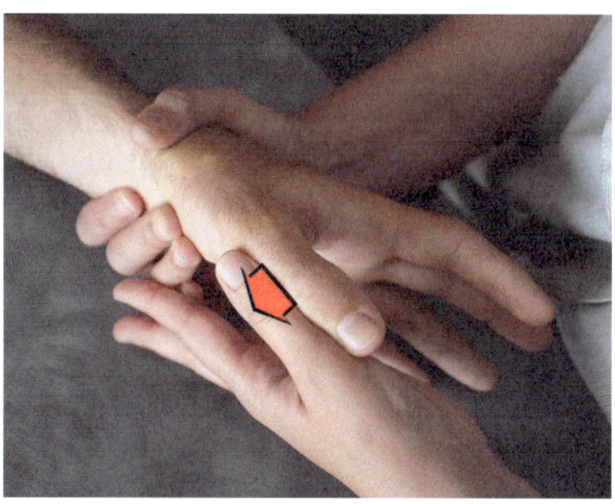

Fig. 10.3 Manual strengthening of the external sesamoid muscles. (Picture by Grégory Mesplié)

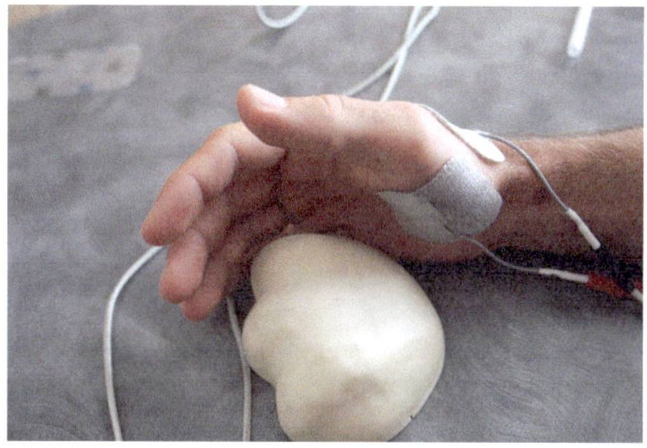

Fig. 10.4 Active electrostimulation of the external sesamoid muscles (placement of the electrode of reference). (Picture by Grégory Mesplié)

- ***Global exercise for the intrinsic muscles***

This exercise limits the apparition of muscular unbalance, often created by compensations when the patient goes back to his daily activities.

It consists in globally and progressively strengthening the intrinsic muscles of the hand to stimulate the functional synergies essential for the efficiency of the prehensions.

We ask for a contraction against resistance with a "vise" pinch: opposition thumb—fifth finger and separation thumb—fifth finger.

This exercise can also be realized instrumentally, with or without visual feedback (Fig. 10.5).

The electrostimulation of the muscles of the opposition arch (thumb—fifth finger) can be used combined with a voluntary contraction (Fig. 10.6).

Working on the tip-to-side pinch, without participation of the flexor pollicis longus, can also be realized with visual feedback (Fig. 10.7).

To complete the protocol, we can add exercises for the rotatory stability, which have a functional and proprioceptive interest (Fig. 10.8).

- ***Rebalancing the muscle balances***

This strengthening protocol must allow regaining muscular ratios comparable to the healthy side (or to the literature), especially

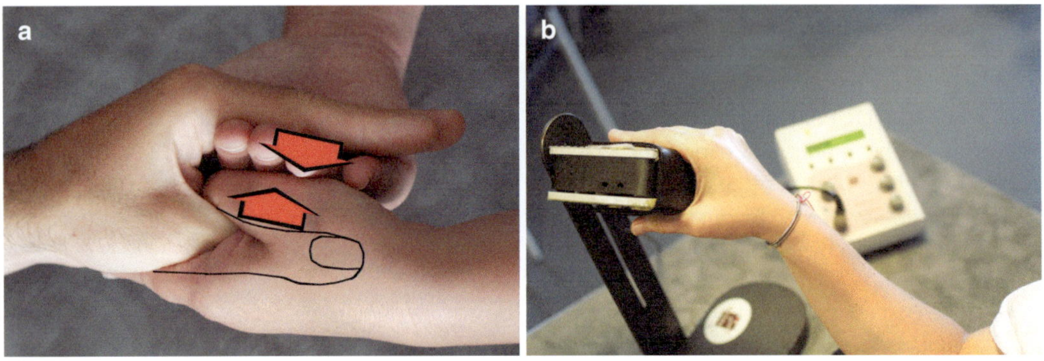

Fig. 10.5 Global manual (**a**) and instrumental (**b**) exercises for the intrinsic muscles. (Picture by Grégory Mesplié)

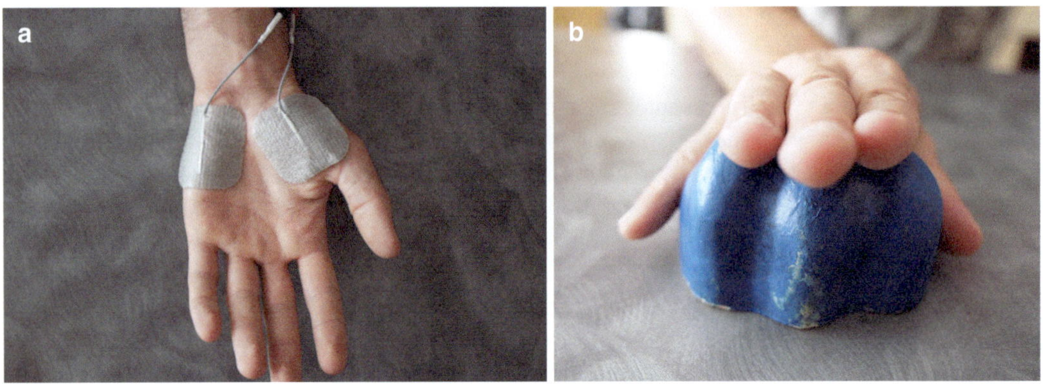

Fig. 10.6 Placement of the electrodes (**a**) for an electroactive exercise of the muscles of the arch of opposition between the thumb and the fifth finger (**b**). (Picture by Grégory Mesplié)

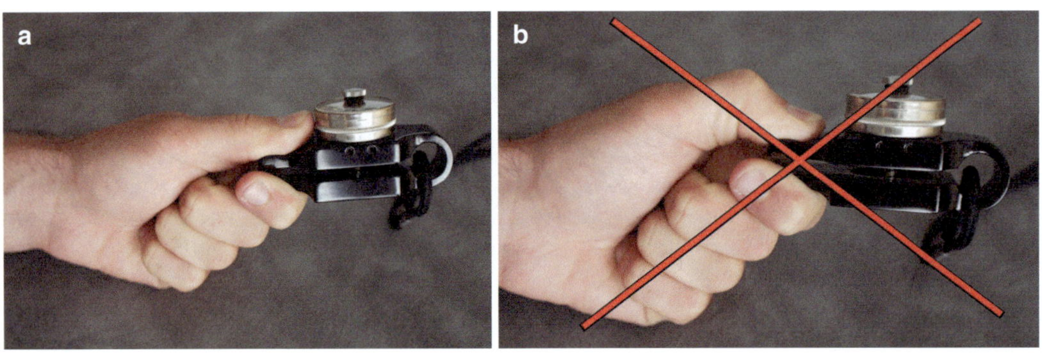

Fig. 10.7 Exercise for the termino-lateral pinch, without compensation from the flexor pollicis longus, which innervation is proximal to the carpal tunnel. This exercise actively stimulates the adductor pollicis longus, innervated by the ulnar nerve. (Picture by Grégory Mesplié)

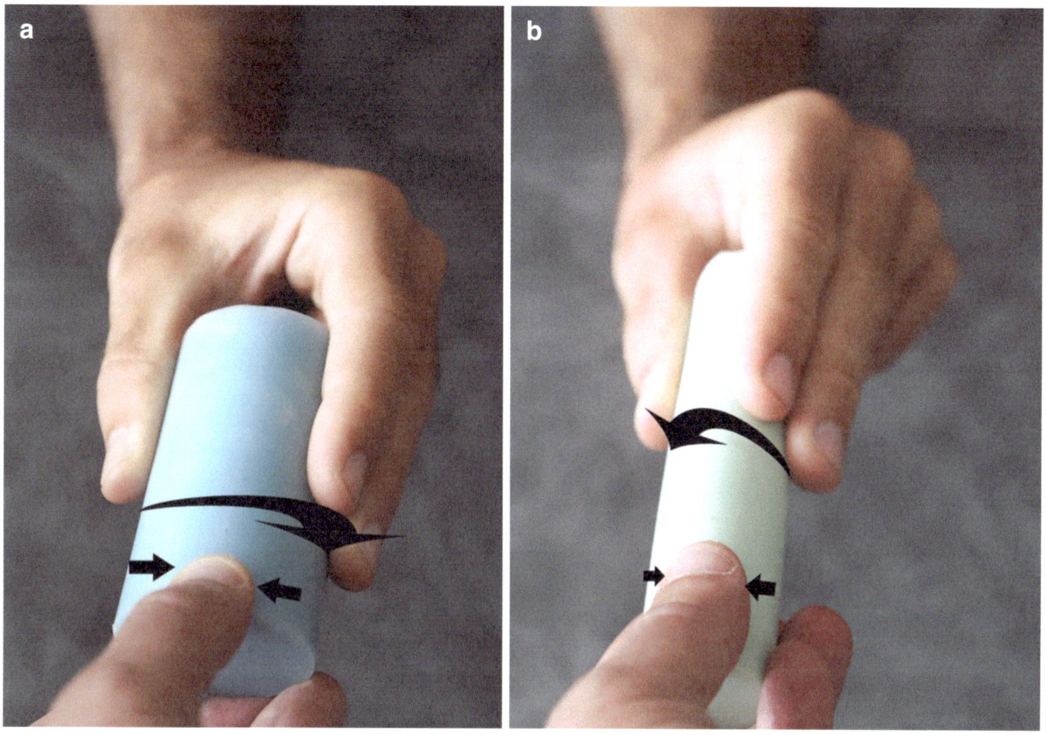

Fig. 10.8 Rotatory stabilization of the thumb, starting with large cylinders (**a**) and progressively decreasing the size of the cylinder (**b**). (Picture by Grégory Mesplié)

between the intrinsic and extrinsic systems, even if all ratios should be controlled.

The measures are controlled during the regular check-ups realized with dynamometers.

Grasp work should be avoided as it increases the risk of developing tenosynovitis and significantly increases pressure in the carpal tunnel [18].

- **Proprioception, coordination, and dexterity**

We work on simple, then complex prehensions to improve proprioceptive, dexterity, and coordination aspects.

These exercises are adapted to the patient's functional needs.

- **Rehabilitation of sensitivity**

These exercises are realized after defining exactly the patient's sensorial disorders (hypoesthesia, hyperesthesia, paresthesia, dysesthesia, allodynia, etc.).

The rehabilitation is then adapted to these disorders, according to the protocol described in chapter "Physiology and Rehabilitation of Sensorial and Motor Disorders" (Volume 1) [19].

- **Cervical mobilizations and strengthening of scapula fixators**

In the management of entrapment syndromes, work on the nerve must be combined with a more global approach involving stretching the cervical muscles and strengthening the scapula fixators (see chapter "Neurodynamic Mobilizations" in Volume 1) (Fig. 10.9).

➔ Orthotic Treatment

A thermoformed orthosis can delay and even avoid surgery [20] when it is realized at the very beginning of the symptoms.

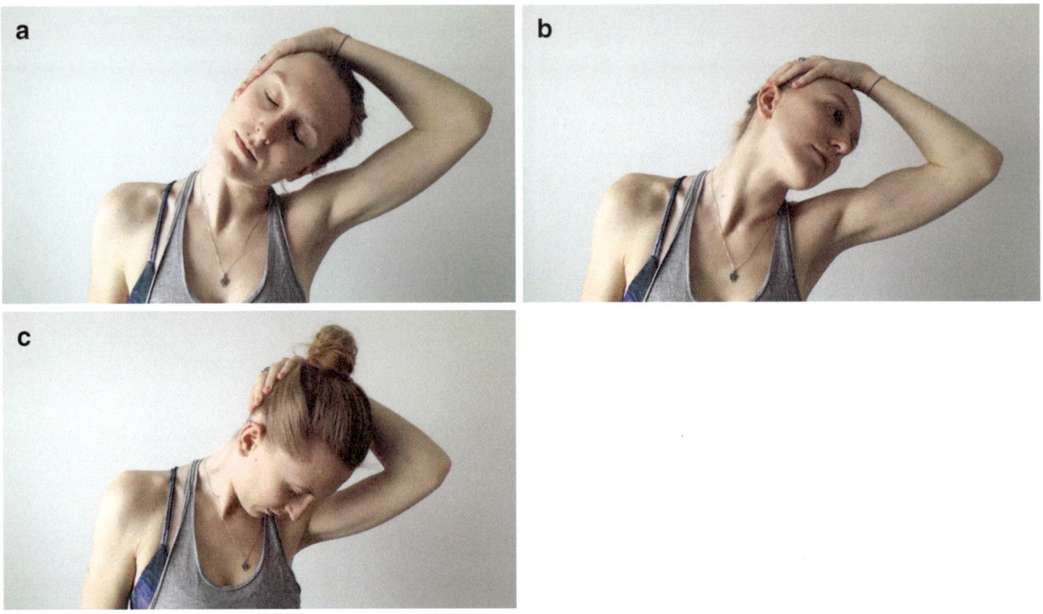

Fig. 10.9 (**a**) Self-stretching of the superior fibers of the trapezius muscle: the patient is seated, the homolateral hand holds the chair to lower the shoulder. The contralateral hand brings the head in flexion, contralateral inclination, and homolateral rotation of the cervical spine. (**b**) Self-stretching of the superior fibers of scalene muscles: the patient is seated, the homolateral hand holds the chair to lower the shoulder. The contralateral hand brings the head in extension, contralateral inclination, and contralateral rotation of the cervical spine. (**c**) Self-stretching of the levator scapulae muscle: the patient is seated, the homolateral hand holds the chair to lower the shoulder. The contralateral hand brings the head in flexion, contralateral inclination, and contralateral rotation of the cervical spine. (Picture by Grégory Mesplié)

Its role is to immobilize the wrist in a neutral position where the pressure in the carpal tunnel is less important [21] and therefore to limit the constraints on the median nerve (Fig. 10.10).

An orthosis worn during the night avoids the nocturnal compression of the median nerve by the lumbrical muscles that get in the carpal tunnel when the fingers are flexed (classical position during the night) (Fig. 10.11).

The orthosis must be worn all the time for 6 weeks, then only during the night until the symptoms disappear… Or until the surgery.

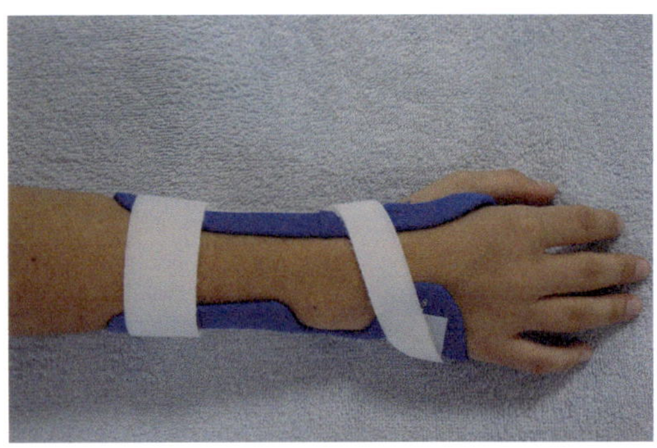

Fig. 10.10 Rest orthosis of the wrist in a neutral position, where the pressure in the carpal tunnel is the least important. (Picture by Coline Geoffroy)

Postoperative

The goal of decompression of the surgery by section of the flexors' retinaculum has several biomechanical consequences:

- Increase of the carpal tunnel volume, allowing the decompression of the median nerve and therefore opposing the ischemic disorders damaging it.
- Decrease of the friction nerve-tendons-synovial sheath inside the tunnel.
- Palmar translation of the flexors by "bow-

string" effect, putting more constraints on the A1 pulley. This phenomenon can lead to a trigger finger after carpal tunnel surgery (Fig. 10.12).
- Loss of the proximal fixing point of the thenar and hypothenar muscles that can cause a loss of strength in these muscles (Fig. 10.13).
- Possibility of hypertrophic healing of the flexors' retinaculum causing pillar pain and perineural fibrosis (Fig. 10.14).
- Relative relaxation of the thenar muscles, which can decompensate a rhizarthrosis that already existed but was not causing any pain.

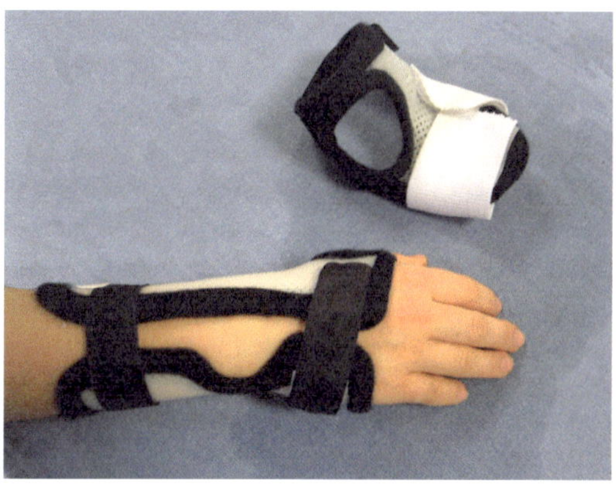

Fig. 10.11 Nocturnal device associated to the rest orthosis. It can be used to limit the compression of the median nerve by the lumbricals when the fingers are flexed. (Picture by Grégory Mesplié)

Other than these mechanical disturbances, the operated patients sometimes have sensorial disorders that must be treated to regain an optimal prehension.

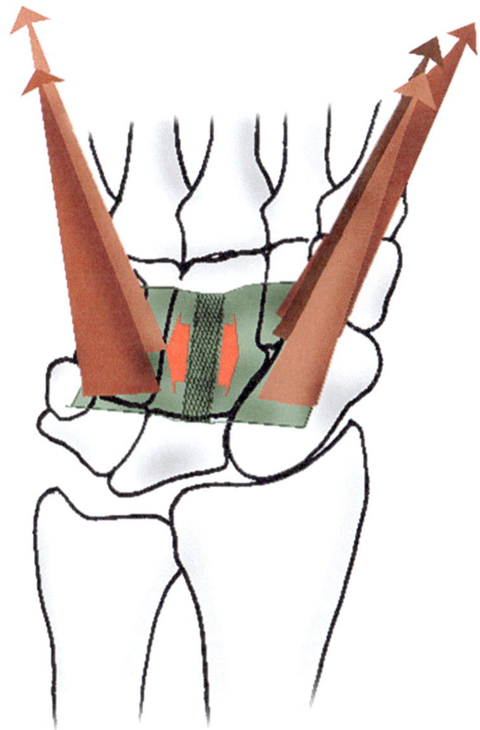

Fig. 10.13 Loss of the proximal fix point of the thenar and hypothenar muscles. (Picture by Josette Mesplié)

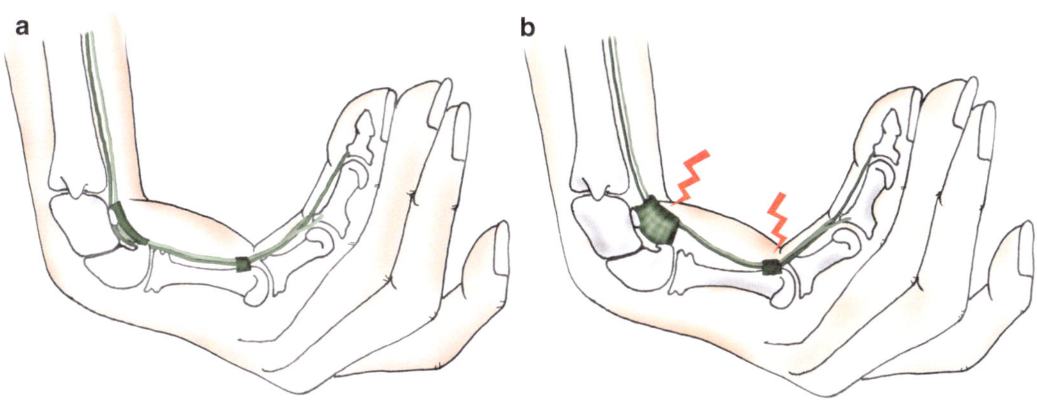

Fig. 10.12 The retinacular ligament opposes to the "bowstring" effect of the flexor tendons at the level of the carpal tunnel (**a**). After surgery, we can observe a palmar translation of the flexors leading to a transfer of the constraints on the A1 pulley (**b**). (Picture by Grégory Mesplié)

➔ Rehabilitation (Fig. 10.15)

The rehabilitation aims to limit the negative impact of these biomechanical modifications on the patient's functions. However, it is not systematic, as the postoperative evolution is usually positive without rehabilitation.

- **Immediate postoperative phase (D3–D21)**

Rehabilitation is not essential in most cases and is reduced to guided self-rehabilitation exercises and advice sheets.

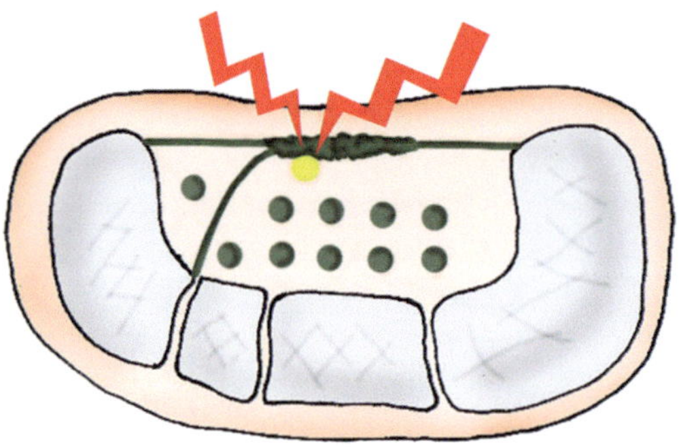

Fig. 10.14 Hypertrophic healing of the flexors retinacular ligament causing perineural fibrosis and "pillar pain." (Picture by Josette Mesplié)

These exercises consist in putting ice on the operated hand, mobilizing passively then actively the fingers and the wrist without resistance, and stimulating the tips of the three radial fingers with various objects (tissue, soft brush, etc.). Strength activities are strictly forbidden as they disturb the healing process and increase the risks of complications.

In some cases (important preoperative fibrosis, important risks of CRPS, important pre- or postoperative sensorial disorders), the rehabilitation starts in this phase with gaseous cryotherapy, disto-proximal pressotherapy, draining massages around the scar, and transcutaneous vibratory stimulations (100 Hz).

- **Healing phase (after D21)**

From D21, the scar is closed, and the hand is usually less inflammatory and painful. In this phase, we fight against healing disorders that can cause fibrosis around the median nerve, mobilize the median nerve, and work for the progressive recovery of the grip. The sensorial rehabilitation will also be key if there are disturbances in the sensitivity of the median territory.

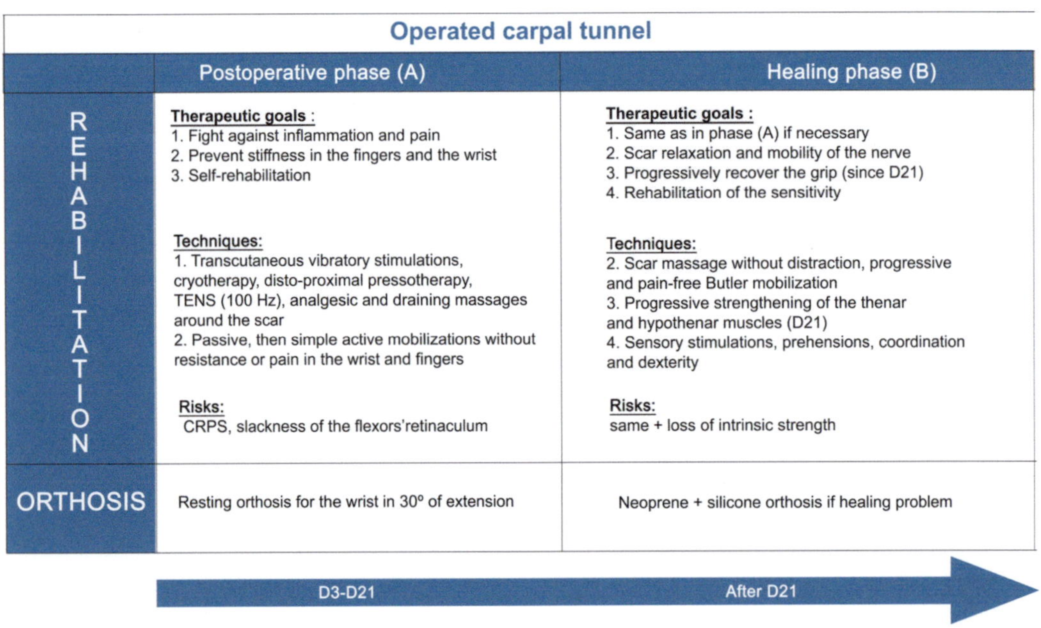

Fig. 10.15 Rehabilitation protocol after carpal tunnel surgery. (Picture by Josette Mesplié)

- ***Fight against healing disorders***

  Healing disorders after a surgery of the carpal tunnel can cause important fibrosis, with consequences that can disturb the hand's functions.

  The cutaneous scar usually causes few problems, but the healing of the flexors' retinaculum can cause pillar pain or "trap" the median nerve, leading to symptoms like the ones observed before the surgery.

  - *Massages around the scar and in fibrosis areas*: their goal is to improve trophicity around the treated area and to relax the scar. We realize disto-proximal glided pressures following the orientation of the fibers of the flexors' retinaculum, thenar, and hypothenar muscles. This helps remodeling the scar tissue. We also use sanding on indurations to relax the areas with the most fibrosis. These techniques are described in chapter "Scar Massage and Treatment" in Volume 1.
  - *Ultrasounds*: once the scar is closed, we use ultrasounds to fight against adherences around the scar. The ideal frequency is 1 MHz as it has a deeper effect than 3 MHz. We prefer using the pulse mode that has a "fibrolytic" effect.
  - *Depressotherapy*: its application must be cautious and progressive. We start using it when the scar is closed. First, when the scar is still inflammatory, we apply the head of the device far from the scar in a disto-proximal direction. When the scar is not inflammatory anymore, we apply the head of the device directly on it, first with the alternative mode and then with the continuous mode if the patient tolerates it well.
  - *Mobilization of the median nerve*: these techniques are realized if the patient presents paresthesia without any other neurologic disorders on the median territory. We use the same techniques as the ones described for the rehabilitation without surgery.
  - *Longitudinal massage*: it is first applied far from the operated area, then getting closer to the wrist, according to the same modalities as the ones described for the rehabilitation without surgery.

- ***Strength recovery***

  The carpal tunnel surgery is meant for compressive nervous injuries not exceeding the stage of the axonotmesis or stage 2 of Sunderland, but that can cause motor disorders often rated between 2 and 4 on the Daniels and Worthingham's scale described in chapter "Physiology and Rehabilitation of Sensorial and Motor Disorders" (Volume 1).

  - *Stage 2*: this stage corresponds with the ability to mobilize the concerned segment in all its amplitude without gravity or in part of its amplitude against gravity. We ask the patient to realize simple active mobilizations if the mobilization is not against gravity, and active-assisted contractions against gravity. The interest here is to improve the trophic state of the muscle and to maintain the glidings in different anatomic planes.
  - *Stage 3*: this stage corresponds with the ability to mobilize the concerned segment in all its amplitude against gravity. The interest is the same as in stage 2, but here we can start an intermittent static exercise against gravity to alternate the contractile modes, depending on the patient's abilities.
  - *Stage 4*: this stage marks the beginning of the strengthening protocol, progressively putting charge on the flexors' retinaculum, as the motor ability of the thenar muscles allows us to use manual or instrumental resistances.

The strength loss in this stage is constant, even if the muscles' motor ability is normal, because of the incision of the flexors' retinaculum that weakens the proximal fixing point of the thenar muscles, which is an essential element for the efficiency of the grabs between the thumb and fingers (Fig. 10.13).

Working with the external thenar muscles is part of a global strengthening protocol for the intrinsic muscles of the hand. It must be progressive until 8 weeks in order not to damage the flexors' retinaculum, which would distend it and limit the strength recovery, or favor the appearance of fibrosis around the scar that could compress the median nerve.

The maximal contraction of the extrinsic muscles is forbidden until the end of healing as it multiplies by 3 the pressure in the carpal tunnel and tends to relax the flexors' retinaculum because of the "bowstring" effect.

The exercises proposed in this phase are the same as the ones for the rehabilitation without surgery.

- ***Rehabilitation of sensitivity***

Sensory disorders after a carpal tunnel surgery can appear when the nerve is a lot damaged before the intervention, or in the case of hypertrophic healing of the flexors' retinaculum that "traps" and compresses the median nerve.

Rehabilitation is not always needed but is essential in the case of sensory disorders on the median territory, which corresponds with the precise functions of the hand and needs an exceptional discriminative sensitivity.

This rehabilitation is realized following the modalities described in chapter "Physiology and Rehabilitation of Sensorial and Motor Disorders" (Volume 1).

- ***Prehensions***

Manipulation exercises allowing improving dexterity and coordination are realized, insisting on the precision of the thumb-index pinch.

➔ Orthotic Treatment

Its benefits are still debated [22], but the orthosis places the wrist in 30° of extension to maintain the flexors and median nerve in contact with the carpal floor and therefore:

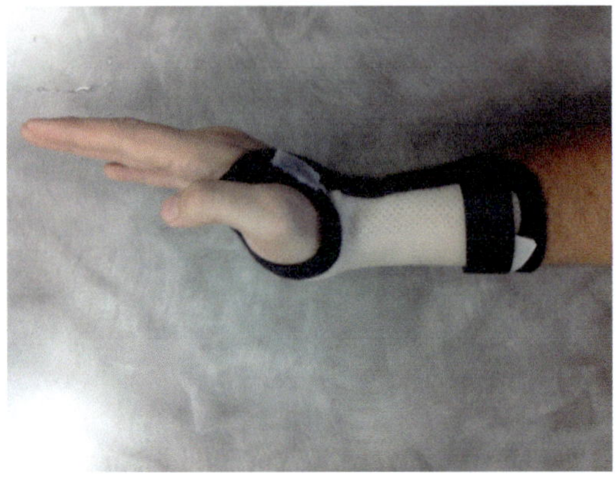

Fig. 10.16 Postoperative orthosis after carpal tunnel surgery, with a wrist extension to limit the risks of adherences between the median nerve and the flexors' retinaculum. (Picture by Josette Mesplié)

- Improve the flexors' retinaculum healing, limiting the "bowstring" effect of the finger flexors during the flexion of the wrist (especially in active flexion).
- Limit the risk of adherence between the median nerve and the flexors retinaculum (Fig. 10.16).

In the case of hypertrophic healing with pillar pain, a neoprene orthosis with a silicone pad on the scar can be realized once the scar is closed.

This orthosis allows progressively getting back to professional activities while protecting the scar from painful contacts. It also improves healing with the silicone pad.

Other Entrapment Syndromes of the Median Nerve (Fig. 10.17)

Even if the carpal tunnel syndrome is, by far, the most common entrapment syndrome of the median nerve, other locations are possible, and several compression sites can be associated to generate a double crush syndrome that is a proximal compression of the nerve causing positive clinical signs distally on a second less important compression site.

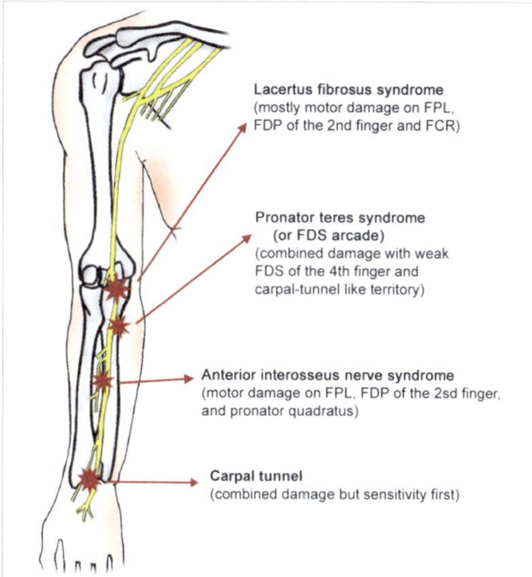

Fig. 10.17 Other compression sites of the median nerve and observed symptoms for each site. (Picture by Grégory Mesplié)

Arcade of Struthers

The ligament of Struthers, very inconstant, forms an inextensible arch between the medial epicondyle and the supra-epicondyle apophysis, where injuries of the median nerve can occur.

Its compression at this level causes muscular and sensorial disorders in all its innervation territory, as there are no collateral branches yet.

Under the Lacertus Fibrosus

The lacertus fibrosus is an accessory bicipital aponeurosis on the ulnar side of the principal biceps tendon that can be the source of compression of the median nerve, which symptomatology corresponds to a motor impairment with weakness and loss of endurance of the flexor digitorum profundus of the index, and the flexor carpi radialis [23].

Sensory disorders linked to a compression at this level are rare [24] and reserved to severe forms.

Between the Two Fascicles of the Pronator Teres

The pronator teres syndrome is a compression of the median nerve between the two heads of the pronator teres, causing symptoms close to the ones we observe in the carpal tunnel syndrome.

However, the symptoms decrease during the night and the Tinel sign is positive at the level of the pronator teres, which helps localize the injury.

If the clinical signs are triggered by an elbow flexion against resistance + forearm pronation (elbow positioned between 100° and 135°), the site of compression is probably the lacertus fibrosus.

If the clinical signs are triggered by a pronation against resistance + elbow flexion between 0° and 45°, the site of compression is probably the pronator teres.

If clinical signs are triggered by a flexion against resistance of the proximal interphalangeal joint of the middle finger + elbow in extension, the site of compression is probably the arcade of the flexor digitorum superficialis.

Under the Arcade of the Flexor Digitorum Superficialis

The compression of the median nerve at this level is the source of a compression of the anterior interosseous nerve, which is a branch of the median nerve formed at the level of the pronator teres.

The anterior interosseous syndrome causes motor deficit in the flexor pollicis longus, flexor indicis profundus, and pronator quadratus. There is no associated sensory disorder.

At an advanced stage, the pinch between the thumb and the index is in the shape of a "duck beak" (Fig. 10.18).

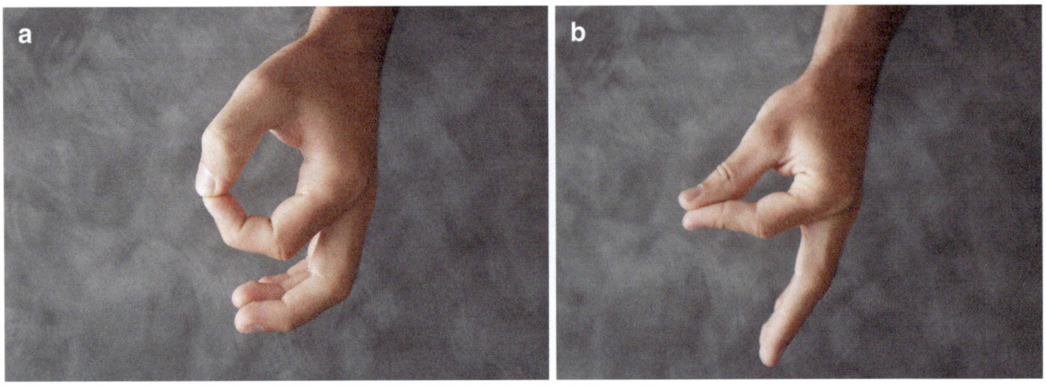

Fig. 10.18 The syndrome of the anterior interosseous nerve leads to a motor damage of the flexor pollicis longus and the flexor digitorum profundus of the second finger. The pinch between the thumb and the index is not normal (**a**), but in the shape of a "duck beak" (**b**). (Picture by Josette Mesplié)

Rehabilitation and Orthotic Treatment

The rehabilitation of the entrapment syndromes of the median nerve only concerns the early stages of compression of the nerve; more severe stages require surgery.

It aims to improve tissue glidings around the nerve and sensitivity in the damaged areas and to maintain (and even recover) trophicity of the concerned muscles in the most advanced cases.

➔ Fight Against Trophic Disorders and Pain

It is based on a combination of cryotherapy, pressotherapy, analgesic vibrotherapy, and draining massages that can improve symptomatology.

In the case of neurogenic pain (mechanosensitivity) and neuropathic pain (without allodynia), fasciatherapy techniques combined with taping can have very interesting effects. The therapist moves the skin in different directions and, if an improvement in symptoms is observed, applies a tape reproducing the maneuver performed.

➔ Longitudinal Massage

They are realized on the accessible areas of the median nerve.

The median nerve goes along the internal side of the arm until it reaches the arcade of Struthers where it is easily accessible. We realize longitudinal massages along the nerve and transversal and dot-shaped massages on the areas with fibrosis.

The nerve then passes in the anterior part of the elbow under the lacertus fibrosus and passes between the two heads of the pronator teres, then under the flexor digitorum superficialis.

Here we also use longitudinal massages on areas where the nerve is reachable and transversal and dot-shaped massages on areas with fibrosis.

➔ Decontracting Massages

They are realized on the internal side of the arm and the anterior side of the forearm and based on glided pressures and kneading to improve local trophicity and muscular relaxation.

➔ Improving Tissue Glidings Around the Nerve

The goal is to realize differential glidings between the nerve and the adjacent tissues, mobilizing the nerve directly or indirectly with myo-aponeurotic stretchings or muscular contractions.

The mobilizations of the median nerve are realized following the modalities described in previous paragraphs, and contractions—rest—stretchings can concern the biceps, flexor digitorum superficialis, or pronator teres depending on the localization of the compression. Each stage of pumping is maintained 4–6 s to avoid risks of ischemia.

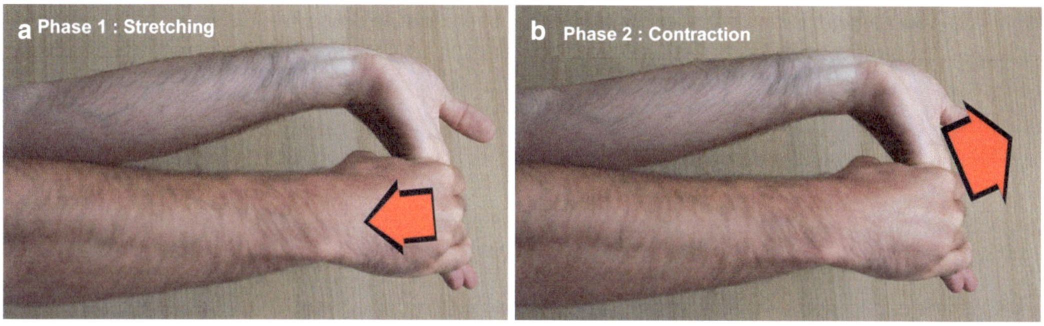

Fig. 10.19 Alternating stretching (**a**) and contraction (**b**) of the flexor digitorum superficialis to mobilize it in relation to the median nerve. (Picture by Grégory Mesplié)

- **Flexor digitorum superficialis**

The stretching is realized with the elbow extended, extending the wrist and fingers except the distal interphalangeal joint, in order not to put tension on the flexor digitorum profundus that is not a compressive element for the median nerve (Fig. 10.19).

The contraction is realized in external race and closed chain to get a decompressive effect in the arcade of the flexor digitorum superficialis (Fig. 10.20).

- **Pronator teres**

Contraction-relaxation of the pronator teres are realized to create a "pumping" effect around the median nerve, improving local trophicity. These maneuvers are realized with the elbow at 90° of flexion, which is the position where the pronator teres is solicited the most.

- **Biceps**

We alternate contraction—rest—stretching in every elbow position to favor glidings of the lacertus fibrosus.

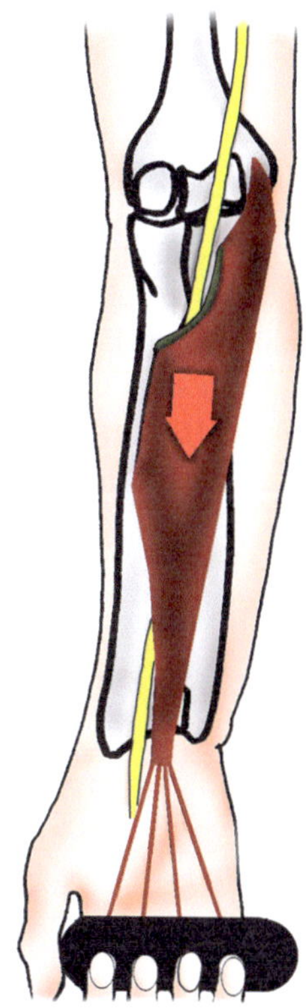

Fig. 10.20 Working in a closed chain for the flexor digitorum superficialis decompresses the median nerve at the level of its arcade. (Picture by Josette Mesplié)

➔ Strength Recovery

This part of the treatment is adapted to the Daniels and Worthingham's scale, following the same steps as in the rehabilitation after carpal tunnel surgery.

➔ Rehabilitation of Sensitivity

These exercises are realized following the modalities described in chapter "Physiology and Rehabilitation of Sensorial and Motor Disorders" (Volume 1).

➔ Self-Rehabilitation

Self-rehabilitation exercises based on mobilizations, longitudinal self-massages, and cryotherapy are explained to the patient.

The mobilizations are realized several times a day in all the amplitudes of the wrist and elbow to improve perineural glidings.

Longitudinal massages are realized three times a day during 1–2 min (until there is a modification of the perception) at the level of the median nerve, depending on the compression site.

We put ice on the compression area after all the other exercises during 20 min, depending on pain.

➔ Cervical Mobilizations and Strengthening of Scapula Fixators

In the management of entrapment syndromes, work on the nerve must be combined with a more global approach involving stretching the cervical muscles and strengthening the scapula fixators (see chapter "Neurodynamic Mobilizations" in Volume 1).

Important Points

Diagnosis

The diagnosis of these injuries is difficult as the different possible locations are close from each other and the clinical signs can be unclear with a mixed or incomplete clinical picture.

For example, the anterior interosseous syndrome only affects the flexor pollicis longus and therefore can be confused with a rupture of this tendon.

We can also find a clinical picture that reminds us of a pronator teres syndrome, when the compression is really at the level of the arcade of the flexor digitorum superficialis. Or we can find a clinical picture of anterior interosseous syndrome with a compression at the level of the pronator teres or even more proximal.

For these reasons, the surgical approach is the same for compressions related to the lacertus fibrosus, the pronator teres, and the arcade of the flexor digitorum superficialis, which allows the surgeon to evaluate the nerve state and specify the compression site.

There are also double crush syndromes, in which the nerve is compressed in several places.

Therefore, we must not stay focused on just one location, and it is essential to control the state of the nerve in its entire pathway. A painful area can correspond with another compression site of the nerve.

Some symptoms are close to the ones we can observe in entrapment syndromes and yet are due to completely different causes.

For example, the radicular compressions, referred pain, systemic pathologies, etc.

Therefore, it is essential to take a complementary medical advice if the symptoms do not evolve.

Rehabilitation Techniques

Nervous compressions are complex and need a precise and adaptive treatment.

Some techniques, like nerve mobilizations and longitudinal massages, can worsen the symptomatology if they are not realized well. When in doubt, it is better to delay their application.

Bibliography

1. Uchiyama S, et al. Current concepts of carpal tunnel syndrome: pathophysiology, treatment, and evaluation. J Orthop Sci. 2010;15(1):1–13.
2. Adler JA, Wolf JM. Proximal median nerve compression: pronator syndrome. J Hand Surg Am. 2020;45(12):1157–65.
3. Novak CB, et al. Provocative testing for cubital tunnel syndrome. J Hand Surg. 1994;19:817.
4. Cheng CJ, et al. Scratch collapse test for evaluation of carpal and cubital tunnel syndrome. J Hand Surg Am. 2008;33(9):1518–24.
5. Jimenez I, Delgado PJ. The scratch collapse test in the diagnosis of compression of the median nerve in the proximal forearm. J Hand Surg Eur Vol. 2017;42(9):937–40.
6. Huynh MNQ, Karir A, Bennett A. Scratch collapse test for carpal tunnel syndrome: a systematic review and meta-analysis. Plast Reconstr Surg Glob Open. 2018;6(9):e1933.
7. Lange J. Carpal tunnel syndrome diagnosed using ultrasound as a first-line exam by the surgeon. J Hand Surg Eur Vol. 2013;38(6):627–32.

8. Futami T. Natural history of the carpal tunnel syndrome. J Jpn Soc Surg Hand. 1992;9:128–30.
9. Ortiz-Corredor F, et al. Natural evolution of carpal tunnel syndrome in untreated patients. Clin Neurophysiol. 2008;119(6):1373–8.
10. Léger O. Influence de la technique opératoire sur le coût du traitement chirurgical du syndrome du canal carpien. Chir Main. 2000;19(2):95–9.
11. Janssen RG, Schwartz DA, Velleman PF. A randomized controlled study of contrast baths on patients with carpal tunnel syndrome. J Hand Ther. 2009;22(3):200–7; quiz 208.
12. Fernandez-de-Las-Penas C, et al. The effectiveness of manual therapy versus surgery on self-reported function, cervical range of motion, and pinch grip force in carpal tunnel syndrome: a randomized clinical trial. J Orthop Sports Phys Ther. 2017;47(3):151–61.
13. Wolny T, et al. Effect of manual therapy and neurodynamic techniques vs ultrasound and laser on 2PD in patients with CTS: a randomized controlled trial. J Hand Ther. 2016;29(3):235–45.
14. Le Roux P. Syndrome du canal carpien et mobilisation des nerfs. Kinésithérapie, la Revue. 2007;7(68–69):49–52.
15. Lundborg G, Rydevik BL. Effects of stretching the tibial nerve of the rabbit: preliminary study of the intraneural circulation of the barrier function of the perineurium. J Bone Joint Surg Br. 1973;55:390–401.
16. Coppieters MW, Butler DS. Do "sliders" slide and "tensioners" tension? An analysis of neurodynamic techniques and considerations regarding their application. Man Ther. 2008;13(3):213–21.
17. Echigo A, et al. The excursion of the median nerve during nerve gliding exercise: an observation with highresolution ultrasonography. J Hand Ther. 2008;21(3):221–7; quiz 228.
18. Goss BC, Agee JM. Dynamics of intracarpal tunnel pressure in patients with carpal tunnel syndrome. J Hand Surg Am. 2010;35(2):197–206.
19. Mesplié G. Thérapie de la main, examen clinique et outils de prise en charge rééducative avancée du poignet et de la main. Montpellier: Sauramps Médical; 2021.
20. Graham B. Nonsurgical treatment of carpal tunnel syndrome. J Hand Surg Am. 2009;34(3):531–4.
21. Weiss N, et al. Position of the wrist associated with the lowest carpal-tunnel pressure: implications for splint design. J Bone Joint Surg Am. 1995;77(11):1695–9.
22. Shalimar A, et al. Splinting after carpal tunnel release: does it really matter? Malays Orthop J. 2015;9(2):41–6.
23. Hagert E, et al. Lacertus syndrome: a ten year analysis of two hundred and seventy five minimally invasive surgical decompressions of median nerve entrapment at the elbow. Int Orthop. 2023;47:1005.
24. Lalonde D. Lacertus syndrome: a commonly missed and misdiagnosed median nerve entrapment syndrome. BMC Proc. 2015;9(Suppl 3):A74.

11 Entrapment Syndromes of the Ulnar Nerve

Grégory Mesplié and Olivier Léger

Compression of the Ulnar Nerve in the Elbow

The vulnerability of the ulnar nerve, because of its anatomical path, has been known since the beginning of the twentieth century. A traumatic origin, or one secondary to a degenerative damage, was frequently found, and in 1957 Osborne described the concept of the cubital tunnel syndrome. He showed that opening this tunnel has positive effects on the symptomatology.

Etiology

- Primitive forms in a context of hyper-use
- Traumatic forms by direct contusion, fracture of the inferior extremity of the humerus, elbow dislocation, or prolonged compression
- Secondary forms, nontraumatic with arthrosis, rheumatoid polyarthritis, osteochondromatosis, or tumor
- Anconeus muscle [1]

Clinical Assessment

It must search for traumatic or nontraumatic factors that could be causing the symptoms. Instability of the ulnar nerve in its groove may be caused by a hypertrophic medial head of the triceps or groove dysplasia [2].

The symptomatology depends on the fibers concerned by the compression; it can be sensory or motor.

Paresthesia occurs in the fifth finger and the ulnar side of the fourth finger; they can be more important during the night as the elbow is flexed (around 90°) and become permanent over time.

For the motor function, we must look for a global loss of the clamping strength and an ulnar paralysis with Froment's sign, revealed by a flexion of the interphalangeal joint of the thumb when pinching a sheet of paper between the pulps of the thumb and index. This compensation is related to the contraction of the flexor pollicis longus (innervated by the median nerve) that compensates the weakness of the adductor pollicis (innervated by the ulnar nerve) (Fig. 11.1).

The weakness of the interossei is brought to light by Wartenberg's sign, which is a permanent abduction of the fifth finger (Fig. 11.2).

Tinel's sign has a sensitivity of 62%–70% but is not enough to unsure the nerve suffering, as it is also present in patients with no neurological damage [3, 4].

G. Mesplié (✉) · O. Léger
Institut Sud Aquitain de la Main et du Membre Supérieur (ISAMMS), Biarritz, France

G. Mesplié (ed.), *Hand Functional Anatomy and Therapy*,
https://doi.org/10.1007/978-3-031-92505-4_11

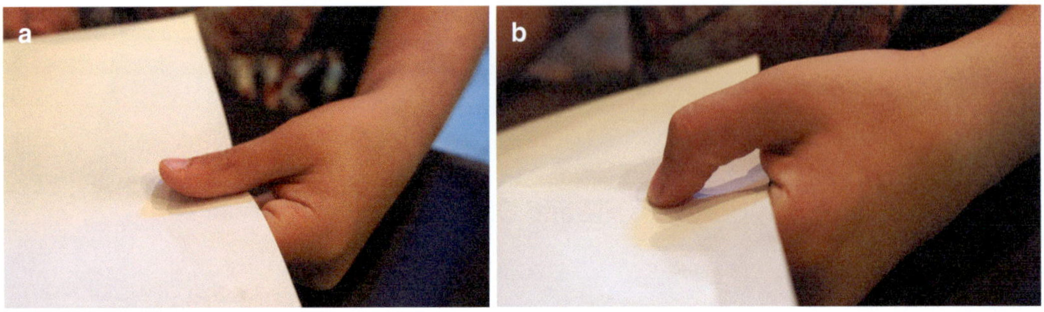

Fig. 11.1 Froment's test: maintain a sheet of paper being pulled away is impossible without compensating with the flexor pollicis longus (innervated by the median nerve) as the adductor pollicis (innervated by the ulnar nerve) is inefficient. (**a**) Negative test. (**b**) Positive test. (Picture by Grégory Mesplié)

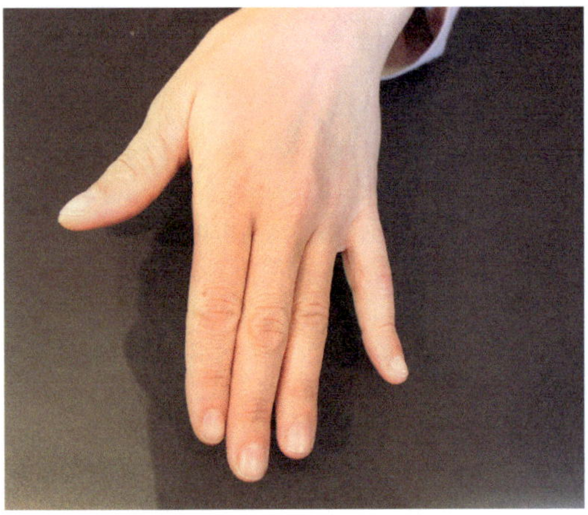

Fig. 11.2 Wartenberg's sign, meaning the fourth palmar interosseous is weak. The abduction of the fifth finger is permanent because of the effect of the extensor digiti minimi. (Picture by Grégory Mesplié)

Additional Exams

We look for signs of arthrosis or traumatic aftereffects with X-rays of the elbow.

The electromyogram is part of the systematic assessment in every entrapment syndrome and determines the seriousness and level of the injury.

Medical and Surgical Treatment

Medical Treatment

When the symptomatology is intermittent with a minimal damage on the electromyogram, the medical treatment combines anti-inflammatories with a nocturnal orthosis in 30° of elbow flexion, as well as an adapted rehabilitation [5].

Compression phenomena must be reduced by adapting the workstation.

Surgical Treatment

Extra-articular neurolysis improves symptomatology in most of the cases. Epicondylectomy and transposition of the ulnar nerve are used in the case of relapse, nervous instability, or bony deformity.

➔ Extra-articular Neurolysis

Realized with a plexus block and a pneumatic tourniquet. It consists in successively lifting every compression site, with the section of the retinaculum of the ulnar canal, the Osborne's fascia, and the arcade of Amadio and Beckenbaugh while checking that there is no nervous subluxation that would require an anterior transposition [6] or a medial epicondylectomy.

➔ Medial Epicondylectomy

Proposed by King and Morgan, it consists in removing the medial epicondyle to decrease the path of the nerve and the intracanal pressure during the movements of flexion-extension.

➔ Subcutaneous Transposition

It consists in modifying the path of the nerve, placing it under the medial epicondyle and therefore decreasing the tension and stretching during the movements of flexion-extension of the elbow.

This transposition can be subcutaneous or submuscular and is realized when the simple neurolysis has failed and in the case of degenerative or post-traumatic deformities.

Compression of the Ulnar Nerve in the Wrist

Damage of the ulnar nerve in the wrist is less frequent than in the elbow. It requires a paraclinical assessment with electromyogram and echography to look for the various possible causes of damage of the nerve in this anatomical area.

The ulnar nerve gets into the palm of the hand through Guyon's canal, which has a triangle shape and is limited by the flexors' retinaculum in its superior part, the hook of the hamate laterally, and the insertion of the piso-hamate ligament and the pisiform medially.

There are several etiologies, from a tumorous or vascular pathology to a traumatic or degenerative origin.

The medical treatment consists in wearing a resting orthosis for 3–6 weeks, followed by rehabilitation. However, most of the times the patients seek a consultation when they are already in an advanced stage and need surgery liberating the sensory branches and the motor branch.

Rehabilitation and Orthotic Treatment

Without Surgery

As for the median nerve, this treatment concerns moderate damages of the nerve without important sensory and motor disorders. The patient describes tingling sensations, most often during the night.

The rehabilitation and orthotic treatment can delay and even avoid surgery.

Rehabilitation

The techniques used are the same as for the median nerve, adapted to the anatomical situation of the ulnar nerve.

➔ Fight Against Inflammation and Pain

It is based on a combination of cryotherapy, pressotherapy, and draining massages that can help decrease the perineural inflammation.

In the case of neurogenic pain (mechanosensitivity) and neuropathic pain (without allodynia), fasciatherapy techniques combined with taping can have very interesting effects. The therapist moves the skin in different directions and, if an improvement in symptoms is observed, applies a tape reproducing the maneuver performed.

➔ Longitudinal Massage

This massage is applied at the level of the accessible area of the nerve closest to the damaged area.

It consists in realizing a longitudinal pressure along 3–4 cm of the nerve, to improve its vascularization and restart the axonal flow.

The ideal pressure recreates the distal symptomatology, without producing pain. It is maintained a few minutes, which allows obtaining a variation of the initial symptoms.

In epitrochlear-olecranon compressions, the patient is placed in decubitus with his elbow in a 30° flexion. After locating the groove (sometimes with an area with fibrosis), we realize longitudinal maneuvers along the ulnar nerve. Transversal maneuvers can also be done to relax the retinaculum of the epitrochlear-olecranon groove (or ulnar canal).

For compressions in the wrist, the patient is in the same position. We locate the external part of the flexor carpi ulnaris, where the ulnar nerve passes from the inferior 1/3 of the forearm and realize the longitudinal massage there.

A different way of doing this technique consists in realizing a static pressure at the level of the damaged area and mobilizing the closest joint. The nerve is mobilized, which is sometimes better tolerated by the patient.

We realize this technique on the two possible compression sites, no matter where the "major" compression is.

➔ Fight Against Perineural Fibrosis

It improves glidings between the ulnar nerve and the adjacent tissues, which limits the compressive constraints to which it is exposed and improves its vascularization.

- *Mobilization of the nerve*

  Nerve mobilizations aim to mobilize the nerve with respect to the adjacent tissues to limit the risks of compression and ischemia [7, 8].

  We avoid the Upper Limb Tension Tests, described by Butler in 1991. These maneuvers are diagnostic, not therapeutic.

  In fact, nerves do not tolerate stretching well: an 8% stretching causes venous obstruction, a 15% stretching causes ischemia, and a 20% stretching causes nerve rupture [9].

  We therefore prefer gliding maneuvers, which allow twice more excursion than tension maneuvers, with 8.5 times less tension [10] (see chapter "Neurodynamic Mobilizations" in Volume 1).

  In cases of ulnar nerve damage at the level of the epitrochlear-olecranon groove, we do not perform these exercises, as they are likely to increase stress between the nerve and the groove.
- *Mobilizations of the tissues adjacent to the nerve*

  Alternating contraction-relaxation-stretching of the adjacent muscles allows a perineural pumping that improves local trophicity and maintains the inter-tissue glidings.

  These mobilizations are realized preferentially on the flexor carpi ulnaris for proximal compressions, on the hypothenar muscles for distal compressions, and on the adductor pollicis for exclusively motor damages. Each step is maintained 4–6 s to avoid any ischemic risk (Fig. 11.3).

  Imitation exercises improving movements between the different gliding planes participate in this fight against perineural fibrosis.
- *Massages against fibrosis*

  They are realized along the ulnar nerve, on the internal side of the forearm, around the pisiform, and at the level of the hypothenar eminence.

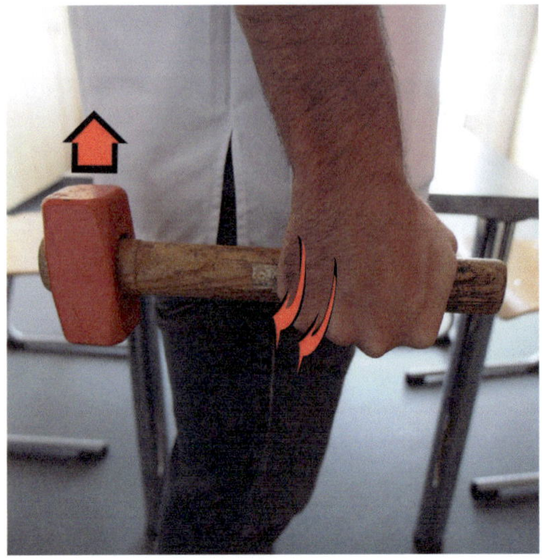

Fig. 11.3 Contraction-release-stretch technique for the flexor carpi ulnaris in case of compression in the forearm. (Picture by Josette Mesplié)

  We use dot-shaped massages, glided pressures, and kneading that improve local trophicity, fight against perineural fibrosis, and relax the muscles adjacent to the nerve.
- *Self-rehabilitation*

  Self-rehabilitation exercises include mobilizations, longitudinal self-massages and cryotherapy.

  The mobilizations are realized several times a day in all the amplitudes of the wrist and elbow to improve the neural gliding.

  The longitudinal massages are realized 3 times a day for 1–2 minutes (until there is a modification of the perception).

➔ Strength Recovery

At this stage of compression, the injuries remain at the stage of neurapraxia or stage 1 of Sunderland. The motor evaluation of Daniels and Worthingham is most often rated 4.

The muscles concerned by the compression of the ulnar nerve in the wrist are the hypothenar muscles, the interossei, the two ulnar lumbricals, the adductor pollicis, and the deep bundle of the flexor pollicis brevis.

In compressions at the level of the elbow, there is also a damage of the flexor carpi ulnaris and the deep flexors of the fourth and fifth fingers.

However, the symptoms can vary and depend on the fibers concerned by the compression.

The strengthening protocol begins with an intermittent static work and progressively evolves towards more intensive exercises depending on the patient's functional needs (see chapter "Rehabilitation of Proprioception" in Volume 1) [11].

- *Flexor carpi ulnaris*

  We ask the patient to realize a flexion and ulnar inclination of the wrist against resistance.
- *Deep flexors of the fourth and fifth fingers*

  The fourth and fifth fingers have a very important role in locking cylindrical prehensions in strength activities.

  We do not strengthen them analytically as the flexion of the distal interphalangeal joint against resistance has no functional interest.

  It is better to realize a more global work of the grasp or exercises based on the locking of cylindrical prehensions during functional activities.
- *Hypothenar muscles*

  We ask the patient to realize a flexion of the metacarpophalangeal joint of the fifth finger against a resistance placed on the palmar side on the first phalanx to strengthen the flexor digiti minimi brevis (Fig. 11.4).

  An abduction of the metacarpophalangeal against a resistance placed on the lateral side of the first phalanx is asked to strengthen the abductor digiti minimi (Fig. 11.5).

  We ask for an anteflexion of the fifth metacarpal against a resistance placed on the palmar side of the metacarpal to strengthen the opponens digiti minimi (Fig. 11.6).
- *Intrinsic muscles*

  We ask the patient to realize a "vise" pinch against manual or instrumental resistance with visual feedback (Fig. 11.7).

  Exercises against resistance for the muscles of the arch of opposition between the thumb and second finger are interesting and can be combined with active electrostimulation (Fig. 11.8).
- *Adductor pollicis*

  We realize an exercise derived from Froment's test.

  The patient realizes an opposition between the tips of his thumb and index with visual feedback, without compensating with the flexor pollicis longus (Fig. 11.9).

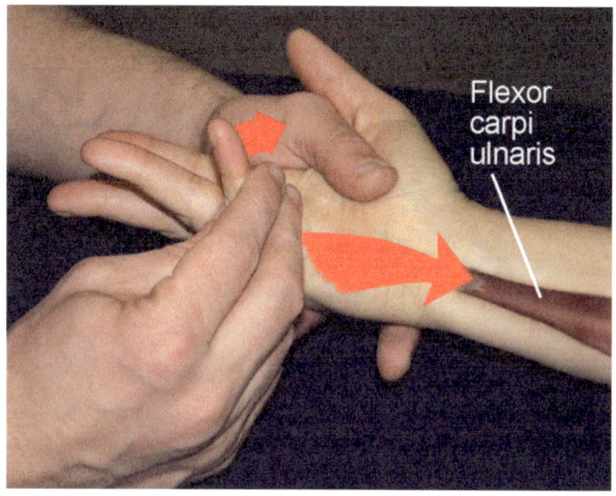

Fig. 11.4 Manual strengthening of the flexor digiti minimi brevis with irradiation towards the flexor carpi ulnaris. (Picture by Josette Mesplié)

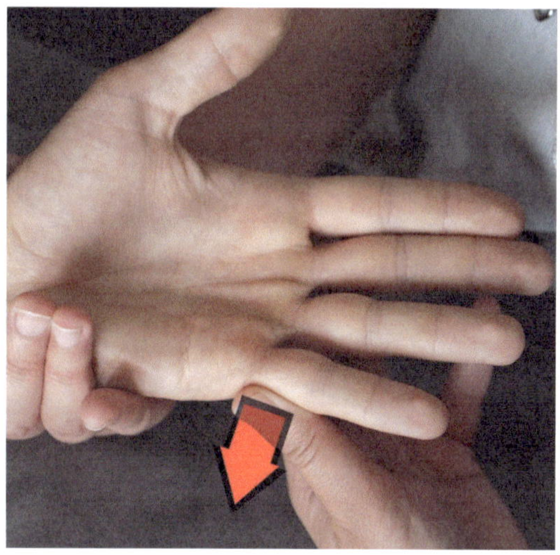

Fig. 11.5 Strengthening of the abductor digiti minimi. (Picture by Josette Mesplié)

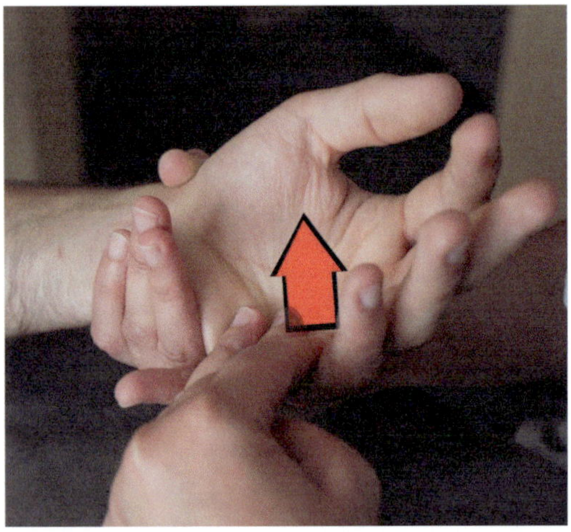

Fig. 11.6 Strengthening of the opponens digiti minimi. (Picture by Josette Mesplié)

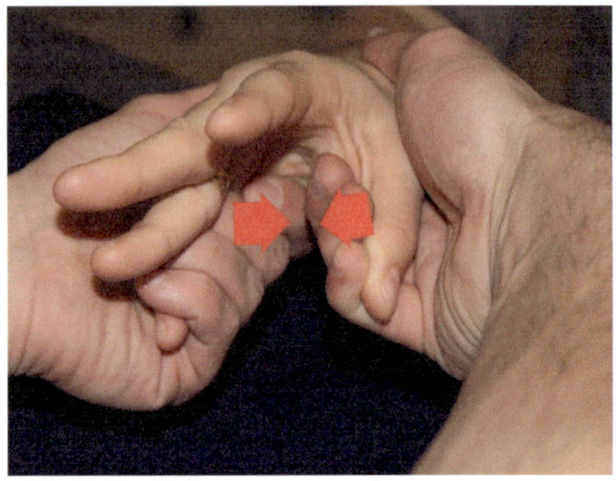

Fig. 11.8 Strengthening of the arch of opposition between the thumb and fifth finger. (Picture by Grégory Mesplié)

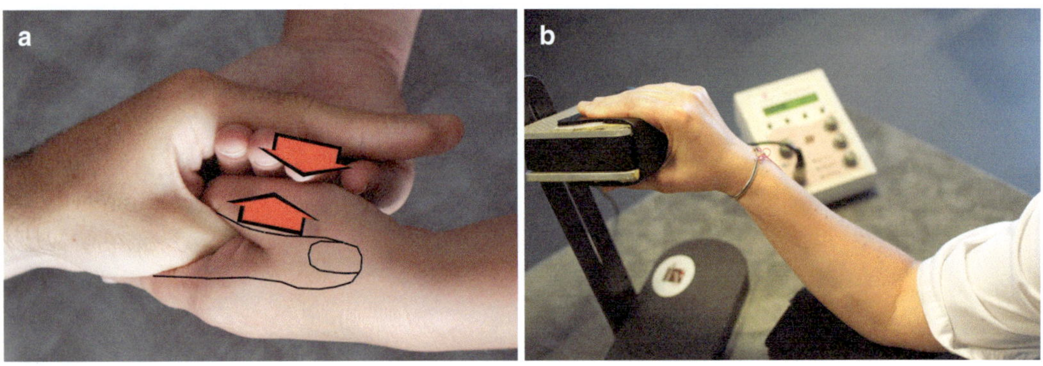

Fig. 11.7 Manual (**a**) and instrumental (**b**) strengthening of the intrinsic muscles with dynamometer and strength captor. (Picture by Grégory Mesplié)

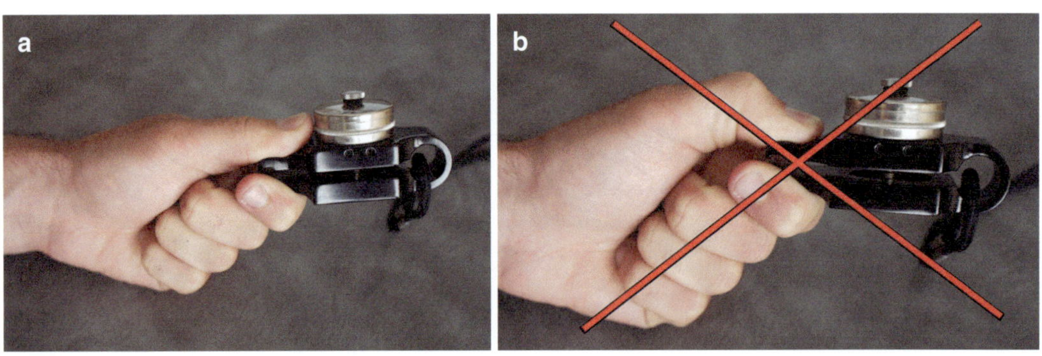

Fig. 11.9 Exercise for the adductor pollicis, derived from Froment's test. The patient must not use the flexor pollicis longus, innervated by the median nerve. (**a**) Correct position using the adductor pollicis. (**b**) Incorrect position using the flexor pollicis longus. (Picture by Grégory Mesplié)

- *Rebalancing the muscle balances*

This strengthening protocol must allow regaining muscular ratios comparable to the healthy side (or to the literature), especially between the intrinsic and extrinsic systems, even if all ratios should be controlled.

The measures are controlled during the regular check-ups realized with dynamometers.

➔ **Rehabilitation of Sensitivity**

Sensory disorders mainly occur on the sensory territory of the ulnar nerve, mostly paresthesia. They are treated according to the protocol defined in the chapter "Physiology and Rehabilitation of Sensorial and Motor Disorders" (Volume 1) [11].

➔ **Proprioception, Coordination, and Dexterity**

Proprioception exercises for the wrist and fingers are realized and improve muscular reactivity as well as coordination in the treated hand.

➔ **Cervical Mobilizations and Strengthening of Scapula Fixators**

In the management of entrapment syndromes, work on the nerve must be combined with a more global approach involving stretching the cervical muscles and strengthening the scapula fixators (see chapter "Neurodynamic Mobilizations" in Volume 1).

Orthosis

Their goal is to rest the nerve when the stage of the injury does not require surgery.

In compressions at the level of the elbow, an orthosis positioning the elbow in a 30° flexion is realized and worn during the night [12]. It avoids a prolonged flexion of the elbow that causes ischemic phenomena and important stretching (Fig. 11.10).

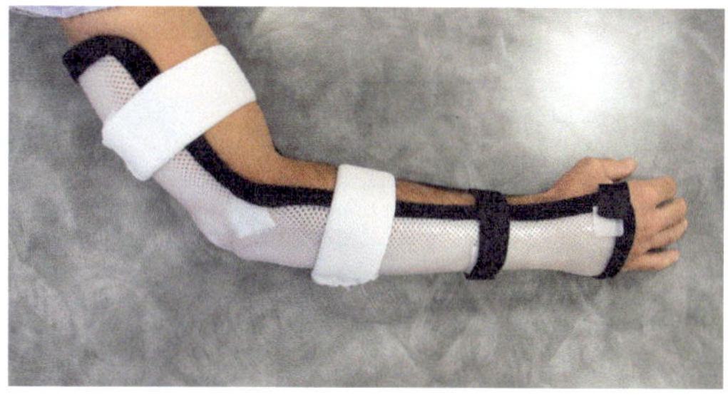

Fig. 11.10 Rest orthosis in case of compression in the elbow, realized in 30° of flexion. (Picture by Grégory Mesplié)

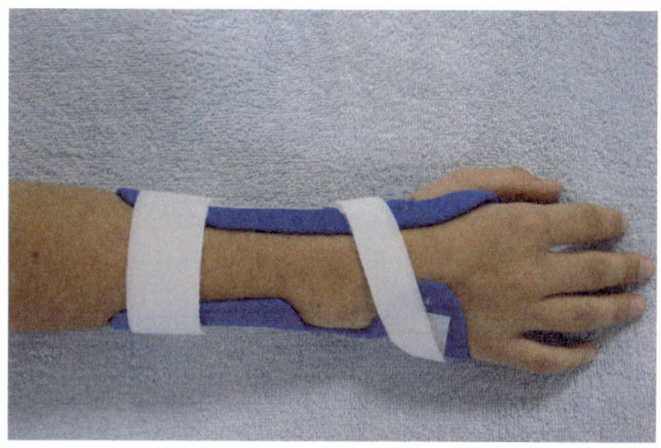

Fig. 11.11 Wrist orthosis in a neutral position in case of compression in the wrist. (Picture by Grégory Mesplié)

In compressions at the level of the Guyon's canal, we realize an orthosis putting the wrist in a neutral position that is kept for 6 weeks (Fig. 11.11).

After Surgery

Rehabilitation (Fig. 11.12)

The main goal of the postoperative rehabilitation is to fight against perineural fibrosis that can have important functional consequences.

Therefore, rehabilitation starts early or even immediately and is based on soft and progressive mobilizations in all the amplitudes of the wrist and elbow.

Operated entrapment syndrome of the ulnar nerve		
	Postoperative phase (A)	Healing phase (B)
REHABILITATION	**Therapeutic goals :** 1. Fight against inflammation and pain 2. Prevent stiffness in the wrist and elbow 3. Self-rehabilitation **Techniques:** 1. Transcutaneous vibratory stimulations, cryotherapy, disto-proximal pressotherapy, TENS (100 Hz), analgesic and draining massages around the scar 2. Passive, then simple active mobilizations without resistance and under the pain threshold for the wrist, elbow and fingers **Risks:** CRPS	**Therapeutic goals :** 1. Same as in phase (A) if necessary 2. Relaxation of the scar and exercises for the mobility of the nerve 3. Progressive recovery of the grasp (from D21) 4. Rehabilitation of sensitivity **Techniques:** 2. Scar massages against fibrosis (± ultrasounds), progressive and pain-free Butler mobilization. 3. Progressive strengthening of the hypothenar muscles, the flexor carpi ulnaris and the adductor pollicis 4. Sensory stimulations, prehension, coordination and dexterity exercises **Risks:** same + lack of intrinsic strength
ORTHOSIS	Resting orthosis for the elbow in 30° of flexion (compression in the elbow) Orthosis for the wrist in a neutral position (compression in the wrist)	Functional orthosis if necessary
	D3-D21	After D21

Fig. 11.12 Postoperative rehabilitation protocol. (Picture by Josette Mesplié)

➔ Immediate Postoperative Phase (D3 to D21)

In this phase, the most important is to fight against trophic disorders and pain, and soft mobilizations of the wrist and elbow.

- *Fight against trophic disorders and pain*

  It is based on the combination of cryotherapy, pressotherapy, analgesic vibrotherapy, and draining and relaxing massages that improve local trophicity and symptomatology.
- *Mobilizations of the elbow, wrist, and fingers*

  Passive then active mobilizations are realized from the joint farther away from the compression site towards the closest joint.

  For example, to liberate the ulnar nerve in the elbow, we mobilize first the fingers, then the wrist, and we end with the elbow in all the amplitudes and without pain.

  It maintains joint mobility and perineural glidings.
- *Self-rehabilitation*

  Self-rehabilitation exercises based on self-mobilizations of the elbow and wrist and icing are described to the patient.

  The mobilizations of the fingers, wrist, and elbow are repeated in all the amplitudes if there is no pain or swelling. We ask for 10 repetitions for each movement of each mobilized segment. Icing is realized for 20 minutes, 3 times a day with an ice bag in a damp cloth. Ideally, the edematous area should be placed in an elevated position for the duration of the icing process.

➔ Healing Phase (After D21)

In this phase we keep fighting against trophic disorders and pain if necessary. We also fight against healing disorders and perineural fibrosis and try to recover strength and sensitivity in the ulnar part of the hand.

- *Fight against perineural fibrosis*

  Healing disorders can cause important fibrosis, with consequences that can disturb the hand's functions.
  - ***Massages around the scar and in fibrosis areas***

    These massages aim to improve perineural trophicity, relax the scar, and limit the risks of fibrosis around the scar.

    They are realized around the scar, along the internal part of the arm and forearm, and at the level of the hypothenar muscles. We use disto-proximal glided pressures and soft kneading in the arm and forearm, and glided pressures at the level of the hypothenar muscles.

– ***Ultrasounds***

Once the scar is closed, we use ultrasounds to fight against adherences around the scar. The ideal frequency is 1 MHz whether the surgery is in the wrist or elbow.

We prefer using the pulse mode that has a "fibrolytic" effect.

The head is applied at the level of the scar and in its immediate vicinity, corresponding to the surgical release zone.

– ***Depressotherapy***

Its application must be cautious and progressive.

We start using it after the scar is closed.

First, when the scar is still inflammatory, we apply the head of the device far from the scar in a disto-proximal direction.

When the scar is not inflammatory anymore, we apply the head directly on it if the patient tolerates it.

– ***Mobilization of the ulnar nerve***

These techniques have already been described in the paragraph about rehabilitation without surgery. They are realized after surgical advice that defines if the state of the nerve observed during surgery allows us to use these techniques.

Clinically, it is most often patients with nocturnal paresthesia without any other neurological disorder.

– ***Longitudinal massage***

It is realized with the same modalities than in the rehabilitation without surgery.

It is first applied far from the operated area, then getting closer to this area if the scar is not inflammatory or painful.

• *Strength recovery*

Surgery in entrapment syndromes of the ulnar nerve concerns nervous injuries that are not beyond stage 2 of Sunderland (axonotmesis) and that can cause motor disorders rated between 2 and 4 on the scale of Daniels and Worthingham described in the chapter "Physiology and Rehabilitation of Sensorial and Motor Disorders" (Volume 1).

– ***Stage 2***

This stage corresponds with the ability to mobilize the concerned segment in all its amplitude without gravity or in part of the amplitude against gravity.

We ask the patient to realize simple active contractions if the mobilization is not against gravity and active-assisted contractions against gravity.

This exercise improves the trophic state of the muscle and maintains the glidings in the different anatomical planes.

– ***Stage 3***

This stage corresponds with the ability to mobilize the concerned segment in all its amplitudes against gravity.

This exercise has the same interest as the one for stage 2, but here we can start an intermittent static exercise against gravity and alternate the types of contraction depending on the patient's abilities.

– ***Stage 4***

In this stage we realize strengthening exercises against increasing resistances, alternating the types of contraction.

The exercises are like the ones realized in the rehabilitation without surgery.

• *Rehabilitation of sensitivity*

Sensory disorders can persist several weeks after surgery, especially in advanced stages.

They can concern the whole sensory territory of the ulnar nerve in compressions at the level of the elbow, but compressions in the Guyon's do not only concern the back of the hand as it is innervated by the dorsal branch that does not pass through this canal (Fig. 11.13).

The rehabilitation protocol is realized according to the modalities described in chapter "Physiology and Rehabilitation of Sensorial and Motor Disorders" (Volume 1).

• *Proprioception, coordination, and dexterity*

Like in the rehabilitation without surgery, these exercises allow the patient to regain coordination and dexterity according to his functional needs.

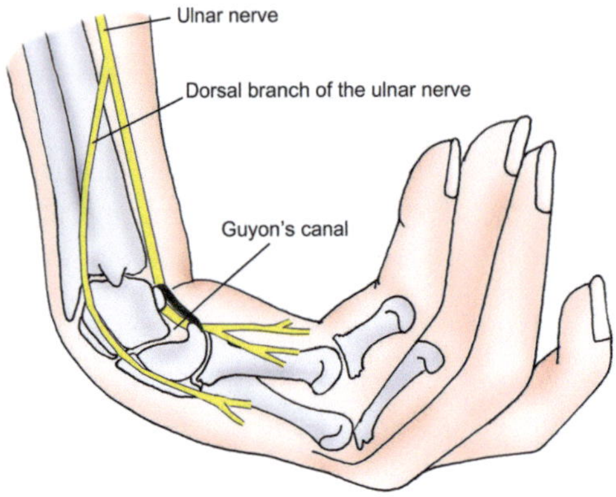

Fig. 11.13 Compressions of the ulnar nerve in Guyon's canal do not cause sensory disorders in the back of the hand, which depends on the dorsal branch. (Picture by Josette Mesplié)

We especially insist on exercises for strong cylindrical grips that suffer a greater deficit in this type of injuries.

Orthotic Treatment

Postoperative orthoses are not systematic but can be useful in case of important pain. As for the conservative treatment, they can be orthoses with the elbow in a 30° flexion or the wrist in a neutral position, depending on the site of surgery.

They are kept for 15 days, but the patient gets self-mobilization recommendations that he must realize every hour to limit the risks of perineural fibrosis and stiffness

Bibliography

1. Park IJ, et al. Cubital tunnel syndrome caused by anconeus epitrochlearis muscle. J Korean Neurosurg Soc. 2018;61(5):618–24.
2. Rioux-Forker D, Bridgeman J, Brogan DM. Snapping triceps syndrome. J Hand Surg Am. 2018;43(1):90.e1–5.
3. Novak CB, et al. Provocative testing for cubital tunnel syndrome. J Hand Surg. 1994;19(5):817–20.
4. Hutchison RL, Rayan G. Diagnosis of cubital tunnel syndrome. J Hand Surg Am. 2011;36(9):1519–21.
5. Palmer BA, Hughes TB. Cubital tunnel syndrome. J Hand Surg Am. 2010;35(1):153–63.
6. Matzon JL, et al. Risk factors for ulnar nerve instability resulting in transposition in patients with cubital tunnel syndrome. J Hand Surg Am. 2016;41(2):180–3.
7. Wolny T, et al. Effect of manual therapy and neurodynamic techniques vs ultrasound and laser on 2PD in patients with CTS: a randomized controlled trial. J Hand Ther. 2016;29(3):235–45.
8. Le Roux P. Syndrome du canal carpien et mobilisation des nerfs. Kinésithérapie, la revue. 2007;2007(68–69):49–52.
9. Lundborg G, Rydevik BL. Effects of stretching the tibial nerve of the rabbit: preliminary study of the intraneural circulation of the barrier function of the perineurium. J Bone Joint Surg Br. 1973;55:390–401.
10. Coppieters MW, Butler DS. Do 'sliders' slide and 'tensioners' tension? An analysis of neurodynamic techniques and considerations regarding their application. Man Ther. 2008;13(3):213–21.
11. Mesplié G. Thérapie de la main, examen clinique et outils de prise en charge rééducative avancée du poignet et de la main. Sauramps Médical; 2021.
12. Lund AT, Amadio PC. Treatment of cubital tunnel syndrome: perspectives for the therapist. J Hand Ther. 2006;19(2):170–8.

12 Entrapment Syndromes of the Radial Nerve

Grégory Mesplié and Olivier Léger

Entrapment syndromes of the radial nerve can occur in the elbow or wrist (Fig. 12.1), with symptoms that can be mistaken for tendon damage.

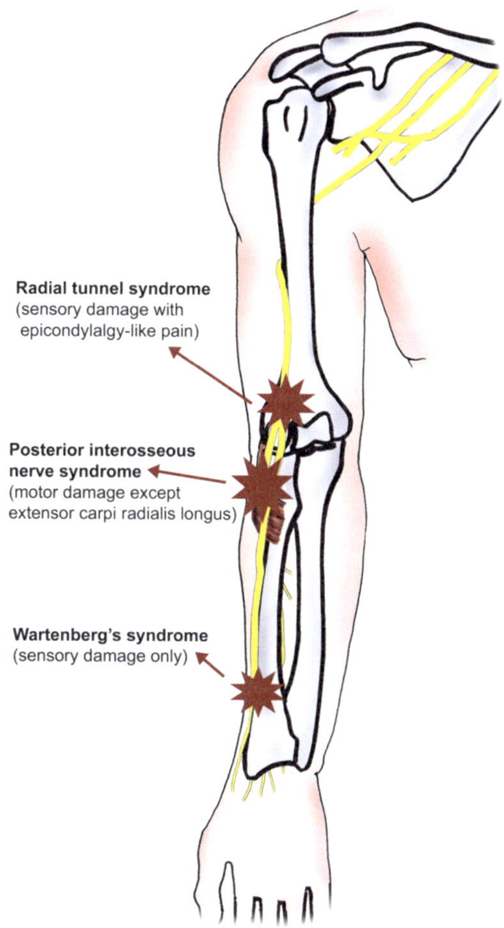

Fig. 12.1 Compression sites of the radial nerve and their symptomatologies. (Picture by Josette Mesplié)

G. Mesplié (✉) · O. Léger
Institut Sud Aquitain de la Main et du Membre Supérieur (ISAMMS), Biarritz, France

G. Mesplié (ed.), *Hand Functional Anatomy and Therapy*,
https://doi.org/10.1007/978-3-031-92505-4_12

Compression in the Humeral Groove

A radial palsy at this level can be secondary to three mechanisms:

- A traumatic damage caused by a fracture of the distal third of the humerus, which requires an exploration during the osteosynthesis.
- An extrinsic compression because of a prolonged pressure or an over-inflated tourniquet kept for too long.
- There are also "spontaneous" palsies corresponding to anatomical structures fixing the nerve to the distal part of the groove and causing mechanical conflicts during prolonged repetitive movements. This could lead to a surgical exploration if the patient does not show signs of recovery after 2 months, with a disturbed EMG.

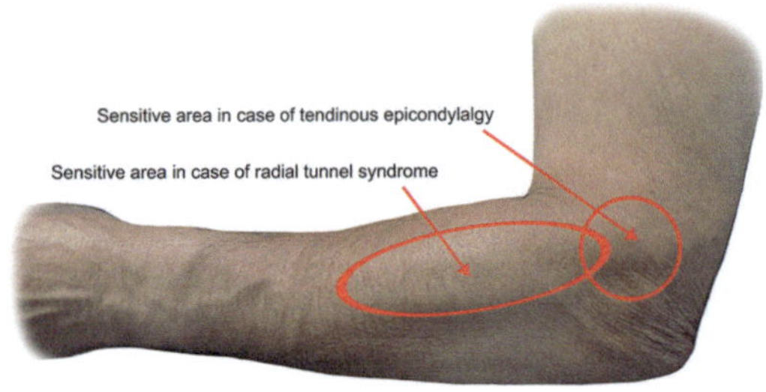

Fig. 12.2 Typical localization of pain with tendinous origin and pain with radial origin in the case of a radial tunnel syndrome. (Picture by Josette Mesplié)

Compression in the Elbow

In the elbow, the radial nerve is subjected to stretching and twisting constraints in flexo-extension and prono-supination.

There are two distinguishable symptomatologies.

Radial Tunnel Syndrome

It corresponds to a compression of the radial nerve in the radial tunnel, between the humeroradial joint and its emergence from the supinator [1].

There is pain at the level of the epicondyle, which can spread until the wrist without sensorimotor disorders (Fig. 12.2).

Pain is increased by movements of extension and supination. The differential diagnosis with epicondylitis requires a meticulous assessment as pain is located at approximately 5 cm below the epicondyle [2].

The Cozen test can be used to make a differential diagnosis. It consists in requesting a contraction against resistance in wrist extension with a closed fist, forearm in pronation, and elbow bent at 90°. It is positive in the case of tendon damage [3], which does not rule out concomitant radial nerve or radicular damage [4].

A conservative treatment will always be recommended at first, along with rest, adaptation of the workstation and orthosis, NSAIDs, and muscle relaxants.

After an observation period of 3 months, surgery will be proposed with opening of the superficial bundle of the supinator and the deep part of the extensor carpi radialis brevis. An orthosis is given to the patient for 2 to 3 weeks, with the wrist in a 20° extension.

Posterior Interosseous Nerve Syndrome

It corresponds to the compression of the posterior interosseous nerve at the level of the supinator arch [5].

It causes a more or less partial loss of the wrist and finger extension that gets worse over time and can be secondary to repetitive movements in patients who have an anatomical predisposition (thick arcade of Fröhse) or a tumor.

An MRI allows the identification of swellings compressing the nerve, and an EMG is always realized to confirm the increase of the distal motor latency and the muscular integrity.

With surgery, we can realize a neurolysis of the posterior interosseous nerve in its entire pathway along the supinator, followed by 15 days of immobilization before starting the rehabilitation.

Compression in the Wrist

Wartenberg's syndrome is the compression of the sensory branch of the radial nerve between the brachioradialis and the extensor carpi radialis longus tendons, in pronation and ulnar inclination of the wrist.

The EMG confirms the diagnosis, comparing the sensorial conduction speed with the opposite side.

The treatment consists in resting the wrist in a 20° extension with an orthosis immobilizing the thumb, removing the watchband, and an adaptation of professional and sports movements, combined with appropriate rehabilitation.

If the medical treatment fails, surgery allows excising at least 6 cm of the fascia between the brachioradialis and the extensor carpi radialis longus.

Rehabilitation and Orthotic Treatment

Without Surgery

As for the median and ulnar nerves, this treatment concerns moderate damages of the nerve without important sensory and motor disorders. Its goal is to delay or even avoid surgery [6].

Rehabilitation

- *Fight against inflammation and pain*

  It is based on a combination of cryotherapy, pressotherapy, and draining massages that can help decrease the perineural inflammation.

  In the case of neurogenic pain (mechanosensitivity) and neuropathic pain (without allodynia), fasciatherapy techniques combined with taping can have very interesting effects. The therapist moves the skin in different directions and, if an improvement in symptoms is observed, applies a tape reproducing the maneuver performed [7] (Fig. 12.3).

  Scottish baths (or contrast baths) have not been shown to be effective, either before or after surgery [8].

- *Longitudinal massage*

  This massage is applied at the level of the accessible area of the nerve closest to the damaged area.

  It consists in realizing a longitudinal pressure along 3 to 4 cm of the nerve, to improve its vascularization and restart the axonal flow.

  The ideal pressure recreates the distal symptomatology, without producing pain. It is maintained a few minutes, which allows obtaining a variation of the initial symptoms.

  For compressions in the humeral groove, the patient is placed in decubitus. The therapist grabs the posterior side of the elbow with one hand and looks for an area of induration in the lateral side of the arm with the other hand. We apply a "coma" movement to follow the path of the radial nerve. The association of internal and external rotations of the arm effectively participates in this exercise.

  For compressions in the elbow, the patient is in decubitus. The therapist maintains the forearm with one hand and places his thumb across, slightly above the flexion crease of the elbow, on its lateral side. He realizes the longitudinal massage with his thumb or alternates flexion/extension movements of the elbow, with the thumb still.

  The radial nerve can also be manipulated 5 cm below the epicondyle, which is a particularly painful area in radial tunnel syndromes. The patient is in the same position as before, and the therapist grabs the forearm with both hands so that his thumbs contact with the painful area and the elbow in a 100° flexion. He applies the longitudinal massage on the radial nerve with his thumbs or alternates flexion/extension movements of the elbow with the thumb still.

  For compressions in the wrist, the patient is in the same position and the therapist realizes longitudinal massages at the level of the emergence of the superficial branch of the radial nerve.

  We can also mobilize the nerve alternating radial and ulnar inclinations, thumb still.

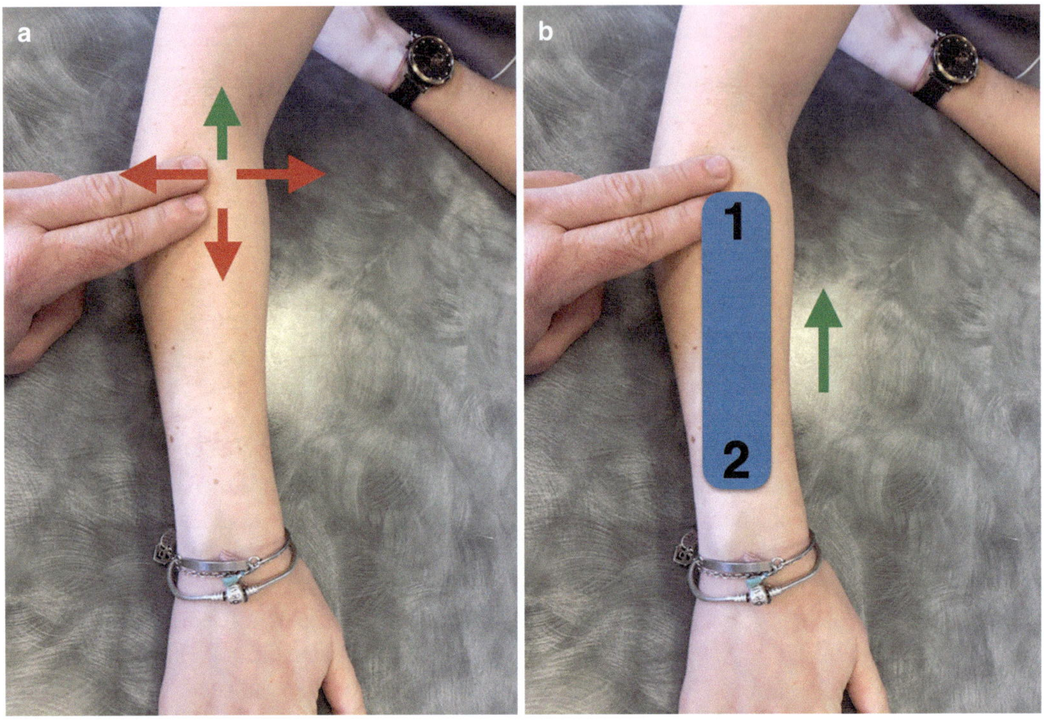

Fig. 12.3 (1) Clock test: the therapist creates cutaneous displacements to improve the symptomatology at rest or during movement (green arrow). (2) The therapist can place a Tape to reproduce the tension applied manually. (Picture by Josette Mesplié)

- *Fight against perineural fibrosis*

  These exercises improve glidings between the median nerve and the adjacent tissues, which limits the compressive constraints and improves vascularization.

  – *Nerve mobilizations*

    The goal of the nerve mobilizations is to mobilize the radial nerve with respect to the adjacent tissues to limit the risks of compression and ischemia [9–11].

    We avoid the Upper Limb Tension Tests, described by Butler in 1991. These maneuvers are diagnostic, not therapeutic.

    In fact, nerves do not tolerate stretching well: an 8% stretching causes venous obstruction, a 15% stretching causes ischemia, and a 20% stretching causes nerve rupture [12].

    We therefore prefer gliding maneuvers, which allow twice more excursion than tension maneuvers, with 8.5 times less tension [13] (Fig. 12.4) (see chapter "Neurodynamic Mobilizations" in Volume 1).

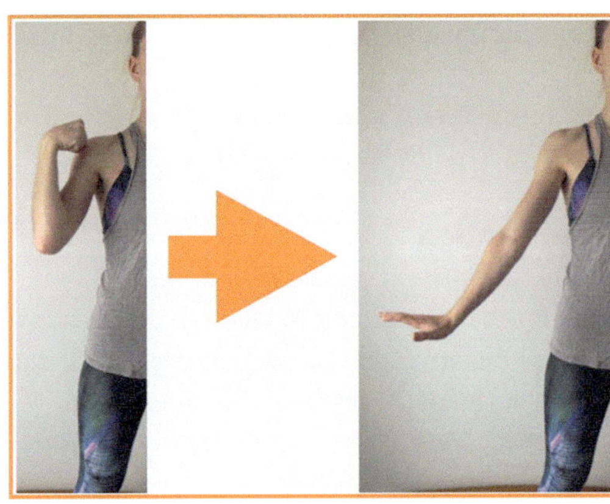

Fig. 12.4 Gliding without tension of the radial nerve. Elbow flexion and supination, wrist and fingers flexion. Elbow extension and pronation, wrist and fingers extension. (Picture by Coline Geoffroy)

  – *Mobilizations of the tissues adjacent to the nerve*

    Alternating contraction-relaxation-stretching of the adjacent muscles allows a perineural pumping that improves local trophicity and maintains the inter-tissue glidings.

These mobilizations are realized preferentially on the supinator muscle in posterior interosseous nerve syndromes, on the brachialis and brachioradialis in radial tunnel syndromes, and on the brachioradialis and extensor carpi radialis longus in Wartenberg's syndromes.

Each step is maintained for 4 to 6 s to avoid any ischemic risk.

Imitation exercises improving movements between the different gliding planes participate in this fight against perineural fibrosis.

- *Massages against fibrosis*

  They are realized along the radial nerve, on the posterior and lateral parts of the forearm and hand.

  We use dot-shaped massages, glided pressures and kneading that improve local trophicity, fight against perineural fibrosis, and relax the muscles adjacent to the nerve.

  Massages are extended proximally to the brachial level and up to the cervical spine.

- *Self-rehabilitation*

  Self-rehabilitation exercises include mobilizations, longitudinal self-massages, and cryotherapy.

  The mobilizations are realized several times a day in all the amplitudes of the wrist and elbow to improve the neural gliding.

  The longitudinal massages are realized three times a day for 1–2 min (until there is a modification of the perception).

• *Strength recovery*

At this level of compression, the injuries are not beyond the stage of neurapraxia or stage 1 of Sunderland. The motor assessment of Daniels and Worthingham is most often 4.

The muscles concerned by the compression of the radial nerve in posterior interosseous nerve syndromes are the extensor carpi radialis brevis, the supinator, the extensor carpi ulnaris, the extensor digitorum, the extensor digiti minimi, the abductor pollicis longus, the extensor pollicis longus, the extensor pollicis brevis, and the extensor indicis. The extensor carpi radialis longus is not damaged in these injuries, which explains why the wrist goes spontaneously to a slight radial inclination in complete palsies of the posterior interosseous nerve.

The radial tunnel syndrome and Wartenberg's syndrome do not cause any motor disorder.

The strengthening protocol begins with an intermittent static work and progressively evolves towards more intensive exercises depending on the patient's functional needs (see chapter "Rehabilitation of Proprioception" in Volume 1).

- *Wrist extensors*

  The main functional role of these muscles is to place the wrist in a 30° extension during strong grips, when the finger flexors are inefficient. This should be considered when realizing strengthening exercises.

  Strengthening protocols will therefore take this element into account, with static or stato-eccentric exercises intensified in this amplitude sector.

  Other contractile modes and amplitude sectors are also targeted, with greater or lesser intensity depending on the patient's functional needs.

  These exercises can be realized against a manual resistance, more on the radial or ulnar side (Fig. 12.5).

  The priority is to strengthen the extensor carpi ulnaris in the case of spontaneous

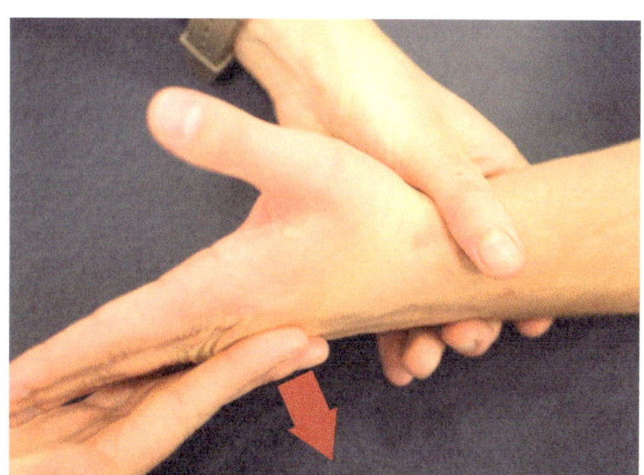

Fig. 12.5 Manual strengthening of the extensor muscles of the wrist. (Picture by Grégory Mesplié)

radial deviation of the wrist, because of the extensor carpi radialis longus that is not damaged in posterior interosseous nerve syndromes related to a compression in the arcade of Fröhse.

Exercises with an elastic band fixed to an espalier allow alternating the contractile modes. We also use visual feedback to control the duration of contraction and rest (Fig. 12.6).

We can favor the radial or the ulnar component in this exercise, but we prefer asking for a "pure" extension for a synergic exercise. Exercises with weights allow the same type of exercises, also working with a strong cylindrical prehension (Fig. 12.7).

– *Extensors of the fingers*

They are not "strong" muscles but participate in cylindrical prehensions as they open the hand and therefore allow the flexors to be efficient.

Exercises for these muscles can be realized manually with a resistance on the dorsal side of the first phalanx of the fingers we work with (a resistance on the second and third phalanges strengthens the interossei, innervated by the ulnar nerve) (Fig. 12.8).

An exercise for the index or the fifth finger only allows working analytically with the extensor indicis or the extensor digiti minimi (Fig. 12.9).

Instrumental exercises are also possible.

– *Global exercises*

Exercises for the fingers with visual feedback are used and are synergic exercises for the wrist and finger extensors (Fig. 12.10).

- *Proprioception, coordination, and dexterity*

Proprioception exercises for the wrist and fingers are realized and improve muscular reactivity as well as coordination in the treated hand.

- *Rehabilitation of sensitivity*

Sensorial disorders only occur if the superficial branch of the radial nerve is damaged (Wartenberg's syndrome). They are treated according to the protocol defined in chapter "Physiology and Rehabilitation of Sensorial and Motor Disorders" (Volume 1).

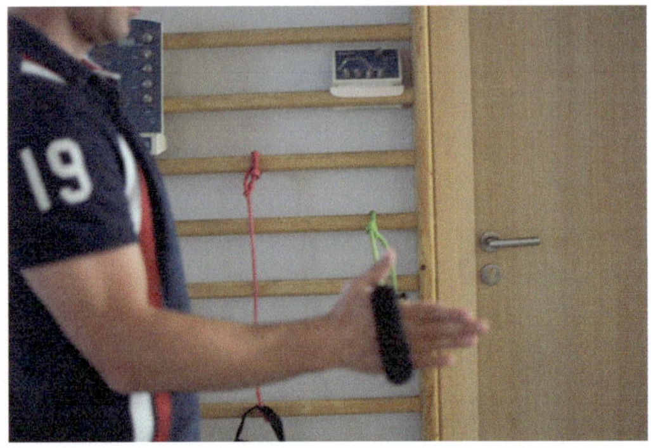

Fig. 12.6 Strengthening of the extensor muscles of the wrist with an elastic band, combined with visual feedback. (Picture by Grégory Mesplié)

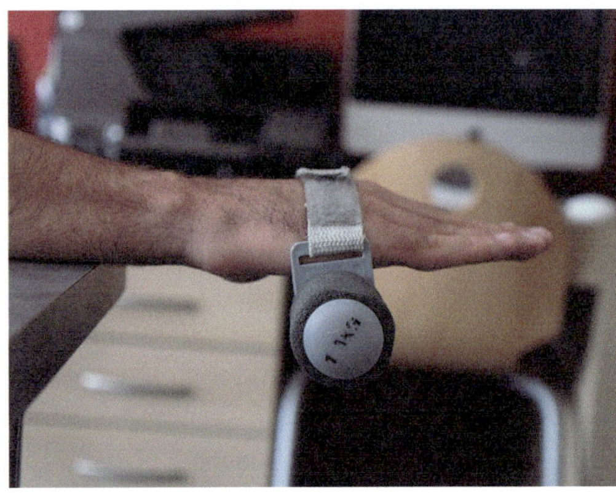

Fig. 12.7 Strengthening of the extensor muscles of the wrist with weight. (Picture by Grégory Mesplié)

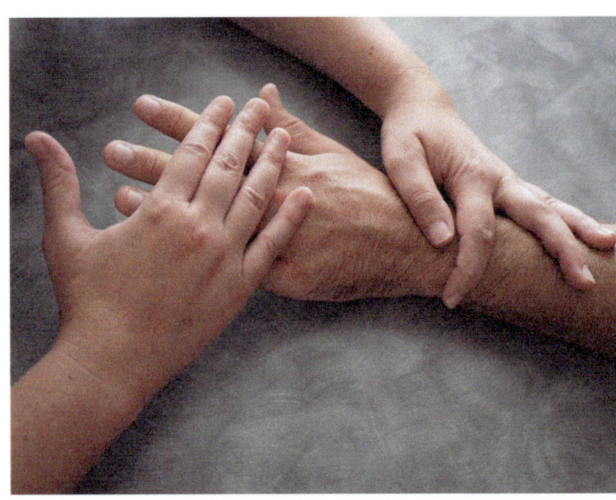

Fig. 12.8 Manual exercise for the extensor digitorum. (Picture by Grégory Mesplié)

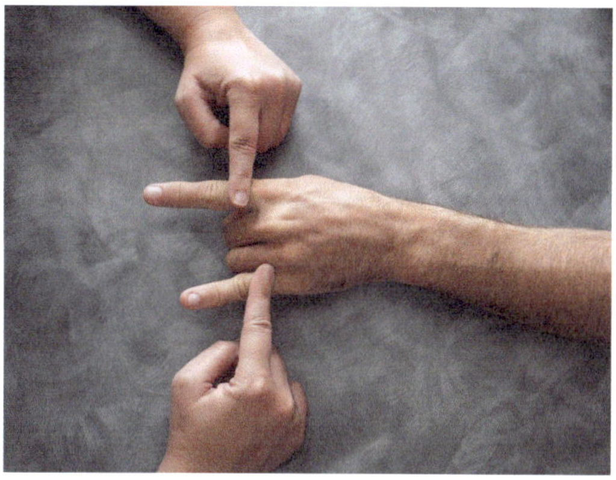

Fig. 12.9 Exercise for the extensor indicis and extensor digiti minimi. (Picture by Grégory Mesplié)

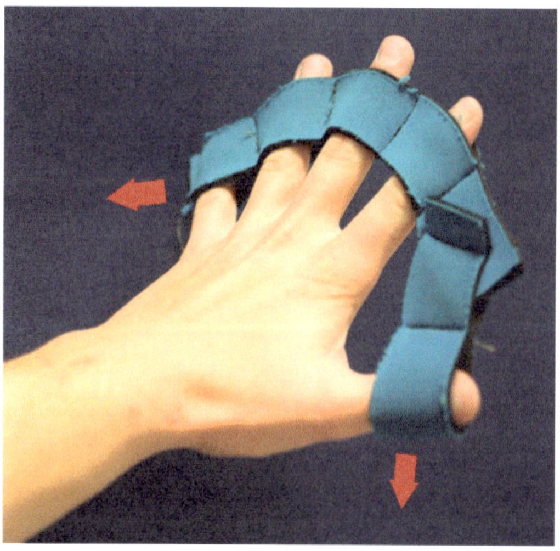

Fig. 12.10 Synergic exercise for the extensors of the fingers and wrist. (Picture by Grégory Mesplié)

- *Cervical mobilizations and strengthening of scapula fixators*

  In the management of entrapment syndromes, work on the nerve must be combined with a more global approach involving stretching the cervical muscles and strengthening the scapula fixators (see chapter "Neurodynamic Mobilizations" in Volume 1).

Orthoses

For compressions in the elbow, resting orthoses are used, placing the wrist in a 20° extension for 6 weeks to 3 months. They are worn at night.

If no clinical improvement is observed within this timeframe, surgery is proposed.

For Wartenberg's syndrome, immobilization orthoses are used for the wrist and thumb (free interphalangeal joint). Particular attention must be paid to the radial side of the cast, to avoid any contact with the superficial branch of the radial nerve.

After Surgery

Rehabilitation (Fig. 12.11)

The main goal is to fight against perineural fibrosis that can have important functional consequences.

Therefore, the rehabilitation starts early or even immediately and is based on soft and progressive mobilizations in all the amplitudes of the wrist and elbow.

- *Immediate postoperative phase (D3 to D21)*
  - *Fight against trophic disorders and pain*

    It is based on the combination of cryotherapy, pressotherapy, analgesic vibrotherapy, and draining and relaxing massages that improve local trophicity and symptomatology.
  - *Mobilizations of the wrist and elbow*

    Passive then active mobilizations are realized from the joint farther away from the compression site, towards the closest joint.

    For example, to liberate the radial nerve in the elbow, we first mobilize the fingers, then the wrist, and we end with the elbow in all its amplitudes, without pain.

    It maintains joint mobility and perineural glidings.
  - *Self-rehabilitation*

    Self-rehabilitation exercises based on self-mobilizations of the elbow and wrist and icing are described to the patient.

    The mobilizations of the fingers, wrist, and elbow are repeated in all their amplitudes if there is no pain or swelling. We ask for 10 repetitions for each movement of each mobilized segment.

    Icing is realized for 20 min, 3 times a day with an ice bag in a damp cloth. Ideally,

Operated entrapment syndrome of the radial nerve		
	Postoperative phase (A)	Healing phase (B)
REHABILITATION	**Therapeutic goals** : 1. Fight against inflammation and pain 2. Prevent stiffness in the wrist and elbow 3. Self-rehabilitation **Techniques:** 1. Transcutaneous vibratory stimulations, cryotherapy, disto-proximal pressotherapy, TENS (100 Hz), analgesic and draining massages around the scar 2. Passive, then simple active mobilizations without resistance and under the pain threshold for the wrist and elbow **Risks:** CRPS	**Therapeutic goals** : 1. Same as in phase (A) if necessary 2. Relaxation of the scar and exercices for the mobility of the nerve 3. Progressive recovery of the grasp (from D21) 4. Rehabilitation of sensitivity **Techniques:** 2. Scar massages against fibrosis (± ultrasounds), progressive and pain-free Butler mobilization 3. Progressive strengthening of the wrist and fingers extensors 4. Sensory stimulations, prehension, coordination and dexterity exercises. **Risks:** same + deficit of the extensors
ORTHOSIS	Resting orthosis for the wrist in 20° of extension (compression in the elbow), Orthosis for the wrist and thumb (compression in the wrist)	Functional orthosis if necessary
	D3-D21	After D21

Fig. 12.11 Protocol after surgery. (Picture by Josette Mesplié)

the edematous area should be placed in an elevated position for the duration of the icing process.

- *Healing phase (after D21)*

  In this phase we keep fighting against trophic disorders and pain if necessary. We also fight against healing disorders and perineural fibrosis and try to recover strength and sensitivity in the radial part of the hand.

  – *Fight against perineural fibrosis*

    Healing disorders can cause important fibrosis, with consequences that can disturb the hand's functions.

    (i) *Massages around the scar and in fibrosis areas*

    These massages aim to improve perineural trophicity, relax the scar, and limit the risks of fibrosis around the scar.

    They are realized around the scar and along the nerve's pathway. We use disto-proximal glided pressures and soft kneading in the arm and forearm, and glided pressures at the level of the posterior and external part of the hand.

    (ii) *Ultrasounds*

    Once the scar is closed, we use ultrasounds to fight against adherences around the scar. The ideal frequency is 1 MHz whether the surgery is in the wrist or elbow.

    We prefer using the pulse mode that has a "fibrolytic" effect.

    The head is applied at the level of the scar and in its immediate vicinity, corresponding to the surgical release zone.

    (iii) *Depressotherapy*

    Its application must be cautious and progressive.

    We start using it after the scar is closed.

    First, when the scar is still inflammatory, we apply the head of the device far from the scar in a disto-proximal direction.

    When the scar is not inflammatory anymore, we apply the head directly on it if the patient tolerates it.

    (iv) *Mobilization of the radial nerve*

    These techniques have already been described in the paragraph about rehabilitation without surgery. They are realized after surgical advice that defines if the state of the nerve observed during surgery allows us to use these techniques.

Clinically, it is most often patients with nocturnal paresthesia without any other neurological disorder.

(v) *Longitudinal massage*

It is realized with the same modalities than in the rehabilitation without surgery.

It is first applied far from the operated area, then getting closer to this area if the scar is not inflammatory or painful.

– *Strength recovery*

Surgery in entrapment syndromes of the radial nerve concerns nervous injuries that are not beyond stage 2 of Sunderland (axonotmesis) and that can cause motor disorders rated between 2 and 4 on the scale of Daniels and Worthingham described in the chapter "Physiology and Rehabilitation of Sensorial and Motor Disorders" (Volume 1).

The radial tunnel syndrome and Wartenberg's syndrome are not associated with any motor disorders, and the muscles involved in posterior interosseous nerve syndrome are described in the "Without Surgery" paragraph.

(vi) *Stage 2*

This stage corresponds with the ability to mobilize the concerned segment in all its amplitude without gravity or in part of the amplitude against gravity.

We ask the patient to realize simple active contractions if the mobilization is not against gravity and active-assisted contractions against gravity.

This exercise improves the trophic state of the muscle and maintains the glidings in the different anatomical planes.

This active-assisted work can be performed on the arthromotor, mobilizing the wrist and/or fingers (Fig. 12.12).

(vii) *Stage 3*

This stage corresponds with the ability to mobilize the concerned segment in all its amplitudes against gravity.

This exercise has the same interest as the one for stage 2, but here we can start an intermittent static exercise against gravity and alternate the types of contraction depending on the patient's abilities (Fig. 12.13).

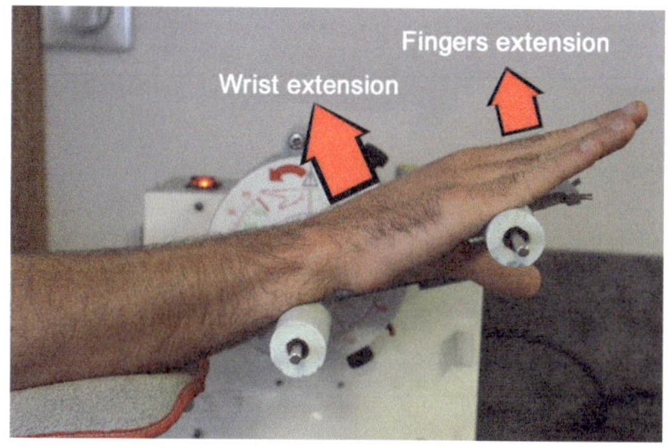

Fig. 12.12 Active assisted exercise in extension for the wrist and/or fingers on an arthromotor device. (Picture by Josette Mesplié)

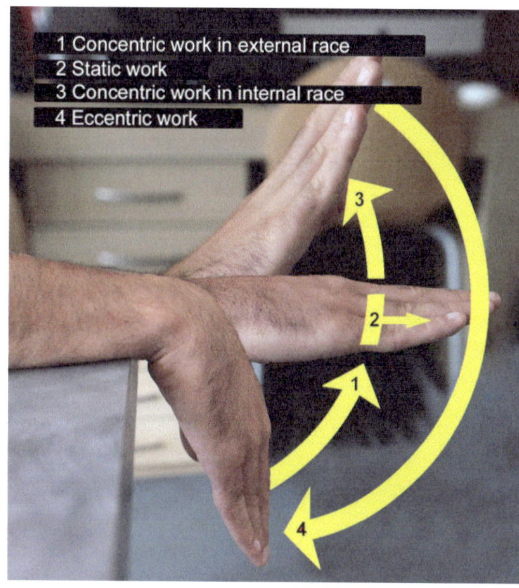

Fig. 12.13 Exercise against gravity for the extensors of the wrist and fingers with different types of contractions. The patient realizes an extension of the wrist and fingers from a wrist flexion (concentric exercise in external race), maintains the neutral position a few seconds (static exercise), keeps extending the wrist (concentric exercise in internal race), then slows down when returning in flexion (eccentric exercise). (Picture by Josette Mesplié)

(viii) *Stage 4*

The exercises are like the ones realized in the rehabilitation without surgery.

– *Proprioception, coordination, and dexterity*

These exercises can be realized when the muscles are graded 4 and are identical to the ones realized without surgery.

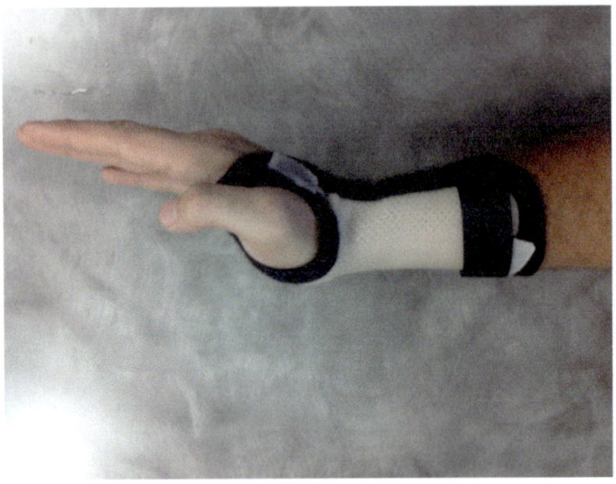

Fig. 12.14 Orthosis after surgery in the elbow, placing the wrist in 20° of extension, kept between 15 days and 3 weeks depending on the associated surgical gestures. (Picture by Grégory Mesplié)

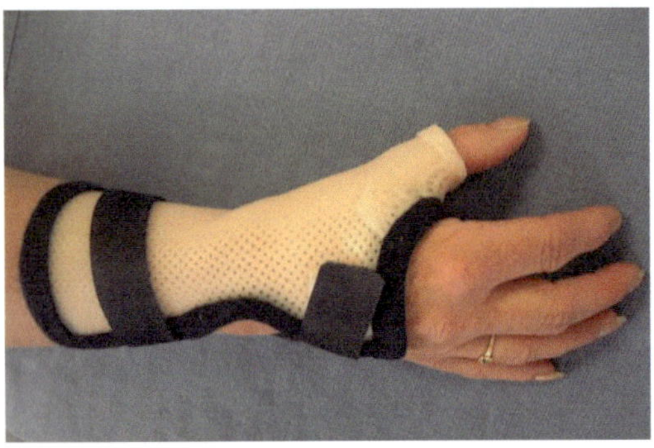

Fig. 12.15 Orthosis after surgery in the elbow, putting the wrist and thumb in a neutral position, kept 1 week. (Picture by Grégory Mesplié)

- *Rehabilitation of sensitivity*

  The sensory rehabilitation only concerns the damages of the superficial branch of the radial nerve in Wartenberg's syndromes. The protocol is realized according to the modalities described in the chapter "Physiology and Rehabilitation of Sensorial and Motor Disorders" (Volume 1) [14].

Orthotic Treatment

After surgery of the radial nerve in the elbow, an immobilization orthosis is realized, placing the wrist between 10 and 20° of extension (Fig. 12.14). It is kept for about 15 days, unless there is also a radial tunnel syndrome (it is then kept 3 weeks).

After wrist surgery, an immobilization orthosis is realized, placing the wrist and the thumb in a resting position (Fig. 12.15). It is kept 1 week before starting rehabilitation.

Bibliography

1. Pratt N. Anatomy of nerve entrapment sites in the upper quarter. J Hand Ther. 2005;18(2):216–29.
2. Markiewitz AD, Merryman J. Radial nerve compression in the upper extremity. J Am Soc Surg Hand. 2005;5(2):87–99.
3. Karanasios S, et al. Diagnostic accuracy of examination tests for lateral elbow tendinopathy (LET) – a systematic review. J Hand Ther. 2021;
4. Stanley J. Radial tunnel syndrome: a surgeon's perspective. J Hand Ther. 2006;19(2):180–4.
5. Sigamoney KV, Rashid A, Ng CY. Management of atraumatic posterior interosseous nerve palsy. J Hand Surg Am. 2017;42(10):826–30.
6. Schmid AB, Fundaun J, Tampin B. Entrapment neuropathies: a contemporary approach to pathophysiology, clinical assessment, and management. Pain Rep. 2020;5(4):e829.
7. Taylor A, Wolff AL. The forgotten radial nerve: a conceptual framework for treatment of lateral elbow pain. J Hand Ther. 2021;34(2):323–9.
8. Janssen RG, Schwartz DA, Velleman PF. A randomized controlled study of contrast baths on patients with carpal tunnel syndrome. J Hand Ther. 2009;22(3):200–7. quiz 208
9. Wolny T, et al. Effect of manual therapy and neurodynamic techniques vs ultrasound and laser on 2PD in patients with CTS: a randomized controlled trial. J Hand Ther. 2016;29(3):235–45.
10. Le Roux P. Syndrome du canal carpien et mobilisation des nerfs. Kinésithérapie, la revue. 2007;2007(68–69):49–52.
11. Cleary CK. Management of radial tunnel syndrome: a therapist's clinical perspective. J Hand Ther. 2006;19(2):186–91.
12. Lundborg G, Rydevik BL. Effects of stretching the tibial nerve of the rabbit: preliminary study of the intraneural circulation of the barrier function of the perineurium. J Bone Joint Surg Br. 1973;55:390–401.
13. Coppieters MW, Butler DS. Do 'sliders' slide and 'tensioners' tension? An analysis of neurodynamic techniques and considerations regarding their application. Man Ther. 2008;13(3):213–21.
14. Mesplié G. Thérapie de la main, examen clinique et outils de prise en charge rééducative avancée du poignet et de la main. Sauramps Médical; 2021.

Part VI

Other Common Hand Pathology

13 Dupuytren's Disease

Grégory Mesplié and Jean-François Chauvet

Dupuytren's disease is a pathology affecting the medium palmar aponeurosis and the digital aponeurosis, leading to the formation of cords and nodules.

It can cause important retractions leading to flexion of the metacarpophalangeal joints, proximal interphalangeal joints, and more rarely distal interphalangeal joints.

History

On December 5, 1831, Baron Guillaume Dupuytren described this pathology during a lecture at the Dieu hospital [1].

He had previously realized a surgery on June 12, 1831, described as follows:

- Transversal incision next to the fourth finger's metacarpophalangeal joint: section of the aponeurosis, easy extension of the fourth finger, nothing on the fifth finger, despite passing subcutaneously the scalpel towards the fifth finger.
- Transversal incision at the level off the fifth finger's proximal interphalangeal joint: unblocks the finger from the palm. Prolonging the incision of the fourth finger's metacarpophalangeal joint and sectioning the aponeurosis does not improve the extension.
- Transversal incision in front of the first phalanx: complete extension.
- Bandage and extension splint, renewed every 48 h.
- Healing phase for 22 days.
- The splint is kept during a month, then "self-rehabilitation" with progressive relaxation, and perfect result on December 5.
- The end of the lecture and his conclusion: "… the cases I've been telling you about, as well as the surgery you've seen yourselves, establish without a doubt that this digital retraction, with the characteristics I've mentioned, is caused by a contracture of the palmar aponeurosis, and mainly of its extensions towards the base of the fingers. This medical condition can be treated by transversal incisions of these expansions and their origin on the palmar aponeurosis."

According to Dupuytren, this pathology was an occupational disease caused by micro-traumas.

Some say this pathology was first described in 1777 by the British surgeon Henry Cline, who recommended a subcutaneous aponeurotomy as treatment.

The surgical treatment does not evolve much in the nineteenth century, except from a proposition from Ferguson in 1842 to do fasciectomies.

G. Mesplié (✉) · J.-F. Chauvet
Institut Sud Aquitain de la Main et du Membre Supérieur (ISAMMS), Biarritz, France

G. Mesplié (ed.), *Hand Functional Anatomy and Therapy*,
https://doi.org/10.1007/978-3-031-92505-4_13

In 1900, Lexer proposes a dermo-fasciectomy of the whole palm, with skin graft.

In 1948, extensive fasciectomy without cutaneous excision would lead to lots of complications and stiffness.

At the same time, Skoog realizes selective fasciectomies, limiting dissections, which improves the results.

Hueston proves that there is no recurrence under a skin graft (1960).

Mac Cash, in 1964, describes an open palm technique, without closing or skin graft, thus updating Dupuytren's technique.

Anatomopathology

Luck describes three evolution stages [2–4]:

- Initial stages: fibroblastic proliferation [5] with nodules
- Intermediate stage: fibroblastic transformation and organization of the collagen with cords
- Terminal stage: organization of a dense mature collagen

Anatomical Expression

There are many different clinical manifestations of Dupuytren's disease, as many different anatomical elements can be affected [6, 7] (Fig. 13.1). However, a few features remain constant:

- The nodules: essentially palmar, they progressively invade the tissues and strongly stick to the skin. They are never responsible for articular retraction.
- The cords: they lead to articular retractions and are the expression of this pathology. We can find pre-tendinous palmar cords and digital cords (median, spiral, lateral, and retrovascular). They cause the retraction of the metacarpophalangeal joint, the proximal interphalangeal joint, and rarely the distal interphalangeal joint (which can even be in hyper-extension because of a boutonnière deformity) (Fig. 13.2).
- Anatomical repartition by order of decreasing frequency for the fingers: V, IV, III, II. The thumb is damaged in 10%–35% of the cases.

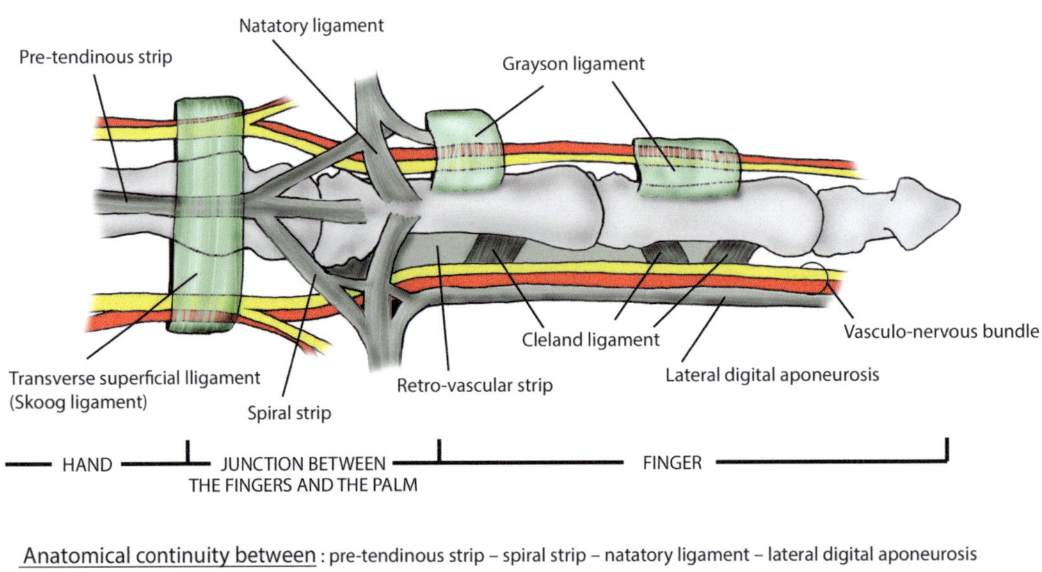

Fig. 13.1 Anatomical elements that may be affected by Dupuytren's disease: pre-tendinous strip, spiral strip, natatory ligament, and lateral digital aponeurosis. (Picture by Josette Mesplié)

Epidemiology

Dupuytren's disease is more frequent in white men from Northern Europe [8].

It is unusual in black people.

In 25% of the cases there is a hereditary factor [9], related to a dominant autosomal recessive gene inherited from Neanderthal [10].

Associated Conditions

Alcoholism doubles the risks, which are even more important in the case of alcoholic cirrhosis.

Diabetes increases the risk, related to the duration of diabetes: after 20 years of evolution, 67% of diabetic patients have Dupuytren's disease. However, it is often limited and almost never needs surgery.

Epilepsy doubles the risks.

About traumas and manual activities, there are no statistic proves, but it could be a triggering factor in patients with a predisposition.

Diathesis

The pathology will be more severe and recurring if it starts early, if it is bilateral, and if there is a hereditary and/or ethnic characteristic.

The association with Peyronie's disease, plantar fibromatosis, and damage in the lateral fingers are pejorative factors.

Clinical and Paraclinical Signs

The diagnosis can be done with a clinical assessment alone.

We systematically observe retractions in flexion of the metacarpophalangeal joints and proximal interphalangeal joints. Because of the anatomical location of the posterior digital aponeurosis, they can cause a hyper-extension of the distal interphalangeal joint (Fig. 13.3).

The spread of the disease to the digital level is linked to the tissue continuity at the level of the metacarpophalangeal joints (Fig. 13.4).

The palpation shows a thickening of the damaged tissues and indurations at the level of the cords and nodules.

The natatory ligament is damaged (or distal commissural ligament in the thumb) so the commissural opening decreases, which can cause maceration.

If the patient cannot put his hand flat on the table (Fig. 13.5), we should take a specialized advice to avoid important tissue retractions that can make the surgery complicated.

Several classifications have been proposed [11], but Tubiana and Michon's grading system remains the most used (Fig. 13.6).

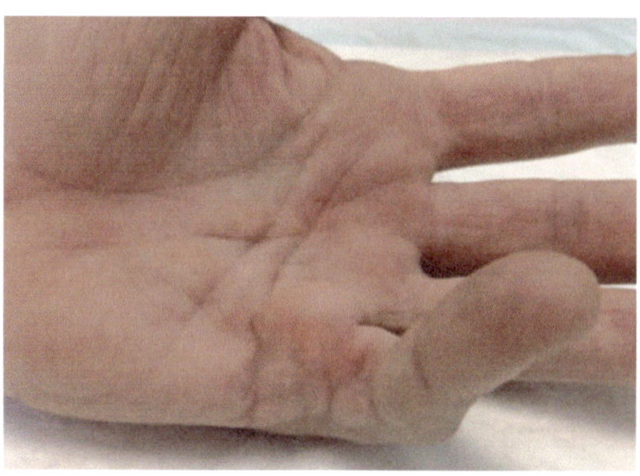

Fig. 13.2 Clinical aspect of a patient with Dupuytren's disease. (Picture by Grégory Mesplié)

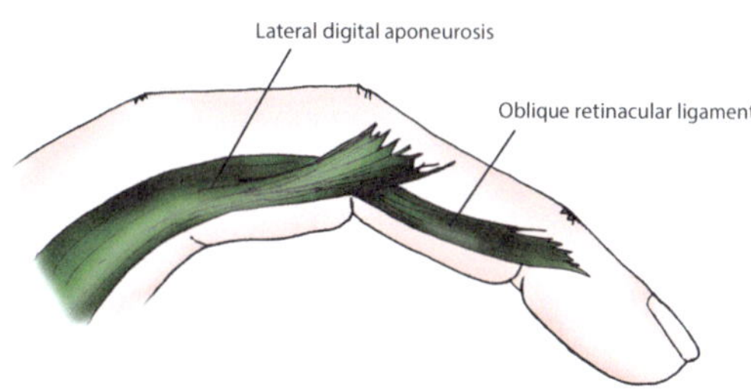

Fig. 13.3 As the digital aponeurosis is palmar in relation to the proximal interphalangeal joint and dorsal in relation to the distal interphalangeal joint, it tends to create a pseudo-boutonnière deformity (flexion of the proximal interphalangeal joint and extension of the distal interphalangeal joint). (Picture by Josette Mesplié)

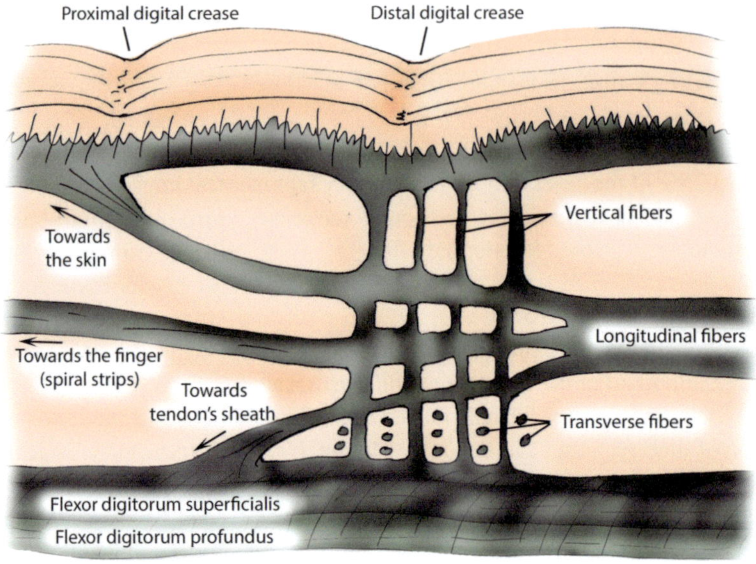

Fig. 13.4 The existence of a digital deformity is explained by the tissue continuity between the pre-tendinous strips and the digital aponeurosis at the level of the metacarpophalangeal joints. (Picture by Josette Mesplié)

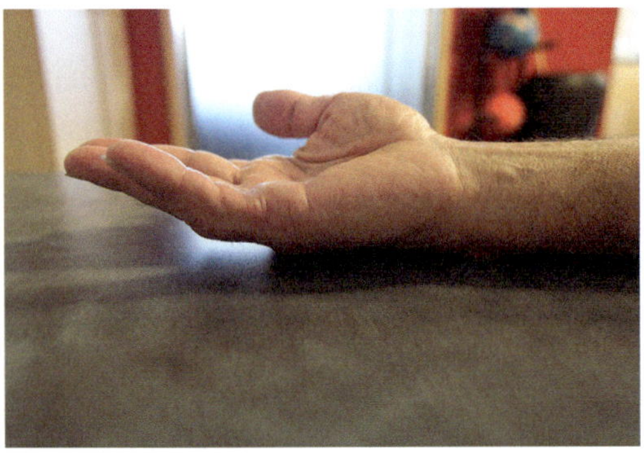

Fig. 13.5 Test of the hand flat on a table, signaling that it is time for surgery. (Picture by Grégory Mesplié)

Some rare manifestations of this pathology are:

- "Knuckle pads" or dorsal nodules located next to the proximal interphalangeal joint that adhere to the skin but not to the extensor system. They can be painful and functionally disturbing.
- Peyronie's disease, retraction of a connective tissue at the level of the albuginea that creates a dorsal angulation in erection.
- Plantar fibromatosis (or Ledderhose's disease): the plantar equivalent of the Dupuytren and Peyronie's diseases.

Fig. 13.6 Grading system of Tubiana and Michon. (Picture by Josette Mesplié)

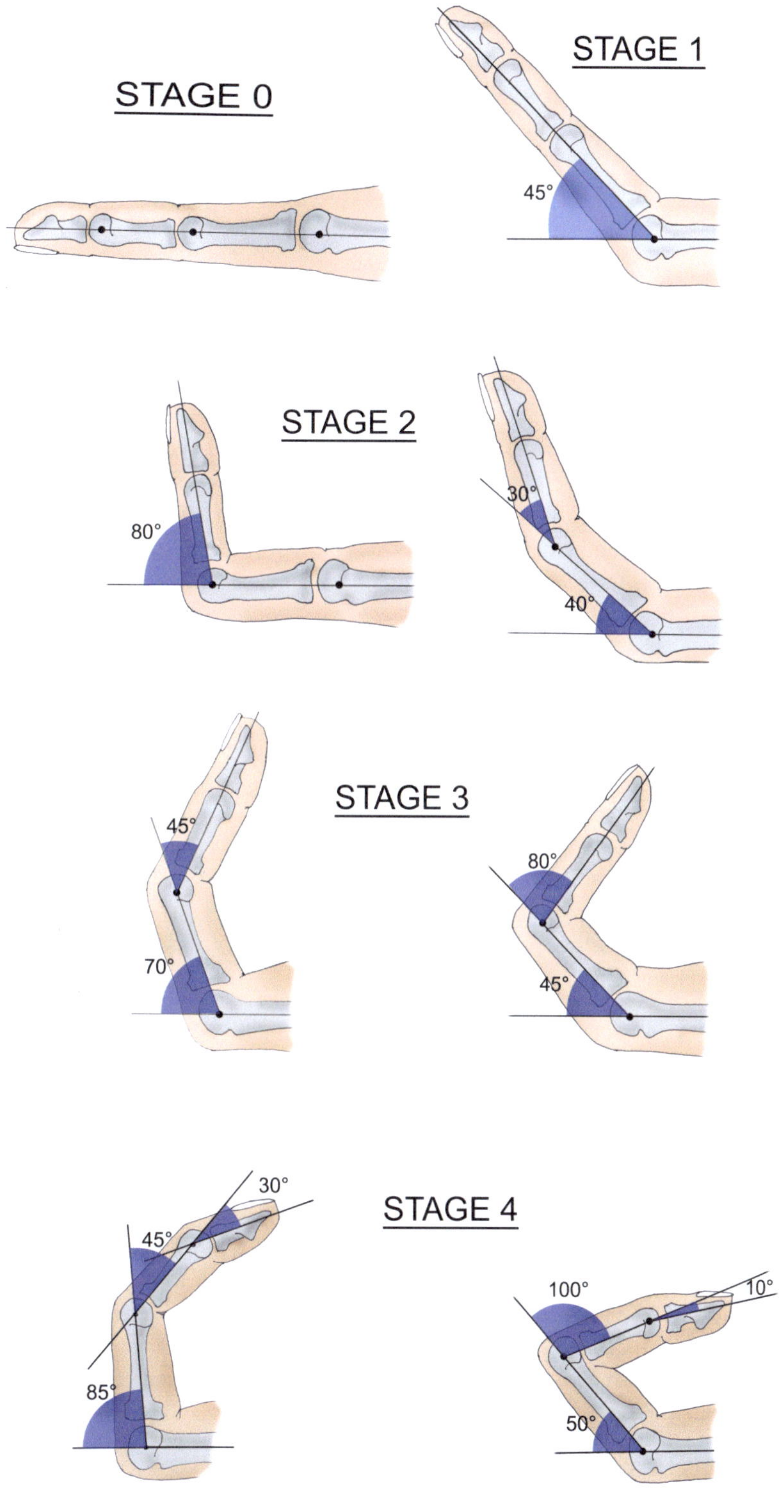

Therapeutic Process and Surgical Treatment

Nonsurgical Treatment

Several treatments have been tried without proving their efficiency:

- Massages with vitamin E, physiotherapy, ultrasounds, corticoids, anti-gout preparations, etc.
- Orthoses: dynamic or static
- Traumatic rupture of the cords
- Corticoid injections
- Interferon: alpha 2β and gamma 5-fluoro-uracil
- Localized radiotherapy in the early stage
- Fibroblastic differentiation inhibitors

Collagenase injection appears to be a promising treatment [12], although cases of secondary tendon rupture have been reported.

Rehabilitation as a preventive treatment is not of major interest [13].

The use of preventive pro-extension orthoses, even if their efficiency appears to be significant in the early stages [13–15], does not seem to be commonly indicated in view of the relationships' constraints for the patient/obtained results/observed recurrences.

Surgical Treatment

Like every hand surgery, the goal is to obtain a hand closer to the functional norm, without after-effects.

This goal, however, can be hard to reach, especially in damages of several fingers and relapses.

General Principles

The surgery must be done with optical magnification (magnifying glasses), and a pneumatic tourniquet in the superior limb previously drained without the help of an elastic band.

It is a precision surgery that requires special attention during the dissection of the neurovascular bundle, especially in the base of the fingers and next to the proximal interphalangeal joints, and of course in case of relapse.

Surgery is carried out under loco-regional anesthesia.

Surgical Techniques

➔ **Aponeurotomy (with Needle)**

Proposed by rheumatologists, this technique has only one indication: a well-individualized palmar cord. It is totally contraindicated for damage to the fingers.

It is mainly indicated for early forms [16].

This technique is a source of vascular, nerve, and tendon complications and has a high recurrence rate, even though it is intended for diseases with a low diathesis.

➔ **Aponeurectomy**

- *Types*
  - ***"Simple" aponeurectomy***
    It is the most complete resection of pathological tissues.
    The excision of the non-pathological palmar aponeurosis has progressively been abandoned in favor of selective excisions of the pathological areas.
    It can be realized with longitudinal incisions in a broken line or transversal incisions.
    We must be particularly careful during the dissection of the neurovascular bundles.
  - ***Dermo-fasciectomy***
    It is the combination of the excision of the aponeurosis and the cutaneous tissue damaged by the disease.
    The cutaneous resection is done according to the functional units, which will later be covered by a total skin graft (Hueston). In some cases, we can let the area exposed for controlled healing, as suggested by Mac Cash [17].
    If the tendons are too exposed, we will choose a more limited excision or a cover with a skin flap.
- *Surgical approach and skin flap*

There are two types of surgical approach:
- Longitudinal incisions: zigzag cuts (Brüner or Palmen) or incisions following the path of the cord associated with a Z-shaped plasty if necessary
- Palmo-digital incisions

These incisions allow realizing a selective aponeurectomy, with an excellent control of the neurovascular structures and without important delamination that causes hematomas.

They have their limitations if the skin is severely damaged, and we should not hesitate to change the technique (skin graft, open palm).

Transversal incisions also allow realizing aponeurectomy, but there is often important subcutaneous delamination that causes hematomas and cutaneous necrosis. They can be directly closed if the skin is flexible and not damaged, but they need draining. When the suture is impossible, we use skin graft or flaps or choose an "open skin" technique.

In some cases, the use of mixed incision will give the best result.

- *Skin closure techniques*
  - ***Direct suture***

    When it is possible, it is the technique that brings the fastest healing.
  - ***Skin grafts***

    There is no relapse of Dupuytren's disease under a skin graft, so we should not hesitate to use them, but they are subject to precise criteria.

    Skin grafts are used in the case of dermo-fasciectomy.

    It is most often a total skin graft that covers the exposed noble structures.

    They must respect the cutaneous functional units of the hand described by Michon.

    The skin grafts must repair the unit in one single piece, reporting the sutures at the level of the neutral lines of their borders.
  - ***Flaps***
  - Their goal is also to cover an exposed area.
    - Jacobsen flap: it avoids the skin graft of the first phalanx of the fifth finger. It is used in evolved and very infiltrating forms. Obtaining the skin sample leaves a loss of palmar substance that will be left for controlled healing like in the Mac Cash technique.
    - Tanzer-Bunnell-Colson flab: taken on the lateral side of the first phalanx, this flap has a commissural base and covers the loss of substances in the base of the finger. The donor site will be covered with a skin graft.
  - ***Open palm techniques***

    Mac Cash described this technique in 1964, which is derived from Dupuytren's technique.

  Principle:
    - Long incision in the distal palmar crease
    - Aponeurectomy
    - Palm left for controlled healing
    - Immediate mobilization and extension orthosis

    There is no skin graft, which avoids maceration, hematoma, and sepsis.
- *Associated gestures*

  Stiffness essentially occurs in the proximal interphalangeal joint. It is the most important problem in the treatment of Dupuytren's disease.

  Sometimes a total surgical resection of the pathological tissue can bring back a complete extension of the proximal interphalangeal joint.

  Otherwise, we will have to do a teno-arthrolysis liberating the flexor tendons, with section of the checkreins and resection of the collateral ligaments.
- *Complications* [18]
  - ***Intraoperative complications: neurovascular wounds***
    - Wounds of the digital nerves that must be immediately repaired with a direct suture.
    - Arterial wounds: if only one artery is damaged and the finger is not devascularized, we realize a hemostasis. If the wounds are bilateral a repartition is obligatory, even if there is a risk of important trophic disorders or necrosis leading to an amputation.

- ***Early postoperative complications***
  - Hematomas could require a draining surgery.
  - Cutaneous necroses that cause shrinking cords must be excised and covered with a skin graft or flap.
  - Infections are rare and require a surgical evacuation, draining, and antibiotic therapy.
- ***Late complications***
  - Algodystrophy and joint stiffness.
  - Relapses and extension of the disease: relapses occur in an operated area, whereas the extension happens in an intact area. They are related to the diathesis of the disease. The extension can be treated by aponeurectomy, but the relapse requires most of the time a dermo-fasciectomy with skin graft avoiding relapse in the grafted area.

Rehabilitation and Orthotic Treatment

Rehabilitation always follows surgery, which is the only efficient treatment for Dupuytren's disease.

Rehabilitation fights against postoperative tissue retractions, regardless of the surgical technique employed (aponeurotomy with needle, aponeurectomy, Mac Cash technique).

Mobilization techniques and deep massages, combined with the nocturnal wear of an extension orthosis, leads to better results.

Rehabilitation Protocol (Fig. 13.7)

Postoperative Phase (D3 to D21)

From D3 to D21, the scar can be spectacular, especially in case of an open palm technique (Mac Cash).

The most important goals in this phase are the fight against pain and trophic disorders and the prevention of finger stiffness and functional exclusion.

No tension should be applied to the aponeurosis during this period, as it may increase the risk of flare reaction [19]. The flare reaction is characterized by a disproportionate reactive erythema, stiffness, and edema in the postoperative period. These symptoms usually appear in the third to fourth week after surgery [20, 21].

Putting tension on the aponeurosis too early also reduces the quality of the results obtained in terms of recovered joint amplitudes.

Self-rehabilitation exercises are described to the patient, without tension, to recover digital flexion. The exercises are repeated every hour, in 3 sets of 10–15 repetitions (passive, then active) if they do not create edema or pain [22].

➔ Fight Against Trophic Disorders

- Draining massages.
- Electrotherapy (1 Hz) on the edematous area.
- Soft active mobilization improving the evacuation of the edema and stimulating the "vis a latere." The mobilizations, if they are too intense and traumatizing for the tissues, can restart the inflammatory process and increase the edema, even triggering a flare reaction.
- Cryotherapy without direct contact with the scar for non-sterile application modes. In this phase the scar is open, so we use two cold bags of cherry stones to "sandwich" the edematous area. The hand is placed higher than the forearm to optimize the draining effect. The patient keeps his bandage to avoid any infection risk. Cryotherapy also has an interesting analgesic effect.
- Pressotherapy, where the device realizes a disto-proximal compression, which drains the edema of the hand and realizes a soft and painless posture in extension during the treatment. In this phase, this technique can be poorly supported by the patient, in which case we delay its application.
- Compressive bandage during the night if the edema is important and resists to treatment.

a

Dupuytren's disease after surgery

	Postoperative (A)	Relative fragility (B)	Consolidation (C)
REHABILITATION	**Therapeutic goals :** 1. Fight against trophic disorders 2. Fight against pain 3. Prevent stiffness 4. Prevent exclusion syndrome **Techniques:** 1. Draining massages, vacuotherapy (drainage), electrotherapy (tonolysis), compressive bandage 2. Cryotherapy, TENS, TVS (100 Hz) 3. Digital mobilization without tension, fluidotherapy after the stitches are gone 4. TVS (70-80 Hz) and various sensory stimulation (without constraint) **Risks:** type 1 CRPS or flare reaction, stiffness and/or pain and /or trophic disorders if maladapted immobilization	**Therapeutic goals :** 1. Same as phase 1, intensify if necessary 2. Complete recovery of the joint amplitudes **Techniques:** 1. Pressotherapy (drainage), vacuotherapy (scar) and defibrosing massage if the scar is not inflammatory (A1), manipulation of light objects (A4) 2. Electrostimulation, soft joint mobilization, defibrosing vacuotherapy, progressive stretching of the intrinsic muscles and tension on the retinacular oblique ligament, soft postures **Risks:** same as phase A + functional exclusion (mainly index)	**Therapeutic goals :** 1. Same as in previous phases, intensify if necessary 2. Complete functional recovery **Techniques:** 1. Intensify specific joint mobilizations, stretching of the intrinsic muscles, postures, electrostimulation (B2) 2. Functional activities adapted to the patient's sporting and professional needs, recovery of normal muscular ratios **Risks:** Same as in phase A and B
ORTHOSIS	Depending on the chosen option (stitches for 15 days): 1. Palmar plate without tension (+ silicone after D15) worn during the night 2. "Anti-extension" orthosis for the fingers (+ silicone after D15) worn all the time	Extension orthosis for 3 to 6 months (palmar plaque or Levame) + silicone	Orthosis to gain amplitude (extension and flexion if necessary), the modalities can be modified if the results are not satisfactory
	D3-D21	D21-D45	After D45

b

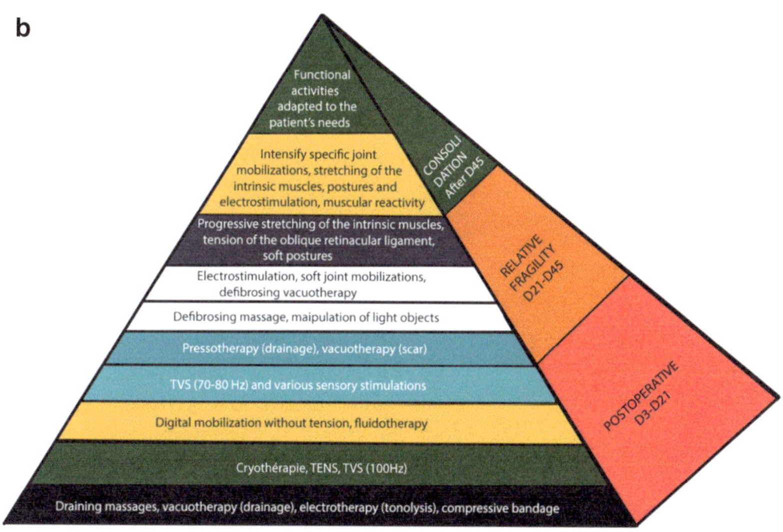

Fig. 13.7 Rehabilitation protocol (**a**) and progression pyramid (**b**). (Picture by Josette Mesplié)

➔ Fight Against Pain

- Analgesic electrotherapy (see chapter "Physical Agents" in Volume 1).
- Transcutaneous vibratory stimulations (frequency 100 Hz, amplitude <1 mm) applied on the painful area, moving along the path of the concerned sensory nerve. If contacting with the device causes pain, we apply it away from the painful area, still along the corresponding nervous path. This type of mechanical vibrations also has a sensorimotor stimulation effect limiting the risks of functional exclusion.
- Infrasounds (frequency >20 Hz, amplitude >1 mm) also fight against pain by relaxing the muscles and improving the local trophic state. They are applied perpendicularly to the area we want to treat.

➔ Prevent Stiffness

Painless passive mobilizations are realized before active exercises [3], which can already be combined with electrostimulation in this phase if it is tolerated by the patient. We must give the patient self-rehabilitation advice, based on passive then active mobilizations of the fingers several times a day, in short and painless series.

Healing Phase (Scar Closed)—D21 to D45

From D21 to D45, the scar is closed, and the hand is usually less inflammatory and painful. The techniques from the previous phase can be prolonged if necessary. The key points are working on the scar, recovering joint amplitudes, and improving the grips.

➔ Fight Against the Edema

We can add cryotherapy with compressed air (−50 °C), as the scar is closed. This quickly lowers the cutaneous temperature until 7 °C (not less than 7 °C as it can cause burning or nervous injury) in 30–60 s and then maintains the temperature around 10 °C for 16 min. It would seem that this modality is the most efficient for the anti-inflammatory and analgesic effects we are looking for.

➔ Work on the Scar

The palmar skin is thick and not very flexible. It is composed of papillary ridges that optimize the efficiency of the mechanoreceptors in the pulp of the fingers. This special organization can make healing difficult, with an important hypertrophy of the scar, and even retractions that greatly impact the grips, limiting the joint amplitudes and disturbing the sensitivity in the area around the scar.

Therefore, relaxing the scar is of particular importance in the treatment of Dupuytren's disease [23].

- *Massages around and on the scar*
  The goal is to improve trophicity around the treated areas and to relax the scar.
  Therefore, we realize glided pressures form distal to proximal, getting closer to the scar. We progressively add sanding and palpating-rolling techniques. These techniques are described in chapter "Scar Massage and Treatments" (Volume 1).
- *Ultrasounds*
  After the closure of the scar, we use ultrasounds to fight against adherences around the scar.
  The ideal frequency is 3 MHz, allowing a superficial effect in accordance with the anatomical location of the cutaneous scar and the superficial palmar aponeurosis. The pulsed mode has a more important "fibrolytic" effect than the continuous mode and should therefore be preferred.
- *Depressotherapy*
  We must be careful and progressive when applying this technique.
  We start to use depressotherapy after the closure of the scar.
  First, when the scar is still inflammatory, we apply the head of the device away from the scar in a disto-proximal direction.
  When the scar is not inflammatory anymore, we apply the head directly on the scar, first in alternative mode and then in continuous mode if the patient tolerates it well (Fig. 13.8).

➔ Recovering Mobility

These techniques, combined with the stretching of the scar, should allow us recovering joint amplitudes in the fingers. When the surgery has been delayed for a long time, the risks of stiffness are higher as the fingers have stayed blocked during months or even years!

- *Electrostimulation*
  This technique helps recovering joint amplitudes in flexion or extension.
  We prefer using currents with a pulse width of 150–200 μs (ideal for the muscles of the superior limb) and a frequency of 20 Hz (stimulations of the slow fibers).
  The patient combines the electric stimulation with a voluntary contraction (electro-active exercise) to stimulate the motor command, sometimes disturbed after a surgical intervention or a prolonged immobilization.
- *Fluidotherapy*
  These techniques participate in the global relaxation of the hand after this kind of intervention. We ask the patient to realize flexion/extension movements and to spread his fingers, in combination with the dry or wet fluidotherapy.
- *Specific mobilizations*
  Decompression and gliding maneuvers in the digital joints help recover a good joint harmony, especially in the case of prolonged preoperative stiffness (see chapter "Hand and Wrist Mobilizations" in Volume 1) (Fig. 13.9).
- *Stretching of the intrinsic muscles*
  The lumbricals and interossei are not stretched the same way.

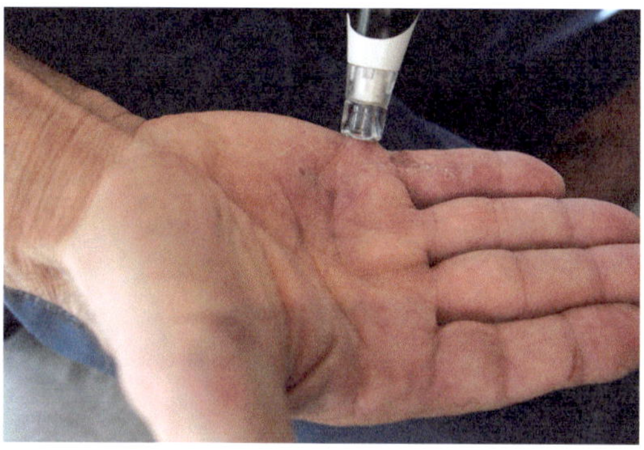

Fig. 13.8 Depressotherapy relaxing the scar tissue. (Picture by Grégory Mesplié)

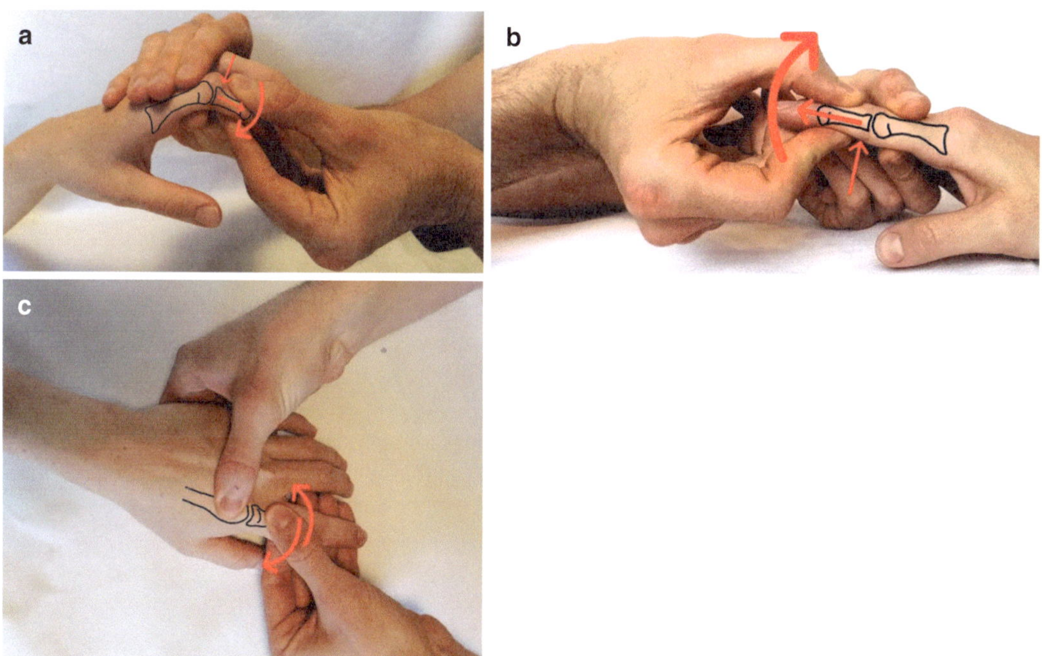

Fig. 13.9 Specific mobilizations of the proximal interphalangeal joint in flexion + anterior gliding (**a**) and extension + posterior gliding (**b**). The metacarpophalangeal joint is mobilized according to the same principles, but we combine abduction/adduction mobilizations (**c**). (Picture by Josette Mesplié)

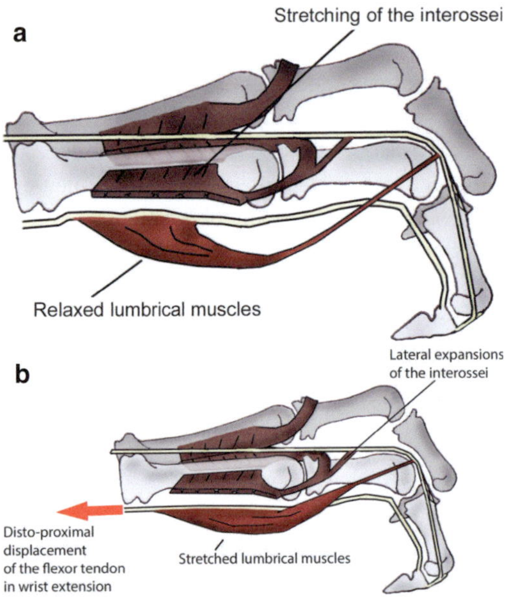

Fig. 13.10 Passive positioning in the extrinsic + position stretches the interossei but not the lumbrical muscles. Extending the wrist stretches the lumbrical muscles by creating a disto-proximal displacement of the flexor tendons. (**a**) Relaxed lumbrical muscles. (**b**) Stretched lumbrical muscles. (Picture by Josette Mesplié)

The interossei are stretched placing the hand in the extrinsic + position, reached actively or passively.

The lumbricals are stretched only if this position is combined with a wrist extension. This is related to the fact that the lumbrical muscles do not have an osseous proximal insertion but insert on the deep flexors that move from distal to proximal when placing the wrist in extension (Fig. 13.10).

➔ Prehension

Manipulating objects improves rapidly and efficiently the coordination and dexterity in the operated hand.

Remodeling Phase (After D45)

After D45, the techniques from phases 1 and 2 are used more intensively (but still painlessly) if the disorders persist.

Progressively recovering strength and starting to do professional and leisure activities again are this phase's goals.

Orthotic Treatment

A static orthosis can be made as early as J3, especially in the most severe cases [24] and according to the individual postoperative assessment [13], although recent publications do not show the benefit of systematically making them [25]. It must create no tension in extension to limit the risks of flare reaction.

At D21, it is remolded if necessary to create a moderate tension in extension, and silicone is added at the level of the scar to improve its evolution (Fig. 13.11).

In our opinion, the advantages of static orthoses are:

- Excellent control of the generated tension, which is especially important in the first 3 weeks.
- Good stress distribution thanks to the large contact surface, with no risk of maceration if perforated plastic is used.
- Easy addition of silicone, regardless of the concerned area.

Dynamic extension orthoses can be used at a distance, in the absence of inflammation, if amplitudes have not been completely acquired [14] (Fig. 13.12).

A winding orthosis can be used when amplitudes in flexion are difficult to recover. This may be a global winding orthosis or a localized flex-

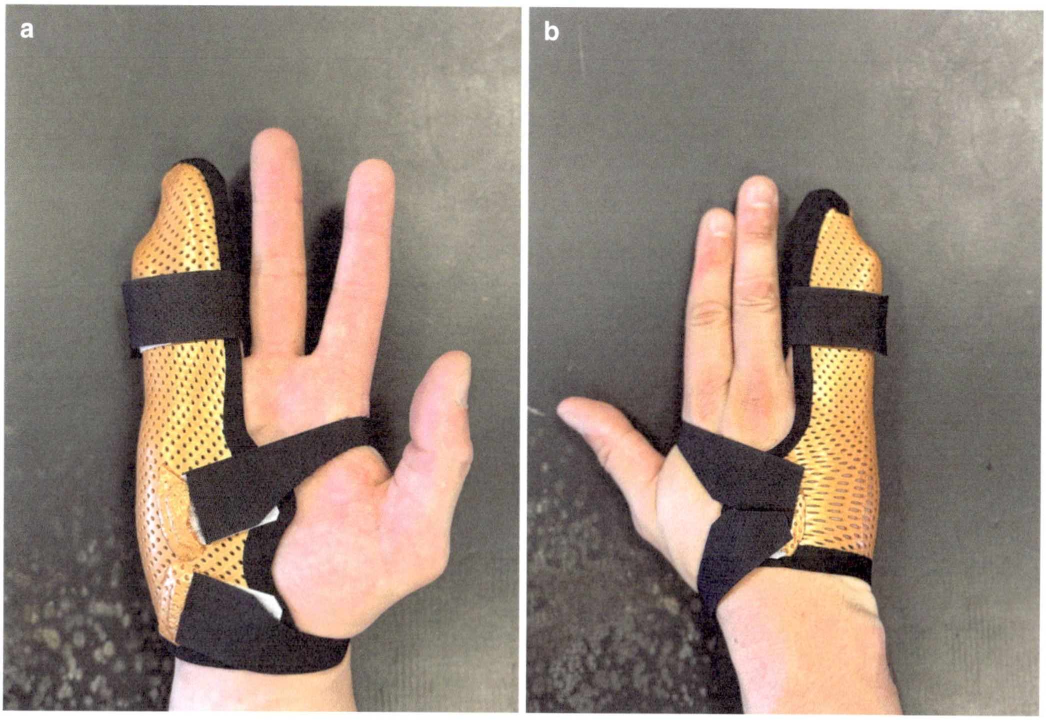

Fig. 13.11 Static orthosis that can be done at D3 in severe cases. (**a**) Palmar view. (**b**) Dorsal view. (Picture by Grégory Mesplié)

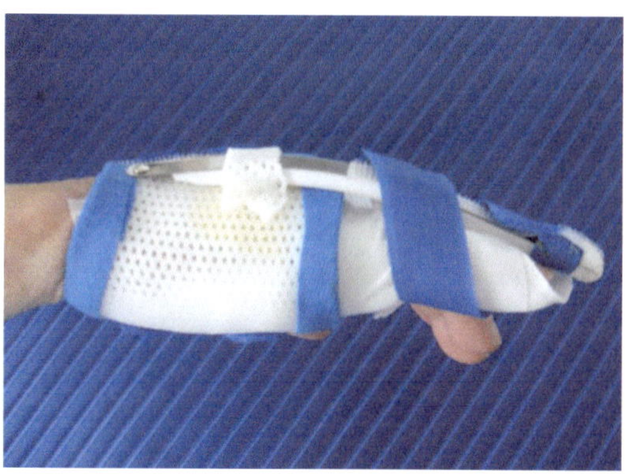

Fig. 13.12 Extension orthosis worn during the night (Levame). (Picture by Grégory Mesplié)

ion orthosis for stiff joints. The duration of the posture is short (around 15 min) to limit the onset of circulatory problems but repeated several times a day (Fig. 13.13).

A Casting Motion to Mobilize Stiffness (CMMS) orthosis can also be proposed, depending on the problems observed during the clinical assessment (see chapter "Common Hand and Wrist Orthoses" in Volume 1) [26] (Fig. 13.14).

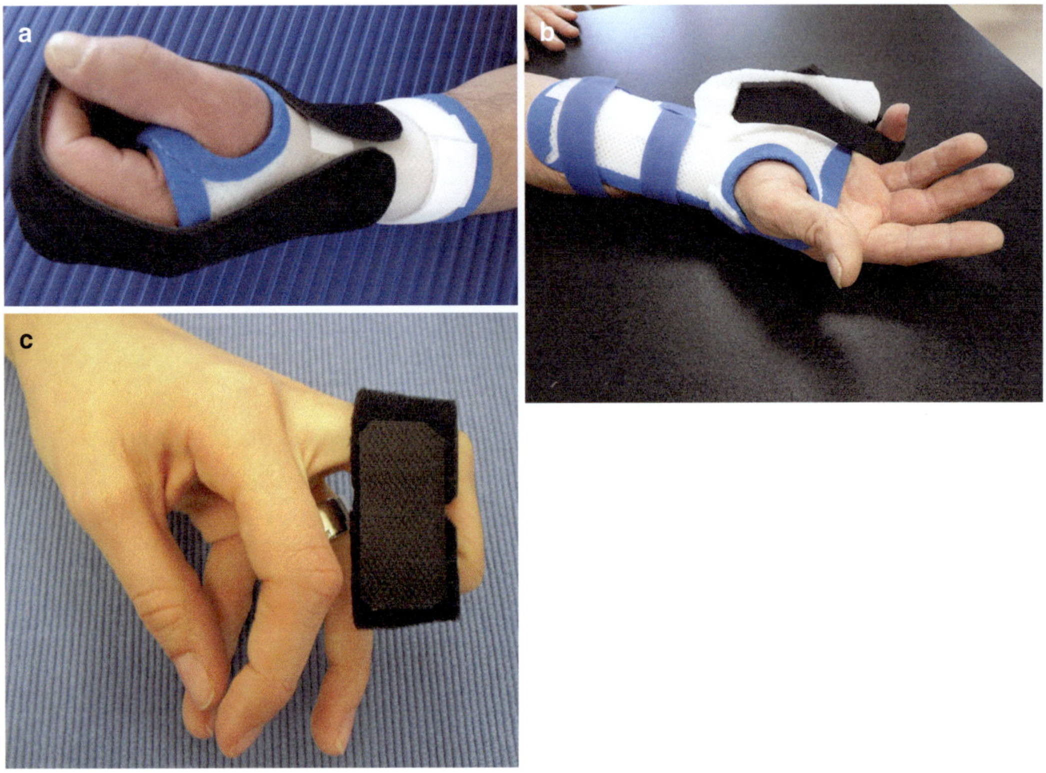

Fig. 13.13 Orthosis for global winding of the fingers (**a**), selective winding of the metacarpophalangeal joint (**b**) and the interphalangeal joints (**c**). (Picture by Grégory Mesplié)

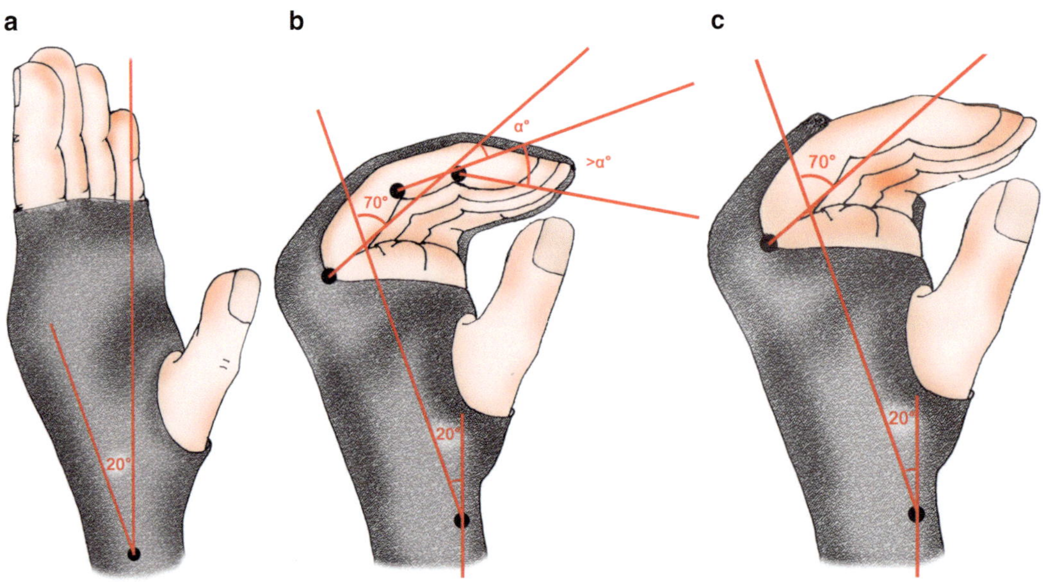

Fig. 13.14 Articular torque transmission orthoses facilitating extrinsic flexor digitorum action and intrinsic muscle stretching (**a**), flexor digitorum profundus action (**b**), metacarpophalangeal joint flexion by their flexed position and proximal interphalangeal joint extension by their resistance against the dorsal part (**c**). (Picture by Josette Mesplié)

Bibliography

1. Glicenstein J. Maladie de Dupuytren, histoire d'un éponyme. Chir Main. 2012;2012(31):107–12.
2. Layton T, Nanchahal J. Recent advances in the understanding of Dupuytren's disease. F1000Res. 2019;8:F1000 Faculty Rev-231.
3. Dutta A, et al. Dupuytren's contracture – current concepts. J Clin Orthop Trauma. 2020;11(4):590–6.
4. Lam W, et al. Re-visiting Luck's classification: a histological analysis of Dupuytren disease. J Hand Surg (Eur Vol). 2010;35(4):312–7.
5. Zhang AY, Kargel JS. The basic science of Dupuytren disease. Hand Clin. 2018;34(3):301–5.
6. Leibovic SJ. Normal and pathologic anatomy of Dupuytren disease. Hand Clin. 2018;34(3):315–29.
7. Shewring DJ, Rethnam U. Cleland's ligaments and Dupuytren's disease. J Hand Surg Eur Vol. 2014;39(5):477–81.
8. Carvalhana G, Auquit-Auckbur I, Milliez PY. Dupuytren's disease: state of knowledge and research in physiopathology. Chir Main. 2011;30(4):239–45.
9. Lee LC, et al. Expression of a novel gene, MafB, in Dupuytren's disease. J Hand Surg Am. 2006;31(2):211–8.
10. Agren R, et al. Major genetic risk factors for Dupuytren's disease are inherited from neandertals. Mol Biol Evol. 2023;40(6):msad130.
11. Akhavani MA, et al. A review of the classification of Dupuytren's disease. J Hand Surg Eur Vol. 2015;40(2):155–65.
12. Hentz VR, et al. Advances in the management of Dupuytren disease: collagenase. Hand Clin. 2012;28(4):551–63.
13. Turesson C. The role of hand therapy in Dupuytren disease. Hand Clin. 2018;34(3):395–401.
14. Gerlac D, et al. Rééducation après maladie de Dupuytren opérée: protocole grenoblois. Kinésithérapie scientifique. 2014;2014(551):17–21.
15. Ball C, Nanchahal J. The use of splinting as a non-surgical treatment for Dupuytren disease: a pilot study. Br J Hand Ther. 2002;2(3):76.
16. Salon A, Cadot B, Marcadet B. Traitement de la maladie de Dupuytren par aponévrotomie percutanée: technique et indications. Kinésithérapie scientifique. 2014;2014(551):11–5.
17. Dacquin P, et al. Rééducation de la maladie de Dupuytren. EMC Kinésithérapie-Médecine physique-Réadaptation 2000:26-220-B-50:7.
18. Eberlin KR, Mudgal CS. Complications of treatment for Dupuytren disease. Hand Clin. 2018;34(3):387–94.
19. Evans RB, Dell PC, Fiolkowski P. A clinical report of the effect of mechanical stress on functional results after fasciectomy for Dupuytren's contracture. J Hand Ther. 2002;15(4):331–9.
20. Emmerich LeDren L. La flare reaction postopératoire de la maladie de Dupuytren. Mémoire présenté en vue de l'obtention du Diplôme Inter-Universitaire européen de rééducation et d'appareillage en chirurgie de la main. 2021.
21. Gerlac D, et al. Rééducation après maladie de Dupuytren opérée: gérer la "flare reaction". Kinésithér Scient. 2017;592:5–11.
22. Sweet S, Blackmore S. Surgical and therapy update on the management of Dupuytren's disease. J Hand Ther. 2014;27(2):77–83; quiz 84.
23. Mesplié G, Chauvet J-F. Dupuytren disease. In: Hand and wrist rehabilitation. Cham: Springer International Publishing; 2015. p. 429–53.
24. Collis J, et al. The effect of night extension orthoses following surgical release of Dupuytren contracture: a single-center, randomized, controlled trial. J Hand Surg Am. 2013;38(7):1285–94 e2.
25. Samargandi OA, et al. Night orthosis after surgical correction of Dupuytren contractures: a systematic review. J Hand Surg Am. 2017;42(10):839 e1–839 e10.
26. Midgley R. Use of casting motion to mobilize stiffness to regain digital flexion following Dupuytren's fasciectomy. Hand Ther. 2010;15(2):45–51.

Part VII

Complications of Hand Pathologies

Complex Regional Pain Syndrome 14

Alexandra Perret

CRPS

Complex regional pain syndrome (CRPS), as its current name suggests, is not a pathology per se, but a set of symptoms whose expression determines a pathological state. The definition of CRPS has evolved over time in line with the recognition and understanding of these symptoms.

First used in 1993, the term CRPS is not yet widely used, but is the subject of an international consensus [1]. The terms algodystrophy (CRPS type 1) and causalgia (CRPS type 2) are still widely used. The term "shoulder-hand syndrome" is also used for the upper limbs as soon as the shoulder is involved.

The current definition of CRPS is that of the International Association for the Study of Pain (IASP) in its 2011 version, known as the "Budapest criteria": "CRPS is a syndrome characterized by continuous regional pain (spontaneous and/or provoked) apparently disproportionate in time and magnitude to the usual course of pain after a trauma or other injury. This pain is regional (not systematized in a nerve territory or dermatome) and usually presents a distal predominance of abnormal sensory, motor, sudomotor, vasomotor sensations and/or trophic aspects" [2] (Fig. 14.1).

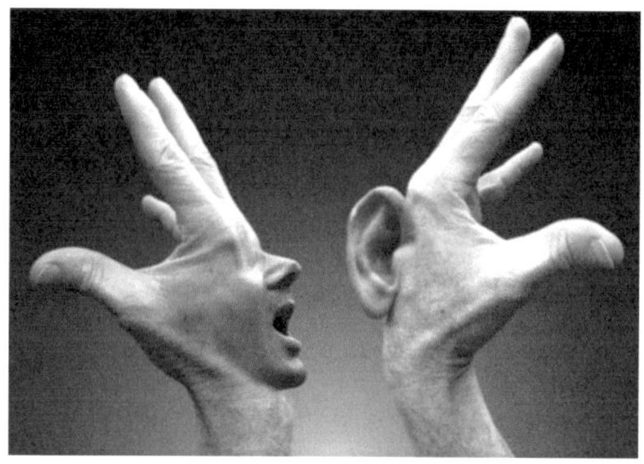

Fig. 14.1 CRPS is a syndrome characterized by continuous regional pain apparently disproportionate in time and magnitude to the usual course of pain after a trauma or other injury

Incidence and Prevalence

Injuries of the extremities, such as fractures, sprains, surgery, and carpal tunnel syndrome, are the most frequently reported events with evolution towards CRPS [2, 3]. In a recent analysis of 1043 patients with CRPS [4], the leading causes were fractures (42%), including 43% of wrist and ankle fractures [5, 6], sprains (21%), surgery (12%), and carpal tunnel syndrome (7%), while 7% had no clear initial event [3].

A. Perret (✉)
Centre Épaule Main, Voiron, France

G. Mesplié (ed.), *Hand Functional Anatomy and Therapy*,
https://doi.org/10.1007/978-3-031-92505-4_14

However, the overall prevalence of CRPS associated with these triggering events remains relatively low. Ranging from 5/100,000 in the USA to 20/100,000 in the Netherlands [4], its incidence is estimated at between 0.19% [1] and 0.64% of CRPS in distal radius fractures with surgical treatment [7]. Although it has been reported to be a common complication of Dupuytren's disease, a recent American analysis found the overall incidence to be 0.31% [8].

Several studies have shown that CRPS is much more common in women, with estimates two to four times higher than in men [3–5, 7, 9]. The average age ranges from 37 to 65 years old, depending on the study [10, 11].

Risk Factors

According to Moseley et al., severe pain (greater than 5 on the visual analog scale) lasting more than 2 days is predictive of CRPS (red flag) [12].

Fibromyalgia increases the risk of progression by up to 2.5 times [1, 13].

Other musculoskeletal conditions, such as rheumatoid arthritis, may also increase the risk [10].

Psychosocial risk factors (referenced as yellow flags) such as stress, post-traumatic stress [6], negative thinking, catastrophism, and dysphoric emotional states have been shown to be poor prognosis factors for recovery, exacerbating CRPS or even promoting its chronicization [14].

Prognosis

According to the various literature reviews, there is no consensus on recovery: some studies report rather short recovery times, with 5.4% of patients recovering within a year [10]. Others report an average of 5.8 years after the injury, in only 64% of cases.

In one study, T. Packham demonstrated that allodynia was strongly correlated (rz.55, $P < 0.01$) with the severity of CRPS and, consequently, its duration [9, 15, 16].

Various Classifications and Subtypes

Although studied for many years, the pathogenesis of this syndrome remains poorly understood. Long clinically identified by aspects of "rubor, calor, tumor, and dolor" (redness, heat, swelling, and pain), the markers of inflammation [17], as well as trophic phenomena such as sweating, mottled skin, and increased hairiness, the inclusion/exclusion criteria have since been refined.

CRPS 1 and CRPS 2

There are two types of CRPS:

- Type 1: in the absence of peripheral nerve damage (old term: algodystrophy)
- Type 2: in the presence of peripheral nerve damage (old term: causalgia)

However, experts agree that there may be peripheral nerve damage in type 1, but that it would be subclinical: when asked whether CRPS is neuropathic pain (PAIN editorial, 2006), Oaklander's team found axonal damage on 29% of the affected side. This would seem to involve preferentially small diameter sensory fibers. They go so far as to suggest that CRPS is sustained by an abnormal activity in the damaged afferent fibers [18].

Recently, a third subtype has also been recognized: not otherwise specified CRPS (NOS), which does not fulfill all the specific features of classic CRPS, but no other diagnosis can explain the pathology found in these patients [4, 19, 20].

Moderate and/or Severe

In the 2023 recommendations of the consortium of international experts, a distinction is made between moderate and severe aspects, with management based on severity: the greater the severity, the greater the need for multidisciplinary management and specific treatments.

They define a moderate CRPS when pain responds favorably to conventional medical and/or neuropathic treatments, and a severe CRPS when there is dystonia, no positive response to treatments within 4 weeks, and/or deterioration or increase in the syndrome despite treatments.

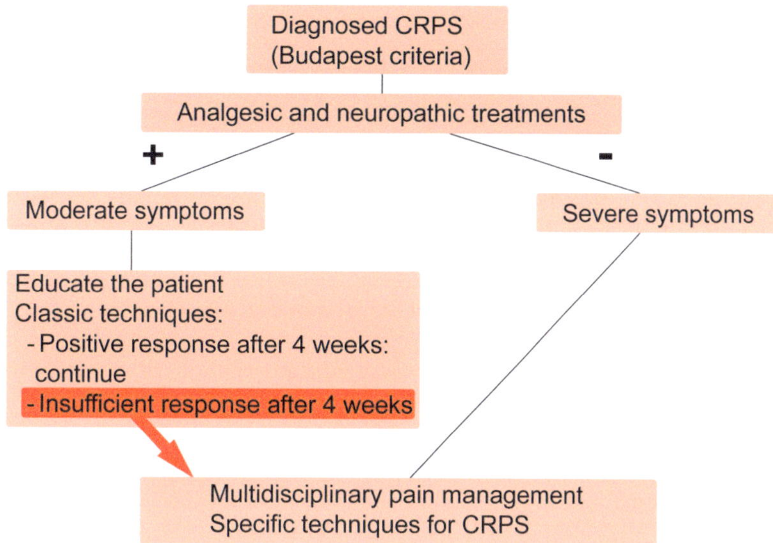

Fig. 14.2 Management algorithm based on UK guidelines

After 4 weeks, the moderate group falls into the severe group, which may suggest more centralized and therefore more complex aspects to management [21] (Fig. 14.2).

Diagnosis

It is a syndrome, and its diagnosis is therefore clinical. Signs and symptoms appear approximately 1 month after a trauma or immobilization [22]. According to the recommendations of the French Society for the Study and Treatment of Pain (SFETD) [23] and the IASP, the clinical criteria according to Budapest should be used clinically.

Clinical Diagnosis According to Budapest

Budapest's criteria are highly sensitive (85%) and relatively specific (68%) [24].

The diagnosis of CRPS is based on a careful questioning and clinical assessment of the patient (Fig. 14.3):

- At least three symptoms reported by the patient.
- At least two signs observed during the clinical assessment [25] (in the context of the research, the inclusion criteria require greater rigor, so 4/4 symptoms must be reported).
- The absence of other diagnoses explaining the symptomatology.

These criteria give rise to the following principles:

- CRPS is characterized by continuous pain, disproportionate to the initial event.
- The diagnosis probability of CRPS increases with the diversity and number of symptoms.
- To be sure that it is CRPS, all other explanatory causes or pathologies must have been ruled out.

Paraclinical Tools for a Differential Diagnosis

- No interest in MRI (little evocative or diagnosis of elimination).
- No interest in EMG (painful, little evocative, or diagnosis of elimination).
- Bone scintigraphy presents too many false positives [26] (Fig. 14.4).

	Check if present
1. Permanent pain, disproportionate to the possible triggering even	
2. The patient must signal at least one symptom in three of the following categories: - Sensory: hyperesthesia (increase in stimuli perception) and/or allodynia (pain in response to stimuli that are normally not painful) - Vasomotor: asymmetry in temperature and/or modification of the skin color and/or asymmetry in skin color - Sudomotor/edema: edema and/or modifications in perspiration and/or asymmetry in perspiration - Motor/trophic: decrease in joint amplitude and/or motor dysfunction (weakness, tremor, dystonia) and/or trophic modifications (hairs, nails, skin)	Clinic: minimum 3/4 OR Research: 4/4
3. During the assessment, we must observe at least one sign in two or more of the following categories: - Sensory: hyperalgesia (to stinging) and/or allodynia (to light touch and/or thermic stimuli and/or deep somatic pressure and/or joint mobilization) - Vasomotor: asymmetry in temperature (>1°C) and/or modifications or asymmetry - Sudomotor/edema: edema and/or modifications in perspiration and/or asymmetry in perspiration - Motor/trophic: decrease in joint amplitude and/ or motor dysfunction (weakness, tremor, dystonia) and/or trophic modifications (hairs, nails, skin)	Minimum : 2/4
4. Absence of other diagnosis that can better explain the signs and symptoms	

Fig. 14.3 Pain—Assessment—Diagnosis—Treatment (Berquin et al. 2015)

	Perfect sensitivity Standard reference (95%CI)	Imperfect sensitivity Standard reference (95%CI)	Perfect sensitivity Standard reference (95%CI)	Imperfect sensitivity Standard reference (95%CI)
No diagnostic criteria	0,933 (0,397;1)	0,933 (0,395;1)	0,72 (0,122;1)	0,829 (0,204;1)
Kozin's criteria	0,814 (0,173;1)	0,806 (0,139;1)	0,931 (0,325;1)	0,946 (0,344;1)
IASP	0,611 (0,005;1)	0,608 (0,008;1)	0,830 (0,026;1)	0,897 (0,045;1)
Budapest criteria	0,543 (0,046;1)	0,551 (0,046;1)	0,89 (0,175;1)	0,935 (0,306;1)

Fig. 14.4 Paraclinical diagnostic tools

Differential Diagnoses

Complex regional pain syndrome requires a comprehensive differential diagnosis [27] (Fig. 14.5), as many symptoms may be caused by other diseases. The differential diagnosis must be made with neurological, vascular, myofascial, inflammatory, infectious, and psychological disorders.

- Local pathology: fracture, arthrosis, arthritis, compartment syndrome, myofascial pain, etc.
- Arterial, venous or lymphatic disease: vasculitis, Raynaud's syndrome, lymphoedema, secondary erythromegaly…
- Central lesion: spinal tumor…
- Peripheral nerve injury and neuropathies: nerve compression, thoracic outlet syndrome, polyneuropathy...
- Malignant tumor: glomus tumor, carcinomas…
- Psychiatric pathology: conversive syndrome (functional neurological disorder), dissociative syndrome, etc. [22, 27].

Assess the Severity of a CRPS

In 2010, Harden et al. proposed a severity score: the CRPS severity score (CSS) [16]. It specifies the diagnosis and makes it possible to assess the evolution for the same patient and to compare results between patients (e.g., for a study). The maximum score is 17 points, with each present criterion counting for 1 point (Fig. 14.6).

Fig. 14.5 Differential diagnosis

Differential diagnosis of complex regional pain syndrome
- Neuropathic pain syndrome - Peripheral polyneuropathy - Nerve entrapment - Radiculopathy - Post-herpetic neuralgy - Post-stroke pain - Plexopathy - Damage to a motor neuron
Others
Vascular disease - Thrombosis - Acrocyanosis - Atherosclerosis - Raynaud's disease - Erythromelalgia
Inflammation - Erysipelas - Inflammation - Bursitis - Seronegative arthritis - Rheumatological disease
Myofascial pain - Overuse - No use - Epicondylitis - Trauma by repetitive movements - Fibromyalgia
Psychiatric issues - Somatoform disorder - Munchausen syndrome

DIAGNOSTIC SIGNS AND SYMPTOMS INCLUDED IN THE CRPS SEVERITY SCORE BY SUBGROUP

Variable	Diagnosis	
	CRPS	Non-CRPS
Self-reported symptoms (%yes)		
Allodynia, hyperpathia	88,6	65,9
Temperature asymmetry	87,7	36,6
Skin color asymmetry	90,4	29,3
Sweating asymmetry	63,2	14,6
Asymmetric edema	88,6	41,5
Trophic changes	75,4	39,0
Motor changes	89,5	46,3
Decreased active range of motion	86,8	34,1
Signs observed on examination (% yes)		
Hyperpathia to pinprick	78,9	43,9
Allodynia	71,1	29,3
Temperature asymmetry by palpation	64,9	14,6
Skin color asymmetry	84,2	34,1
Sweating asymmetry	38,6	12,2
Asymmetric edema	64,9	26,8
Trophic changes	69,3	31,7
Motor changes	78,1	39,0
Decreased active range of motion	86,0	36,6

Fig. 14.6 Severity score according to Harden

Clinical Characteristics and Physiopathology of CRPS

Persistent and continuous pain, disproportionate to the initial injury, is the main complaint, but CRPS also affects other physical and cognitive functions. A summary of these various clinical manifestations, together with their pathophysiological mechanisms, provides a better understanding of the changes in peripheral and cognitive functions in these patients and thus optimizes our management.

Sensory, Autonomic, and Motor Symptoms, Peripheral and Central Mechanisms

The physiopathology of CRPS remains poorly understood. This could be explained by several interrelated phenomena.

The syndrome is characterized by inflammation beyond normal timeframes, leading to vascular changes and a proliferation of fibroblasts, as well as central phenomena such as sensorimo-

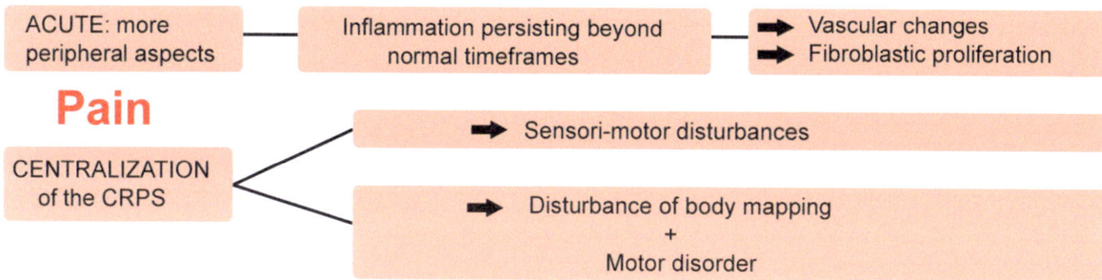

Fig. 14.7 Central and acute pain in CRPS according to Birklein

Fig. 14.8 Peripheral and central changes

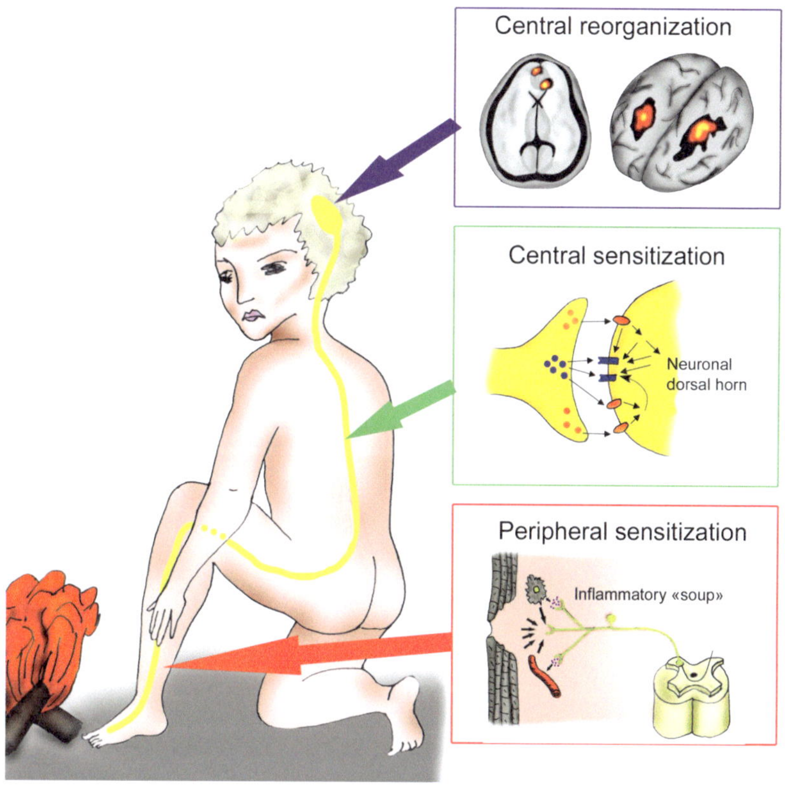

tor disorders, disturbances of perception and body mapping, and motor disorders.

Contrary to popular belief, according to Birklein [28], this phenomenon does not necessarily set in over time, as would be expected in the case of chronic pain, but can be present from the beginning, as early as the acute phase, depending on the patient's characteristics.

These two phenomena, inflammation and centralization, may therefore be concomitant (Fig. 14.7).

In addition, and as in all central phenomena, CRPS deeply alters the neural systems involved in the processing of sensitive and nociceptive information.

These changes affect (Fig. 14.8):

- The primary sensory neurons (first links in the activation and transfer of nociceptive messages)
- The dorsal horn of the spinal cord, where these neurons establish their first synaptic links
- Certain brain structures (functional reorganization of the sensory and motor cortexes through adaptive plasticity)

These are referred to as peripheral and central sensitization phenomena.

Peripheral Phenomena

➔ Local and Neurogenic Inflammation

CRPS is characterized by both a pro-inflammatory immune response and an altered neuropeptide signalization [29]. While one might expect inflammation following surgery or tissue trauma, the activation of the immune system is amplified and persistent in patients with CRPS [5]. This activation triggers a keratinocyte proliferation and the release of pro-inflammatory cytokines [30]. These cytokines trigger an immune cascade that leads to a histamine-induced vasodilation, resulting in the redness, edema, pain, and heat characteristic of CRPS [31, 32]. Pro-inflammatory cytokines also activate osteoblasts and osteoclasts, leading over time to rapid bone turnover and osteopenia (loss of bone density) [33–35].

➔ Peripheral Sensitization

This plays an important role in the development of CRPS. Activation of the free endings of the C-fibers transmits nociceptive signals afferently to the dorsal ganglia and efferently to the affected tissue [36] (axon reflex) (Fig. 14.9). This releases pro-inflammatory neuropeptides (substance P and CGRP). Skin biopsies of patients with CRPS have confirmed that these two peptides bind to their receptors on keratinocytes, leading to their proliferation and neurogenic inflammatory changes with hyperalgesia and primary allodynia [37].

Thus, the nerves themselves can generate a painful experience and without any apparent injury [38]. Peripheral sensitization can make a normal traction of the neural container (the skin) so painful that, in some cases, normal movement becomes impossible [39, 40].

> If pain is an alarm signal, the peripheral sensitization corresponds to a drop in the sensitivity of its sensors. The peripheral system is in orange-red vigilance. If these were guard dogs, they would start barking at the slightest approach to the house.

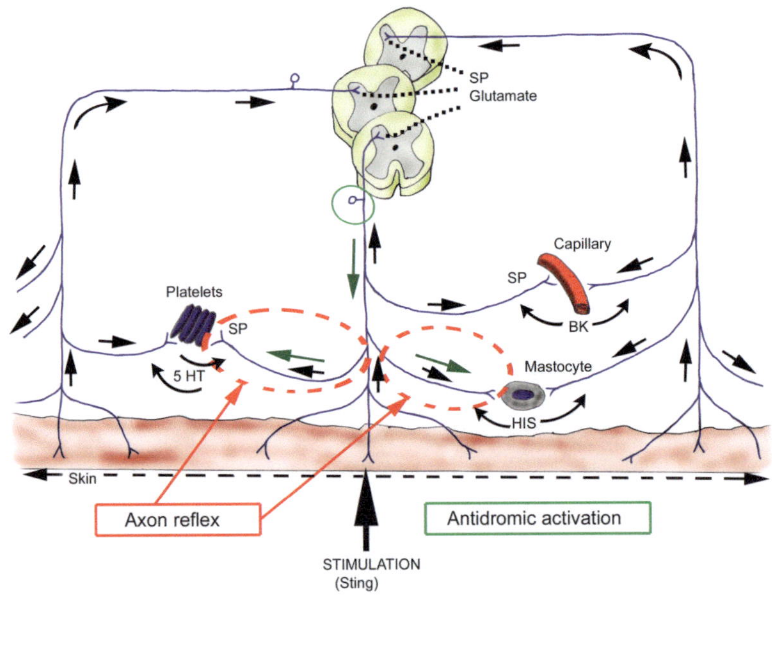

Fig. 14.9 Axon reflex according to L. Fabre

Mechanosensitivity

➔ Characteristics of Mechanosensitivity

It is the name given to the increased sensitivity of a nerve to compression (e.g., palpation) or stretching [41, 42]. It is a nociceptive response conveyed by the nervi nervorum, which are nonmyelinated fibers located in the epineurium of a nerve, whose function is sensory transmission and regulation of all the surrounding structures [43].

We are dealing here with nerve pain (mechanosensitivity), which should not be confused with neuropathic pain (nerve damage or disease) [44–46].

Neural mechanosensitivity occurs without loss of function, even if it is high.

C-fiber axons may also be affected within the nerve (Fig. 14.10), in which case we speak of axonal mechanosensitivity.

Mixed disorders also occur.

These phenomena are found in the skin and fascia and affect the elements surrounding the sensory fibers. We might think of this as "dermo-mechanosensitivity."

➔ Causes of Mechanosensitivity [39]

- **Vascular disorders**
  Twenty-five percent of the body's total energy [47] is used by the nervous system (2% of the body weight). Neural cells require a great deal of metabolic energy (glucose and oxygen). Nervi nervorum may be activated in the event of ischemia due to mechanical stresses affecting intra- or extra-neural arterial vessels [48, 49] (Fig. 14.11).
- **Loss of venous drainage**
  Capillary permeability and exchange are passive mechanisms. The lymphatic drainage of a nerve is weak [50], hence the importance of venous drainage and the harmful effects of immobilization (Fig. 14.12).
- **Nerve compression**
  It will lead to a local immuno-inflammatory reaction, which may spread to the neuron's body (located in the dorsal ganglion) and, as it worsens, spread to the whole ganglion, also affecting the bodies of other adjacent neurons [41, 51].

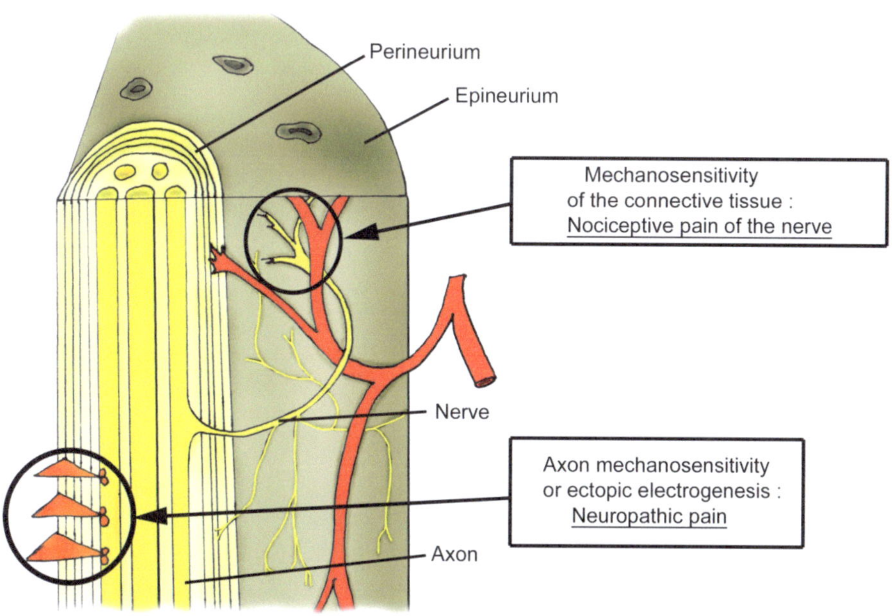

Fig. 14.10 The two types of mechanosensitivity

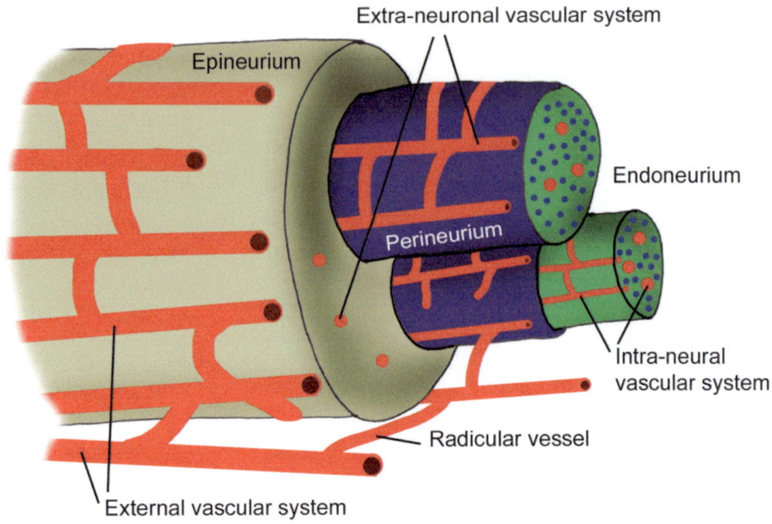

Fig. 14.11 Intra-neural circulation according to D. Jacobs

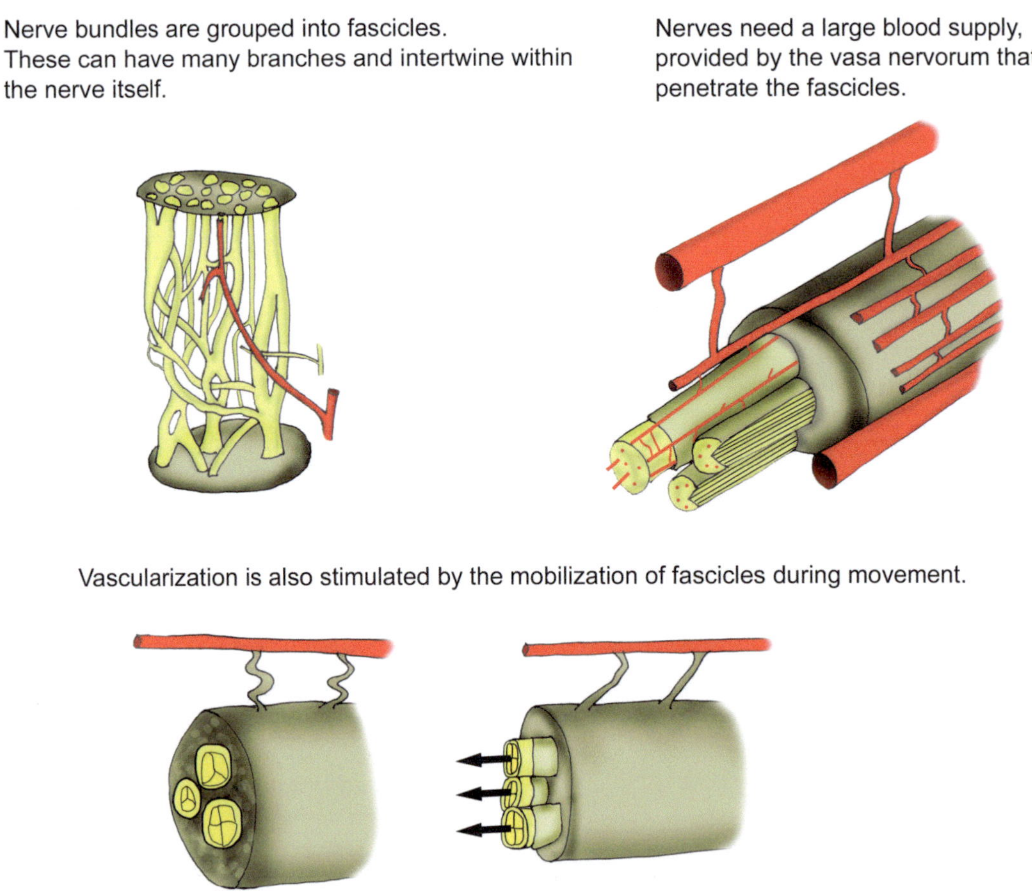

Fig. 14.12 Nerves and their vascularization (D. Jacobs, adapted from Lundborg)

Several sources of compression (subclinical canal syndromes) are possible [40, 52] (Fig. 14.12).

- **Edema**
  Perineurial or endoneurial edema, whether hormonal (pregnancy, menopause, hypothyroidism) or post-traumatic, can cause mechanosensitivity.
- **Pathological dynamics**
  The consequence of canal syndromes [40, 52, 53]: the impeded nerve generates spontaneous or persistent local pain [54], which can be observed directly during movement [55].
- **Mechanical deformations**
  Caused by too much or too little movement (idiopathic canal syndromes) [39].
- **Inflammation**
  It thickens the neural walls and reduces blood supply.
- **Anatomical changes**
  During normal or repetitive movements, they can impair nerve function (osteoarthritis or a cyst rubbing a sensory branch).
- **Diabetes** (Mason 2011)

> Mechanosensitivity is the warning message of the nerve's guardians, who suffer from hunger, lack of oxygen, or obstruction.

➔ Autonomic Nervous System

CRPS patients show a decrease in norepinephrine in favor of catecholamines in the affected limb. Decreased activity of the sympathetic nervous system is thought to result in vasodilation and increased blood flow to the limb with CRPS, leading to warmth and redness [56, 57].

➔ Immunity

Significant quantities of antibodies in the skin and tissues of patients with CRPS have been found in several studies [58]. It is possible that the latter participate in pain phenomena by taking part in the sensitization of nociceptors [59].

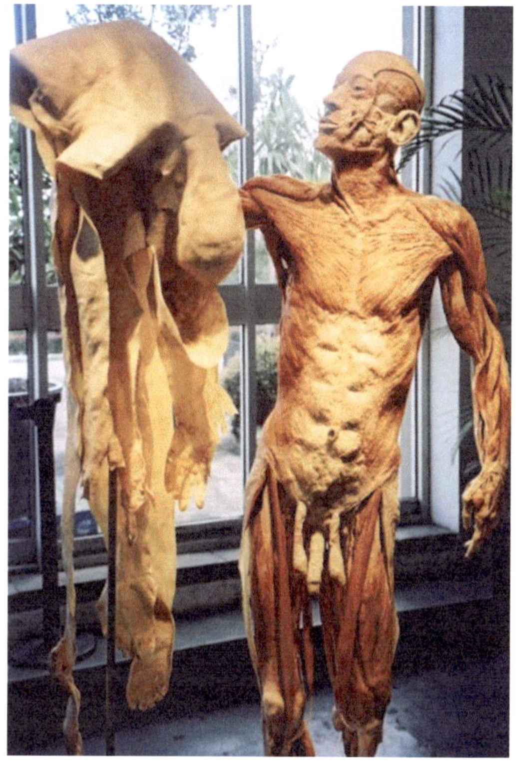

Fig. 14.13 Skin man by Von Hagens

➔ Skin (Fig. 14.13)

Apart from peripheral sensitization phenomena known in CRPS situations, could adherences and scars be a possible cause of neural and/or neuropathic exacerbation?

As we have already seen, edema, inflammation, cutaneous adherences, and adherences of the underlying planes lead to tension, compression, and "loss of cutaneous reserves," affecting the intra- and extra-neural circulation and the mobility of nerve fibers (mostly cutaneous) (Fig. 14.14).

J.P. Guimberteau's beautiful images in "Voyage sous la peau" [60] demonstrate the extent to which the skin, the fascias, and their gliding planes play a role in absorbing mechanical stress. They avoid transmitting the slightest stress to overlying or underlying elements. Professor Stecco's dissection work [61] supports this idea by demonstrating the existence and role of the retinaculum curtis (Fig. 14.15).

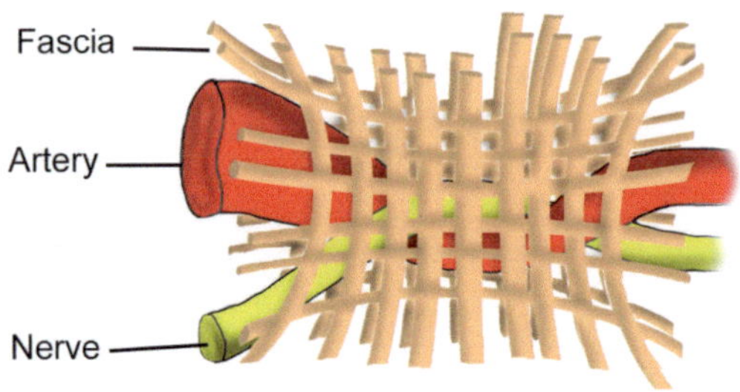

Fig. 14.14 Fascias and gliding planes

Adherences and scars therefore have a significant impact: if the skin loses its role of absorbing internal (muscular contraction) and external (leaning on a table with an elbow) stresses, even though it is itself the container of the sensory system, the latter can easily become stimulated or even irritated.

The skin, directly linked to our brain via the sensory system, also plays a role in absorbing stress.

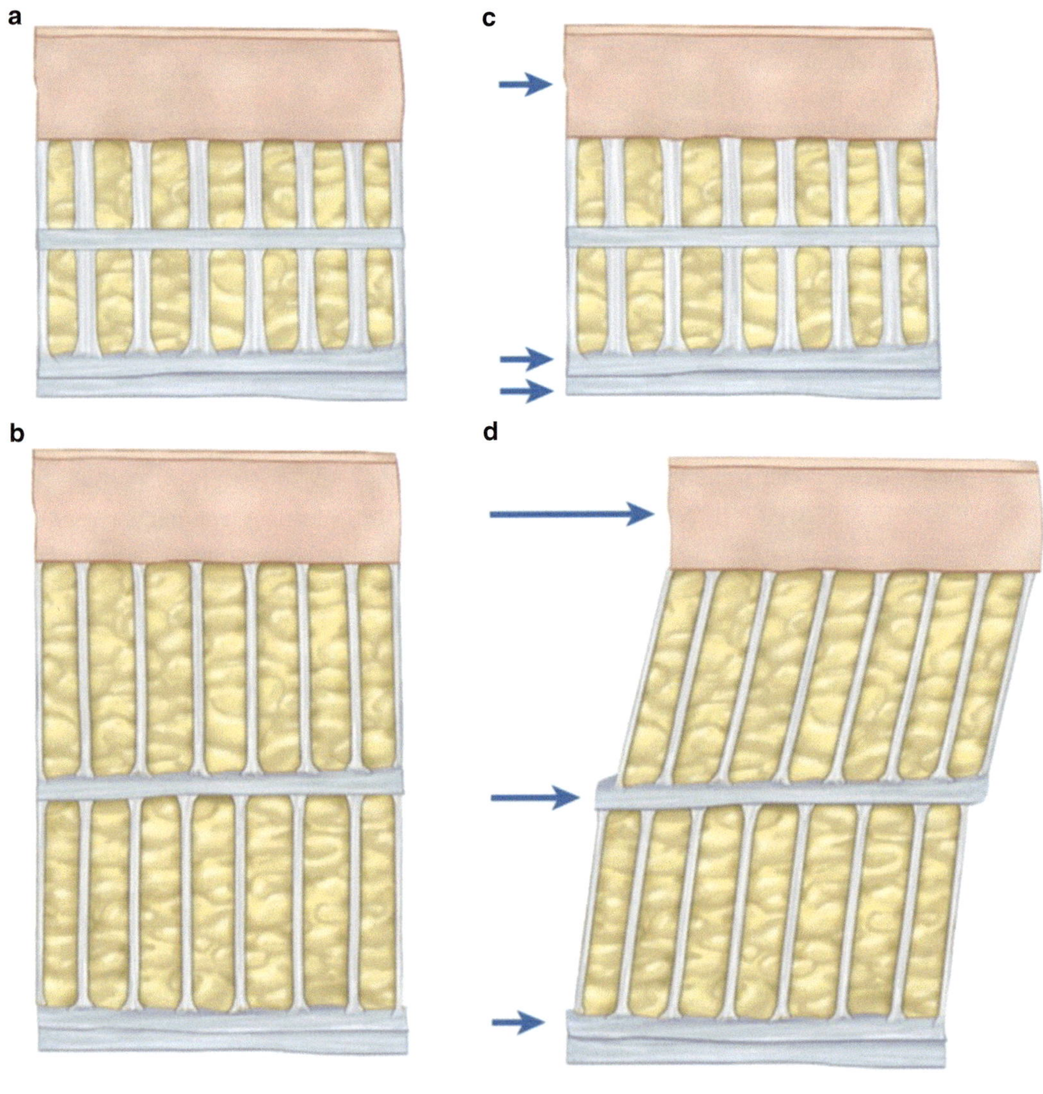

Fig. 14.15 Retinaculum curtis and fascias according to Stecco. (**a**, **c**): when the retinaculum curtis are short and thick, they transmit the least stress to the overlying/underlying elements. (**b**, **d**): long and thin, they can absorb them. They reduce stress from the skin to the muscles and from the muscles to the skin

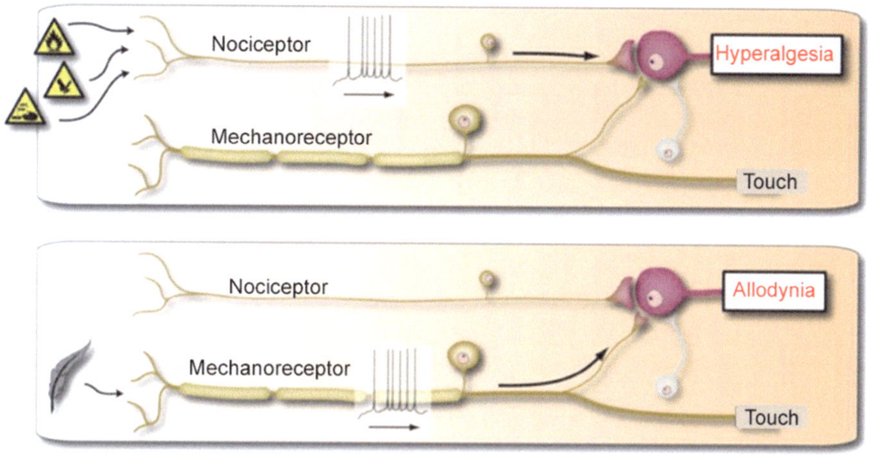

Fig. 14.16 Hyperalgesia and allodynia according to Woolf

Central Phenomena

➔ Central Sensitization

Central sensitization modifies and consequently reorganizes several areas and types of central nervous system (CNS) structures, especially second-order neurons, glial cells, inhibitory interneurons (disappearance), sensory and motor cortex, and endogenous pain modulator [62–64]. It follows intense and prolonged nociceptive stimuli. As a maladaptive plasticity, it increases the CNS response to stimuli of normal or lower intensity than their usual threshold of activation (IASP).

The consequence is an increased response to various stimuli (Fig. 14.16):

- Secondary mechanical hyperalgesia (increased response to a nociceptive stimulus)
- Mechanical allodynia (also secondary)

Another consequence will be an increase in pain surface area and intensity [2] (Fig. 14.17).

> Central sensitization is a maladaptive plasticity in which dogs and house alarms are triggered by nothing. The alert level is at its highest. The whole system is under orange-red vigilance.

➔ Cortical Territories and Pain

There are four main regions involved in pain [65]:

- The primary and secondary somesthetic cortex S1-S2, dedicated to sensory components. Concerning pain, they deal with the physical aspects of nociceptive stimulation: its location, intensity, duration, and qualities (heat, cold, numbness, etc.). S1 has a representation of each part of the body called the somatotopy. It is composed of a surface area proportional to the number of sensory receptors (Fig. 14.18).
- The anterior cingulate cortex (ACC) and insula (Cis), dedicated to the emotional appreciation of pain, influenced not only by the intensity of stimulation but also by other emotions such as anticipation or fear (Fig. 14.19).

"A pathology, whether it has a traumatic or spontaneous origin, leads to a modification of the perceptions of our body and its environment, modifying to a greater or lesser extent the cerebral mechanisms for processing and encoding visual, tactile and proprioceptive information" [66]. These spontaneous modifications, result of cerebral plasticity, include adaptive and maladap-

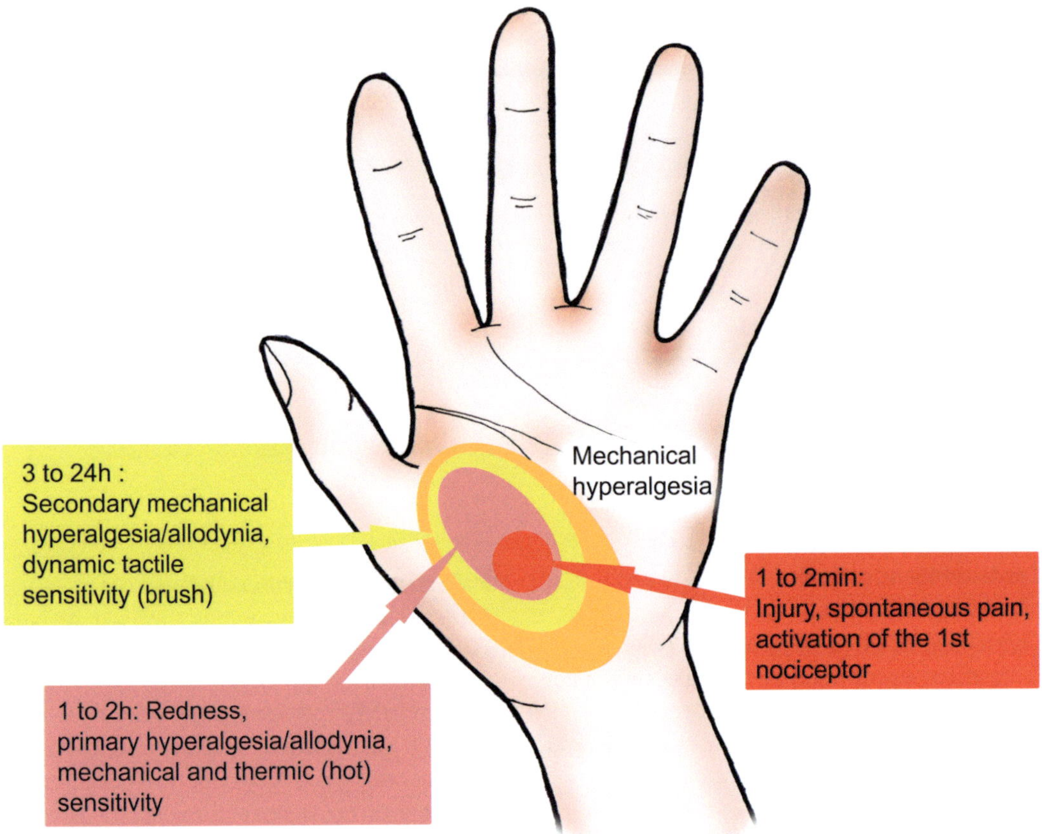

Fig. 14.17 Surface increase in sensitization phenomena, according to Woolf and reviewed by L. Fabre

tive phenomena, which can contribute to the chronicization of pain.

These patterns of cerebral activation are called "neuro-signature" by Melzak, a term later used by Lorimer Moseley as "neurotag."

One of the most accomplished models, which considers all the elements involved in pain, could be Louis Gifford's Mature Organism (Fig. 14.20) where pain is understood as the result of a complex process that enables a biological response to a potential threat to tissues and/or the environment.

> Our growing understanding of the role of the higher centers in pain allows us to realize the complexity of the balance between the sensory and affective (emotional) components of pain... A good understanding of the neural networks of the higher centers allows us to better grasp the nature of certain chronic pains... (S. Marchand).

We understand that pain, the main symptom of our patients with CRPS, needs to be understood, analyzed, and documented during our assessments to optimize our management.

> Pain is the result of a complex process that allows us to respond biologically to a potential threat from the tissues and/or the environment.

➔ Maladaptive Plasticity and Pain

In CRPS, as in all "centralized" pain, the patient presents a modification of the cortical organization of S1 of the affected limb. In their studies, Maihöfner et al. [67], using functional MRI, observed that the areas corresponding to the first

Fig. 14.18 Primary somesthetic cortex

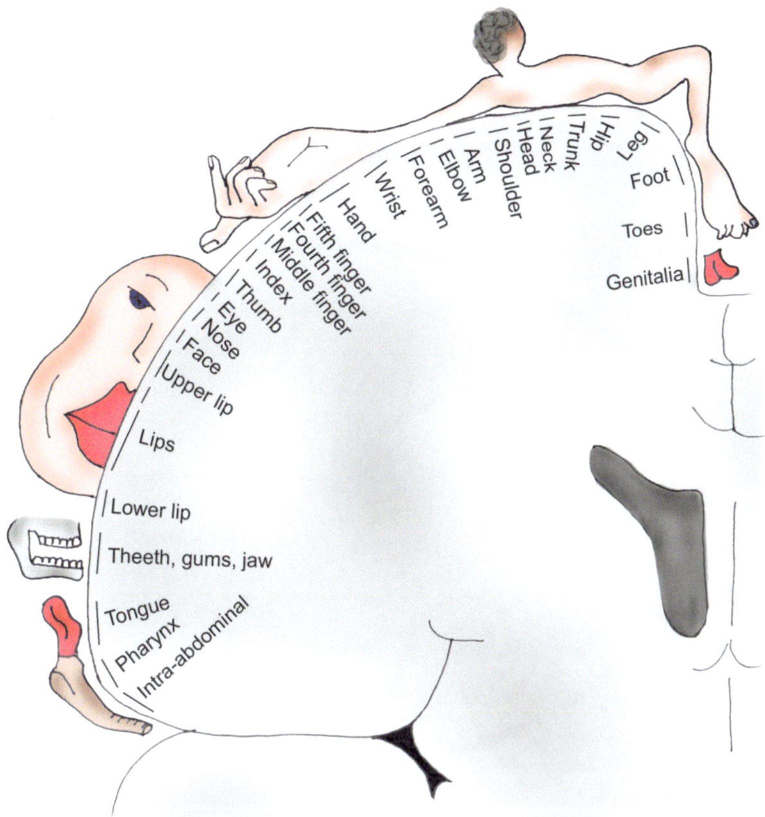

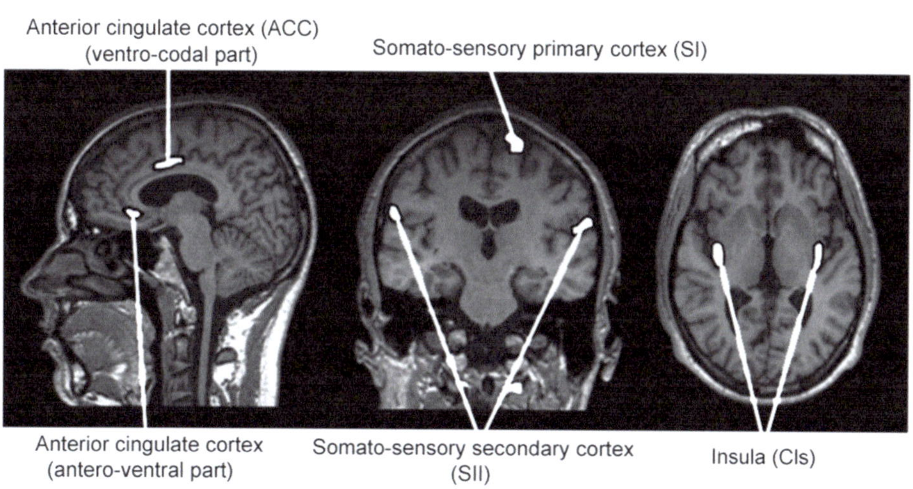

Fig. 14.19 Cortical regions implied in pain [65]

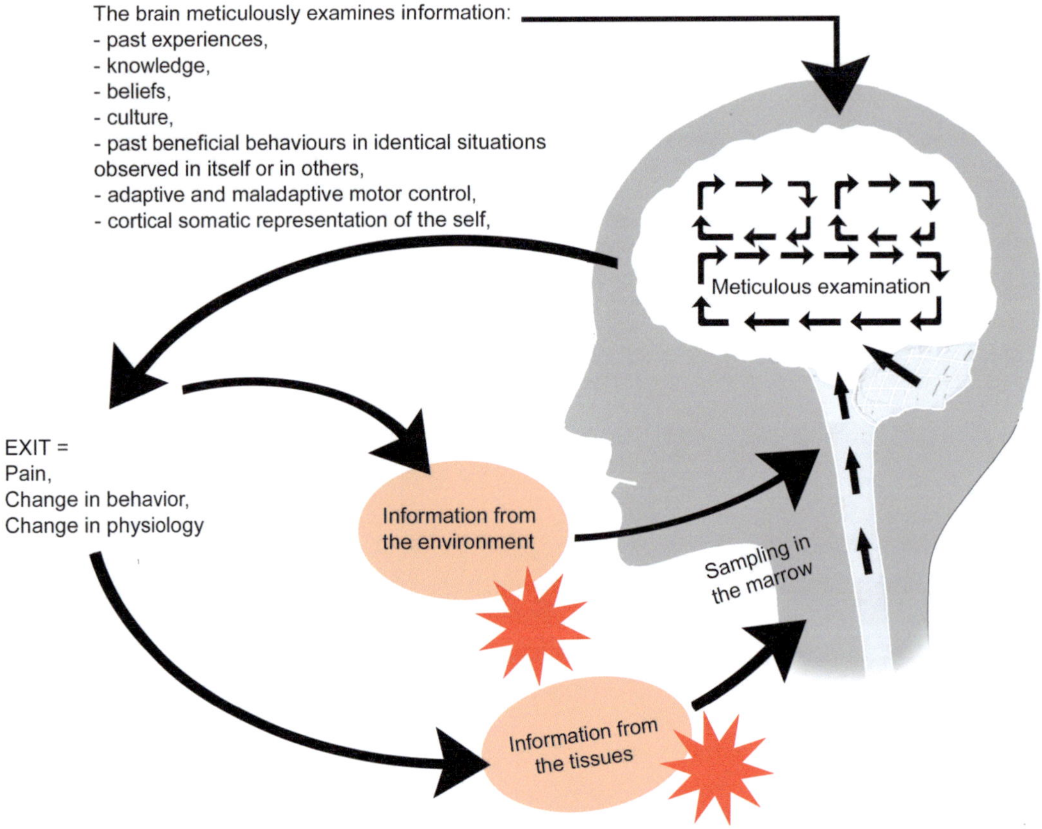

Fig. 14.20 Mature organism (L. Gifford)

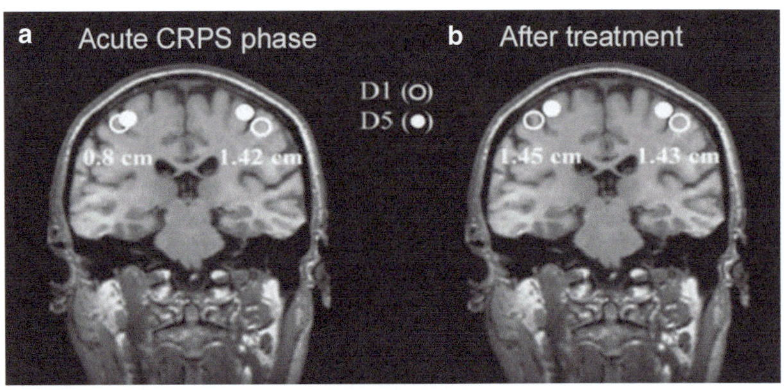

Fig. 14.21 Cortical reorganization in CRPS (Maihöfner et al): (**a**) During the acute phase, the representational area between the first and fifth fingers is reduced compared to the healthy side; (**b**) normalization of the cortical organization after resolution of the problem, 1 year of treatment

and fifth fingers got closer, and the hand area decreased and moved towards the lip area during the acute phase of CRPS. They then observed a re-expansion of the cortical zones after rehabilitation 1 year later. They found a correlation between pain reduction and hyperalgesia with this cortical re-expansion [68, 69] (Fig. 14.21).

➔ Altered Neuropsychological Functions in CRPS

How do we perceive our bodies? The representation of the body could be explained by a perception-action model. On the one hand, a perceptive modality of "what," which would be "body perception," and on the other, a modality

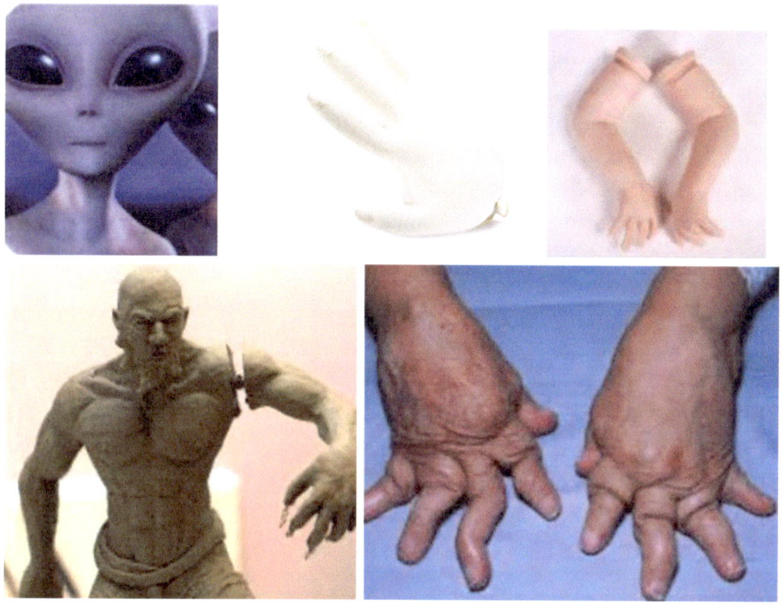

Fig. 14.22 Body perception disorder

of "how," oriented towards motor action, "body mapping" [70].

In a patient with CRPS, disturbances in spatial attention are associated with hypo-attention to proprioceptive and discriminative stimuli of the affected limb, but also of the surrounding space, disrupting the patient's spatial referential [71, 72].

- **Body perception disorders**

One of the symptoms reported by patients with CRPS is an altered perception of the affected limb (Fig. 14.22). According to Lewis et al. [73], it is characterized by sensations of a limb that is deformed, disproportionate, foreign, detached, out of control, a limb that they sometimes reject.

The incidence of this syndrome is not to be underestimated, since it was found to be as high as 84% in the studies by Forderreuther et al. in 2004 and Galer BS and Jensen M in 1999 [74, 75].

It is thought to be the consequence of imprecise peripheral feedback (sensory, especially proprioceptive) [76–79]. Instead, Haggard et al. put forward the notion of "blurring" as the result of the modifications to somatosensory cortical representations [77] (Fig. 14.23).

Cognitive functions linked to altered spatial reference systems could modulate limb perception, with a "top-down" effect that increases pain [45, 73, 80, 81] (Fig. 14.24).

Because of this correlation, correcting disturbances in body perception would improve pain phenomena [82] (Fig. 14.25).

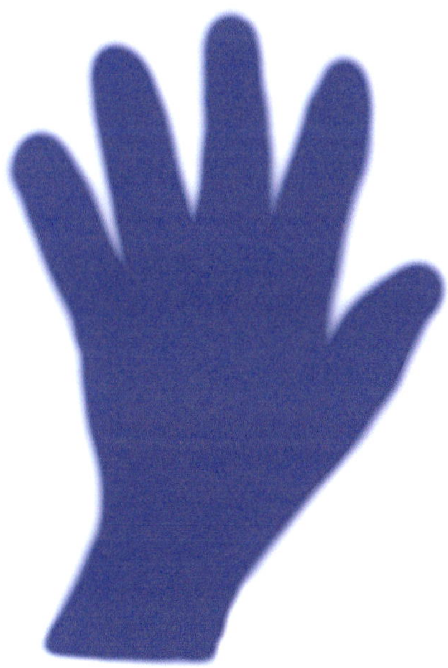

Fig. 14.23 Blurry hand

- **Body and spatial schema disorders**

  Our spatial and bodily representations enable us to locate our body in space and to interact with it. For this purpose, two "points of view," two frames of reference, are recognized: egocentric and allocentric [83].

  – The egocentric viewpoint, centered on the subject: first-person observation, the observer is the frame of reference (Fig. 14.26). It allows a spatial representation of objects depending on their position relative to the observer's body. In this context, right and left are defined in relation to the midline of the body or a part of the body.

  – The allocentric viewpoint: the object is located using an external frame of reference (third-person observation, the observer is independent) (Fig. 14.27).

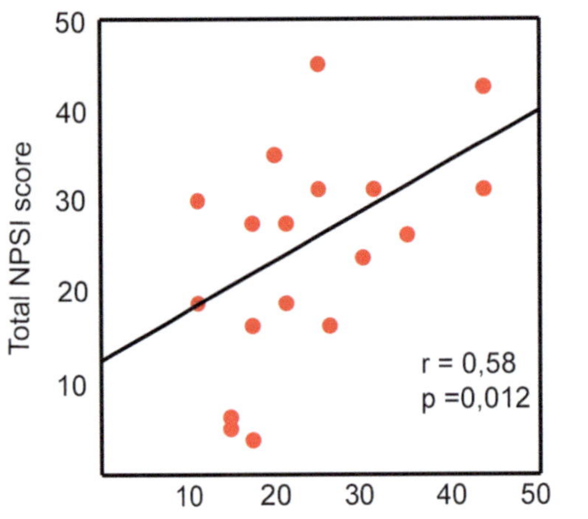

Fig. 14.24 Correlation between body mapping disturbance and pain according to Lewis

The encoding and position of the egocentric frame of reference are the result of a harmonious balance between afferent information from the right and left hemispheres, necessary for the interpretation of sensory information [84].

An altered perception of this egocentric reference and of spatial cognition in general is typically observed in subjects suffering from left-sided spatial neglect, a frequent syndrome following a right-sided stroke (Figs. 14.28 and 14.29).

Patients with CRPS show similarities, especially in the under-use of their limbs and a lack of attention on the affected side.

Fig. 14.25 Correcting the body mapping disturbance decreases pain according to Lewis

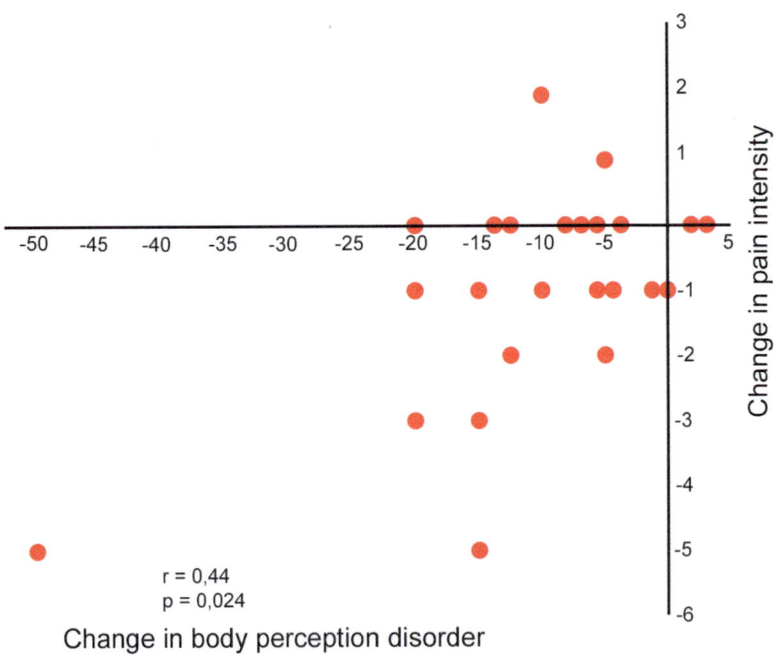

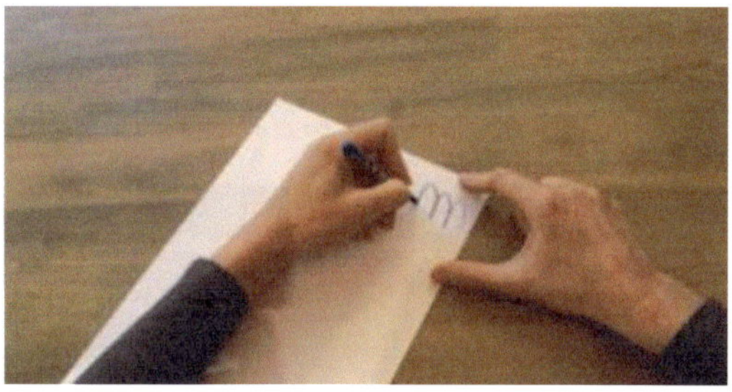

Fig. 14.26 Egocentric representation

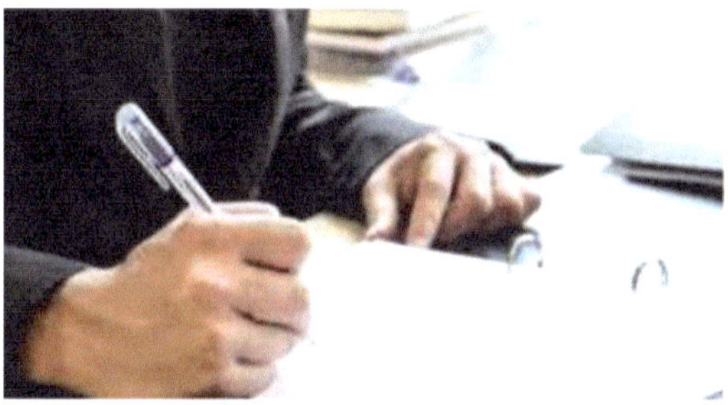

Fig. 14.27 Allocentric representation

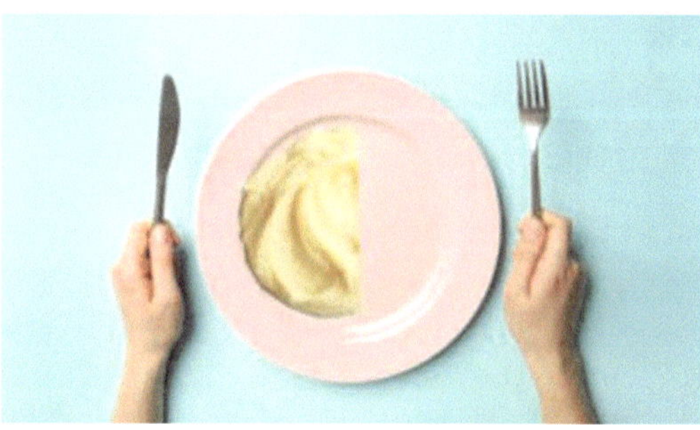

Fig. 14.28 Attention deficit disorder on the right

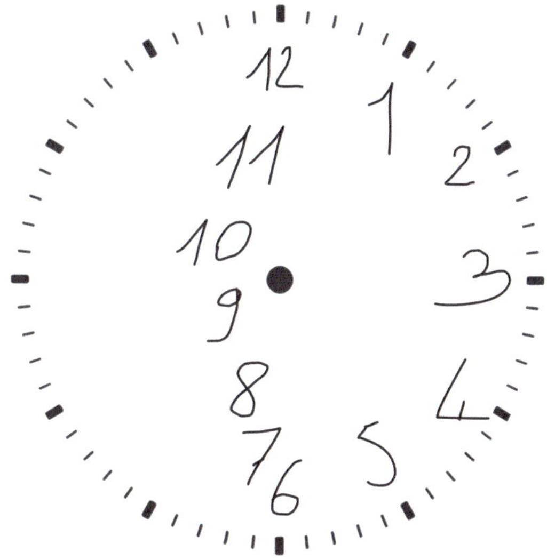

Fig. 14.29 Attention deficit disorder on the left

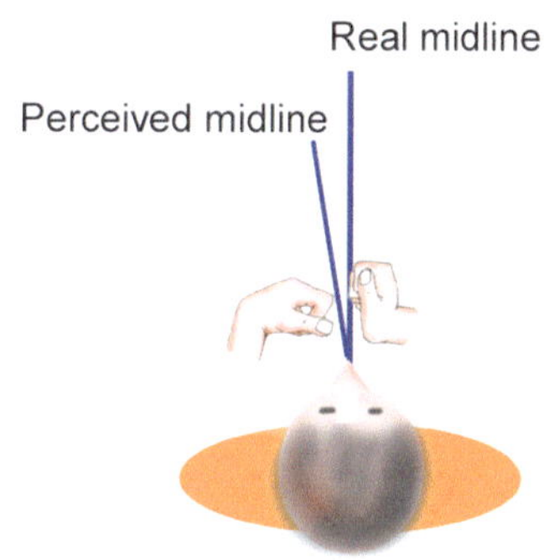

Fig. 14.30 Alteration of the perception of the body midline

- ***Body midline, its perception and effects on pain, homeostasis, and tactile acuity***

In studies where a subject is asked to face a wall 2 meters away (extra-personal space) and to use a laser to indicate where he thinks his body midline is, patients with CRPS tend to shift the midpoint of their subjective body to the symptomatic side [85, 86].

This is the deviation of CRPS patients' egocentric visual frame of reference to the side of the painful limb, which is proprioceptive in post-stroke hemineglect.

The perception of the body midline is altered (Fig. 14.30).

Bultitude points out that there is a difference between the peri-personal space (what is reached by the hand) where attention is directed towards the healthy side and the distant space where attention is directed towards the injured side (Fig. 14.31).

When a CRPS patient is asked to point to the middle of his or her body, the result is shifted to the CRPS side in far space and to the healthy side in personal space.

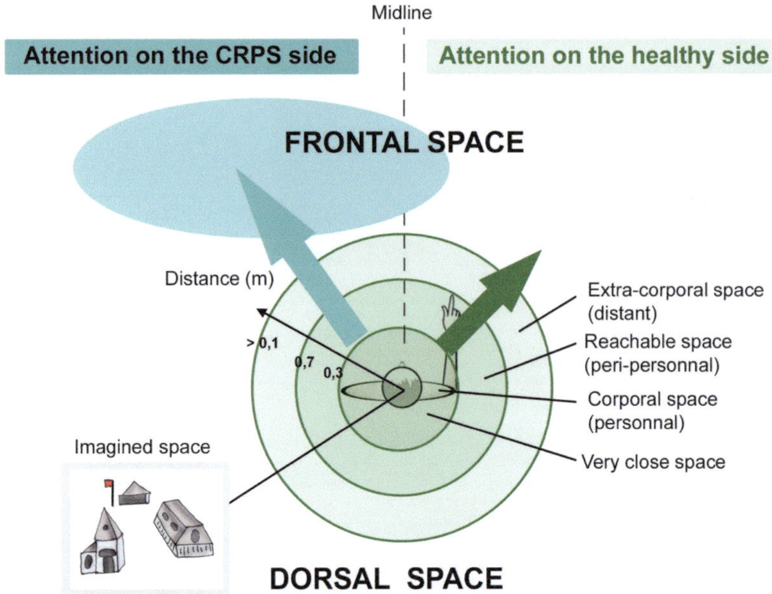

Fig. 14.31 Several bias in different regions of the space

This would seem to be a "somato-spatial attention bias" [87], since, as demonstrated by Filbrich et al. [72], for there to be a significant attentional bias in these visual pointing exercises, the patient's CRPS hands must be in their field of vision.

Lewis' work on body perception disorders is more along the lines of a maladaptive reorganization of the sensorimotor system to avoid triggering a painful experience of the affected limb, thus leading to an altered representation of the limb [81].

Once this hemispace boundary has been reached, this median line also exerts an influence on tactile acuity, homeostasis (such as temperature) [88], and pain. Moving away from or towards this hemispace either decreases or increases results (Figs. 14.32 and 14.33).

Another study by Moseley et al. [89] reported an increase in the CRPS hand temperature when it is visually displaced on the healthy side by prisms (Fig. 14.34).

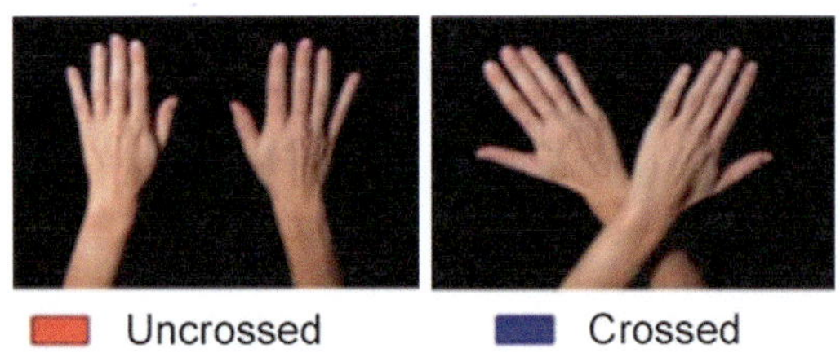

Fig. 14.32 Effect of the midline on tactile discrimination and pain

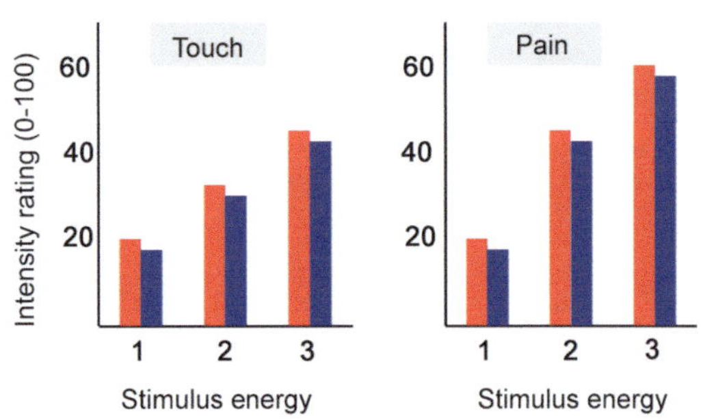

Fig. 14.33 Effect of the midline on tactile discrimination and pain

- ***Slowing down of the information processing on the CRPS side***

In his 2017 studies, Bultitude demonstrated that the patient with CRPS also shows a latency or delay originating from his CRPS hand in processing visual information [90, 91]. On the other hand, when these patients' hands are crossed, latency and delay disappear: their reactivity becomes the same for both sides (Fig. 14.35).

This could be the result of the addition of two biases: visuospatial for the affected limb and

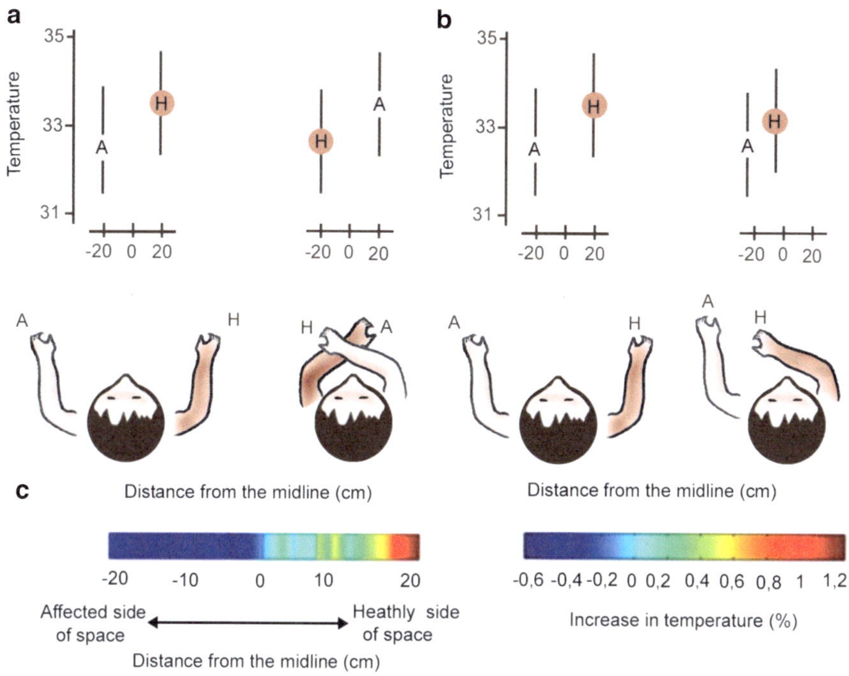

Fig. 14.34 Effect of the midline and temperature

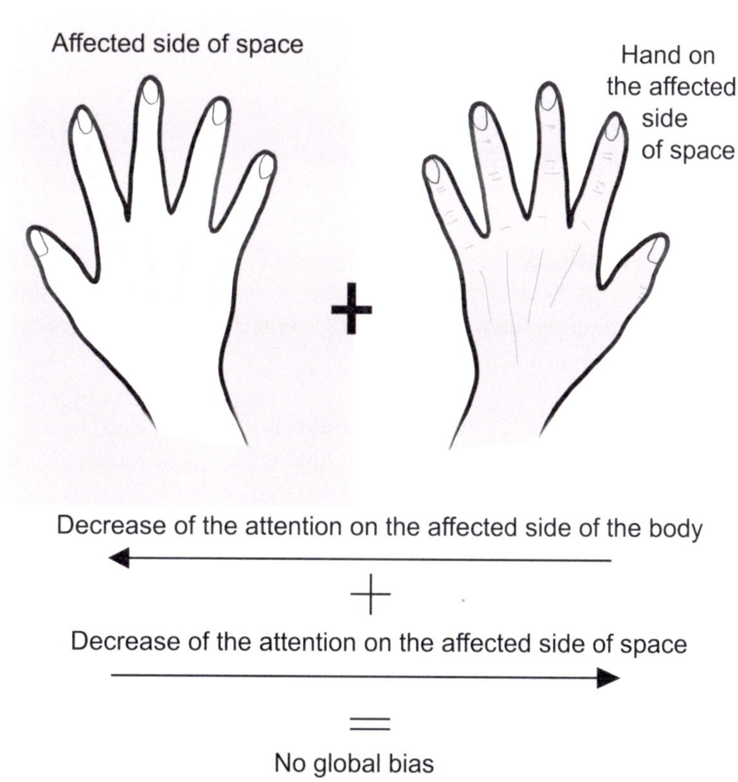

Fig. 14.35 Attention bias in CRPS? A hemispace and/or hemi-body problem? According to Bultitude

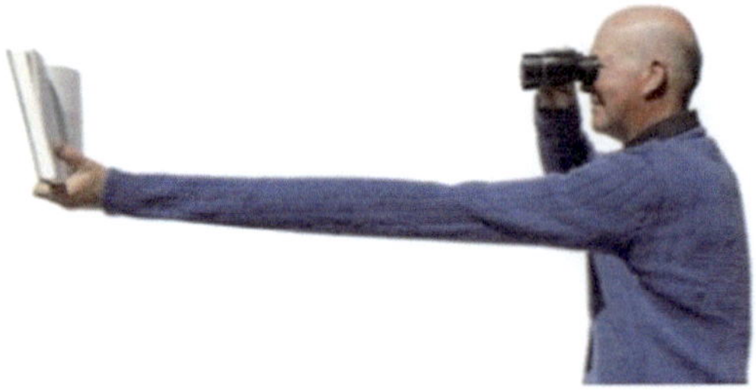

Fig. 14.36 Like myopia

hemispatial for the affected side (proprioceptive), which would cancel each other out (a little like myopia, which helps to compensate for presbyopia) (Fig. 14.36).

> Two concomitant phenomena: impairment of hemisphere information processing and hemispace CRPS.

The results of the study by Reid et al. support this view, but, in agreement with Lewis, they explain errors in spatial information processing because of body perception disorders [87].

How Can We Target Treatments? Depending on the Characteristics of the CRPS

First: Prevention!

This prevention is part of the 2018 United Kingdom recommendations for the management of CRPS.

From 2004 to 2013, audits and evaluations were carried out in Liverpool to study the incidence of Type I CRPS when casts were too tight, restrictive, or flexed. Subsequent corrections were implemented and their impact reassessed.

Results show a significant reduction in the incidence of Type I CRPS in distal radius fractures without surgery, from 25% to a rare event (<1%).

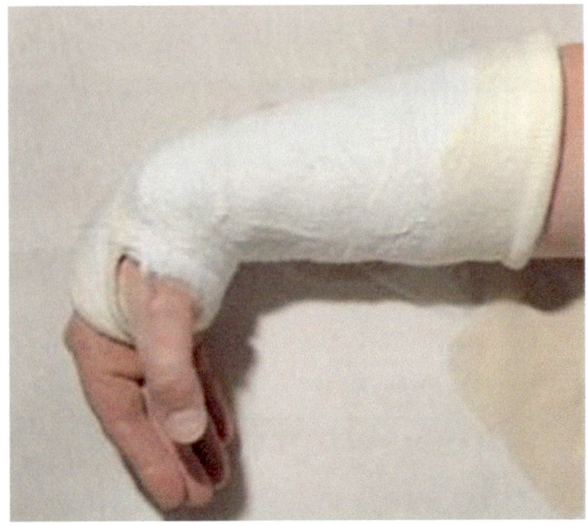

Fig. 14.37 A cast with too much flexion

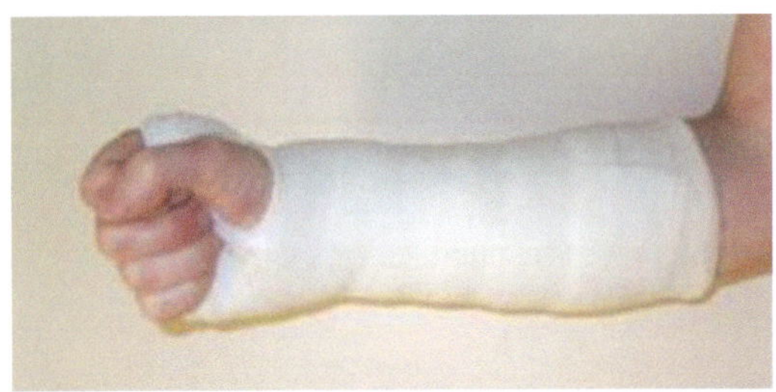

Fig. 14.38 Free the healthy joints

> Several principles were derived from this study [92]:
>
> - Always change a cast if the patient feels tight.
> - Use an orthosis as a good alternative.
> - Avoid orthoses with too much wrist flexion (Fig. 14.37).
> - Free healthy joints (Fig. 14.38).
> - Encourage a light activity.
> - Recognize at-risk patients to act early (Fig. 14.39).

Particular attention should be paid to the following alerts (Liverpool recommendations [93]) to detect at-risk patients as early as possible:

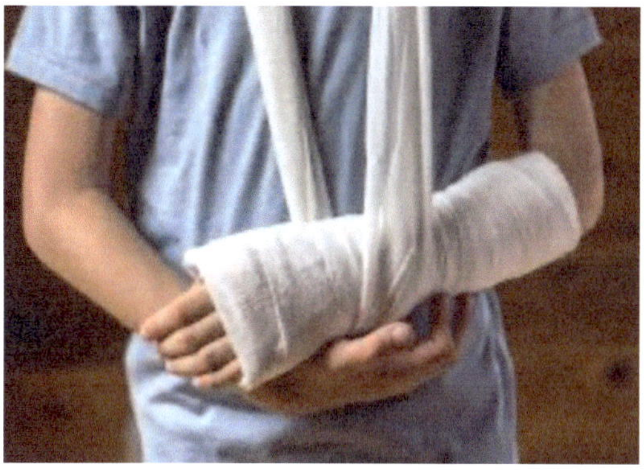

Fig. 14.39 At-risk patients

- Patient repeatedly requests cast changes.
- Patient shows neglect/rejection of the affected limb.
- Patient shows "claustrophobia" in the cast.
- Patient expresses: "the limb seems not to be mine."
- Patient shows allodynia.
- Patient shows uncontrolled pain for more than 2 weeks in the cast.
- Patient shows limitation of the amplitudes of unaffected joints.

With the aim of communicating and improving this prevention, flyers and posters are proposed (Malonet 2017) (Figs. 14.40, 14.41, and 14.42).

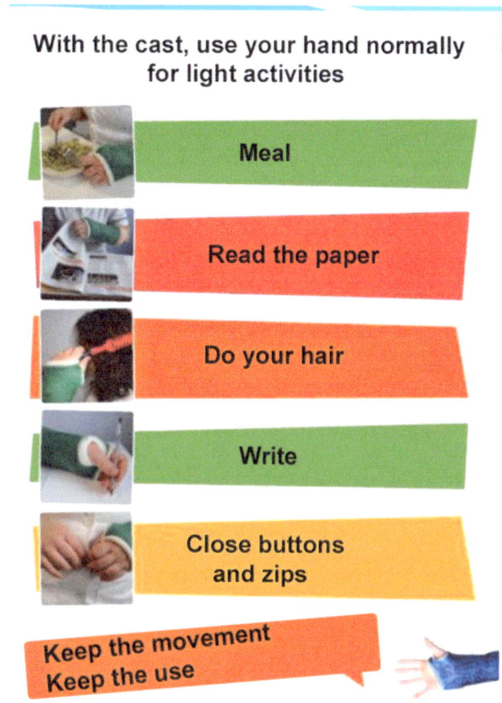

Fig. 14.40 CRPS poster. (© 2024. CRPS Forum)

To begin with, as Alison Taylor reminds us, let's refocus on listening and observing the patient, "no longer treating a simple diagnosis, but our patient's complaint." Thus, an operated carpal tunnel syndrome will not be the only explanation for the pain experienced, but could be, for example, an ulnar nerve suffering as the result of an edema contained in an orthosis.

Our physiotherapy observation will then seek to correlate the signs and symptoms described by the patient with physiopathological elements. Think in terms of: which irritative thorn is responsible for the disproportionate pain or the persistent inflammation? And determine which is the centralized part.

Precise Assessment for a Tailor-Made Treatment

Method

> One of the major causes of therapeutic failure lies in the difficulty of establishing a diagnosis and identifying the mechanisms at the origin of painful symptoms (Dallel 2000).

It is time to differentiate our CRPS patients, by identifying their symptoms to guide our treatments and no longer apply "recipes" that are supposed to be valid for all. Just as the diagnosis of "wrist sprain" is not enough to guide our treatment, distinguishing between the different CRPS enables more effective, tailor-made managements.

➔ Observe and Listen to the Patient

> We need to ask them to describe their sensations, observe the sites and paths they describe, and analyze possible correspondences with nerves, skin territories, muscles, skin, even old scars and joints, and central phenomena (A. Taylor).

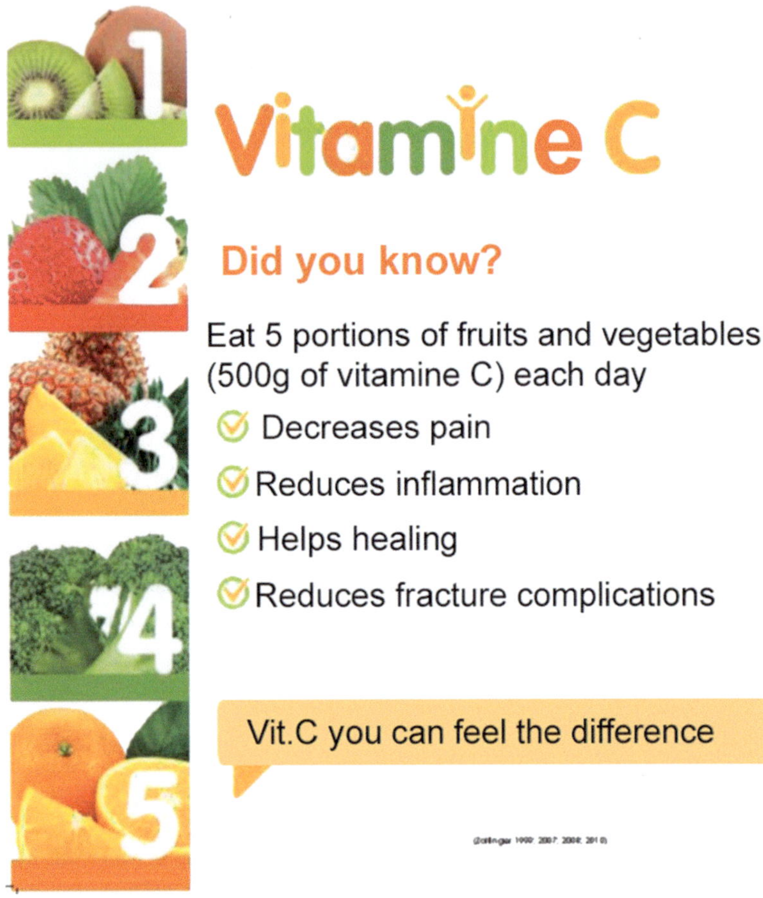
1
2
3
4
5
Vitamine C
Did you know?
Eat 5 portions of fruits and vegetables (500g of vitamine C) each day
Decreases pain
Reduces inflammation
Helps healing
Reduces fracture complications
Vit.C you can feel the difference

Fig. 14.41 CRPS poster. (© 2024. CRPS Forum)

➔ Think in Terms of Irritative Thorns
What are the possible causes of irritative thorns?

- Casts and orthoses, with the consequences of the immobilization: mechanosensitivity (is it caused/maintained by scar or skin adherences, compressions, etc.), nerve or cutaneous axon distress (which can cause pain along a path between several joints, with features such as vicelike sensations, stiffness, and the whole cohort of neuropathic symptoms such as tingling, burning, electric discharges, etc.), circulatory problems, "plaster phobia" (a patient who cannot stand being contained in a cast)
- A peripheral nerve injury generating hypoesthesia, allodynia
- The osteosynthesis material that could irritate nerves, arteries, tendons
- A lack of bone consolidation, with possible undocumented fractures
- Joint instability, leading to tension, conflict, and loss of proprioceptive information (regularly found in wrist injuries)

Assessing Central Sensitization (Fig. 14.43)

Various tools allow us to specify and assess central sensitization and its characteristics.

As we have seen, the severity of pain and other signs of CRPS (mechanical hyperalgesia, impaired tactile discrimination, reduced grip strength) is proportional to the extent of the functional reorganization of the primary sensory and motor cortexes [68, 69, 94–96]. Reducing this functional reorganization [68, 95] would improve CRPS symptoms.

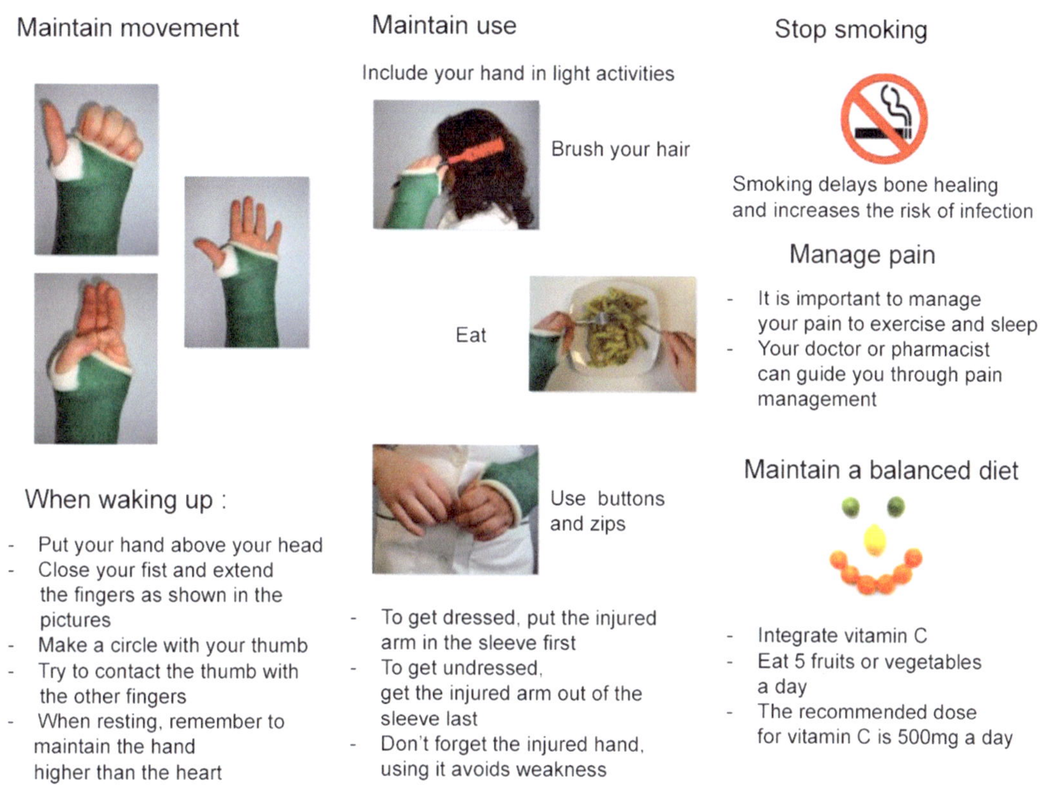
Maintain movement
When waking up :
- Put your hand above your head
- Close your fist and extend the fingers as shown in the pictures
- Make a circle with your thumb
- Try to contact the thumb with the other fingers
- When resting, remember to maintain the hand higher than the heart
Maintain use
Include your hand in light activities
Brush your hair
Eat
Use buttons and zips
- To get dressed, put the injured arm in the sleeve first
- To get undressed, get the injured arm out of the sleeve last
- Don't forget the injured hand, using it avoids weakness
Stop smoking
Smoking delays bone healing and increases the risk of infection
Manage pain
- It is important to manage your pain to exercise and sleep
- Your doctor or pharmacist can guide you through pain management
Maintain a balanced diet
- Integrate vitamin C
- Eat 5 fruits or vegetables a day
- The recommended dose for vitamin C is 500mg a day

Fig. 14.42 Suggested sheet for promoting movement with a cast or orthosis, according to Malonet

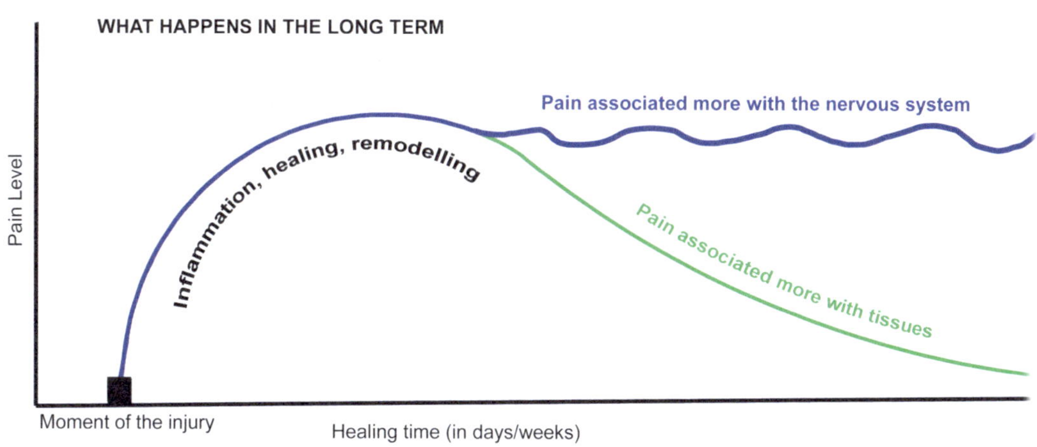

Fig. 14.43 Central sensitization

➔ Is It Centralized?

- **Central sensitization inventory (CSI)**
  It is a self-report instrument that helps to better assess symptoms of central sensitization in patients suffering from chronic pain [97–99]. Today, it has been validated in its French-language version [99].
- ***Description of the CSI***
- The CSI is a two-part questionnaire:
  - Part A measures 25 somatic and emotional symptoms associated with central sensitization, rated on a 5-point Likert scale from 0 (never) to 4 (always), with a possible total score of 100 (Fig. 14.44).
  - Part B presents possible alternative diagnoses related to central sensitization or associated disorders, such as anxiety and depression. It does not test central sensitization but helps us to determine whether we are dealing with an "at-risk" patient (Fig. 14.45).

  The CSI does not appear to diagnose central sensitization on its own and must be used along with other tests.
- ***How to interpret the CSI?***
  The higher the results, the more symptomatology is linked to central sensitization, with a threshold of 40 or more where central sensitization is confirmed [98–101].
  Levels of severity have been proposed for clinical interpretation [102] (Fig. 14.46).
- ***Central sensitization reasoning algorithm***
  Nijs proposes a reasoning algorithm for musculoskeletal pain to determine whether central sensitization is present or not (Fig. 14.47).
- **Windup ratio (WUR): assessment of temporal summation**
  The progressive activation of central neurons following an intense and sustained stimulation by C-fibers is known as the "windup" phenomenon. Only C-fibers can cause windup. The windup phenomenon of central nociceptive neurons, which become easily "irritated," is in fact a phenomenon of amplification of the response to the stimulus and is a sign of hyperalgesia or central sensitization [103] (Fig. 14.48). This phenomenon can take on such proportions that "spontaneous" activity can become observable in these neurons.
  The WUR is a test that evaluates the temporal summation of pain. It is one of the many tests in the Quantitative Sensory Testing (QST). It requires 10 "pinprick" stimuli (Fig. 14.49) of constant force and is performed at 1-second intervals on the same site (1 cm^2) [104]. It is positive if, after four to five stimulations, a disproportionate pain appears. It is measured using a visual analog scale (VAS).

➔ How Is It Centralized?

- **McGill pain questionnaire and "Questionnaire de la Douleur de Saint Antoine" (QDSA)**

The QDSA is the validated French-language version of the McGill pain questionary. Either of these questionaries must be used in the patient's native language. It consists of a therapist-guided self-evaluation of the sensory pain (35 qualifiers) and the affective-emotional pain (23 qualifiers) (Fig. 14.50).

It gives 3 scores out of 100 points: total score, sensory pain, and affective-emotional pain. It allows us to find the words to describe the pain with the patient and to assess the emotional aspect of the pain. This makes it a choice questionnaire for centralized pain.

It should be carried out once a month to assess the evolution in sensations.

- **In this centralized situation, is there a disturbance in perception and body mapping?**

It should be remembered that in this situation, the patient is no longer able to localize his body, but also its limits in space, and therefore has difficulty in directing it.

- ***"Finger perception" and "body mapping report"***

"Finger perception" measures the duration and success rate of patients who must recognize

Please indicate for each suggestion the most suitable proposal	Never	Rarely	Sometimes	Often	Always
1- I feel tired and unrefreshed when I wake from sleeping	☐	☐	☐	☐	☐
2- My muscles feel stiff and achy	☐	☐	☐	☐	☐
3- I have anxiety attacks	☐	☐	☐	☐	☐
4- I grind or clench my teeth	☐	☐	☐	☐	☐
5- I have problems with diarrhea and/or constipation	☐	☐	☐	☐	☐
6- I need help in performing my daily activities	☐	☐	☐	☐	☐
7- I'm sensitive to bright lights	☐	☐	☐	☐	☐
8- I'm tired very easily when I'm physically active	☐	☐	☐	☐	☐
9- I'm feel pain all over my body	☐	☐	☐	☐	☐
10- I have headaches	☐	☐	☐	☐	☐
11- I feel discomfort in my bladder and/or burning when I urinate	☐	☐	☐	☐	☐
12- I do not sleep well	☐	☐	☐	☐	☐
13- I have difficulty concentrating	☐	☐	☐	☐	☐
14- I have skin problems such as dryness, itchiness or rashes	☐	☐	☐	☐	☐
15- Stress makes my physical symptoms get worse	☐	☐	☐	☐	☐
16- I feel sad or depressed	☐	☐	☐	☐	☐
17- I have low energy	☐	☐	☐	☐	☐
18- I have muscle tension in my neck and shoulders	☐	☐	☐	☐	☐
19- I have pain in my jaw	☐	☐	☐	☐	☐
20- Certain smells, such as perfumes, make me feel dizzy and nauseated	☐	☐	☐	☐	☐
21- I have to urinate frequently	☐	☐	☐	☐	☐
22- My legs feel uncomfortable and restless when I am trying to go to sleep at night	☐	☐	☐	☐	☐
23- I have difficulty remembering things	☐	☐	☐	☐	☐
24- I suffer trauma as a child	☐	☐	☐	☐	☐
25- I have pain in my pelvic area	☐	☐	☐	☐	☐

Fig. 14.44 Central sensitization inventory, part A

CENTRAL SENSITIZATION INVENTORY (PART B)

Have you been diagnosed by a doctor with any of the following disorders ?
Please check the boxto the right for each diagnosis and write the year of the diagnosis

	YES	NO	Year diagnosed
Restless leg syndrome...........................	☐	☐	....
Chronic fatigue syndrome	☐	☐	....
Fibromyalgia	☐	☐	....
Temporomandibular joint disorder (TMJ) ...	☐	☐	....
Migraine or tension headaches..........................	☐	☐	....
Irritable bowel syndrome	☐	☐	....
Multiple chemical sensitivities	☐	☐	....
Neck injury (included whiplash)	☐	☐	....
Anxiety or panic attacks	☐	☐	....
Depression	☐	☐	....

Fig. 14.45 Central sensitization inventory, part B

SCORES	
0-29	Weak
30-39	Light
40-49	Moderate
50-59	Severe
60-100	Extreme

Fig. 14.46 Assessment of the severity of central sensitization according to the results

which of their fingers is being touched without looking (10 questions for each hand).

The "Representation of body" involves reviewing 21 body areas (eyes closed) and comparing the feelings of the two hemispheres: the patient compares the size, weight, and length of the explored areas. If there is a difference between the two sides, he measures the difference as a percentage of the healthy side [105] (Fig. 14.51).

- ***The Bath CRPS perception disturbance scale*** [73]

This scale calculates a score out of 57 points (57 being the worst score) and aims to obtain an image of the patient's representation of his/her affected limb (Fig. 14.52).

- ***Laterality recognition***

Borrowed from the graded motor imaging protocol, it can be used as a test. The patient looks at the images and must recognize the laterality of the represented limb. A high error rate and response latency can be used to assess the presence and severity of body mapping disorders [106] (Fig. 14.53).

- ***Localization exercises***

With his/her eyes closed, the patient must localize the stimulus (performed on the CRPS limb) and bring it into contact with the contralat-

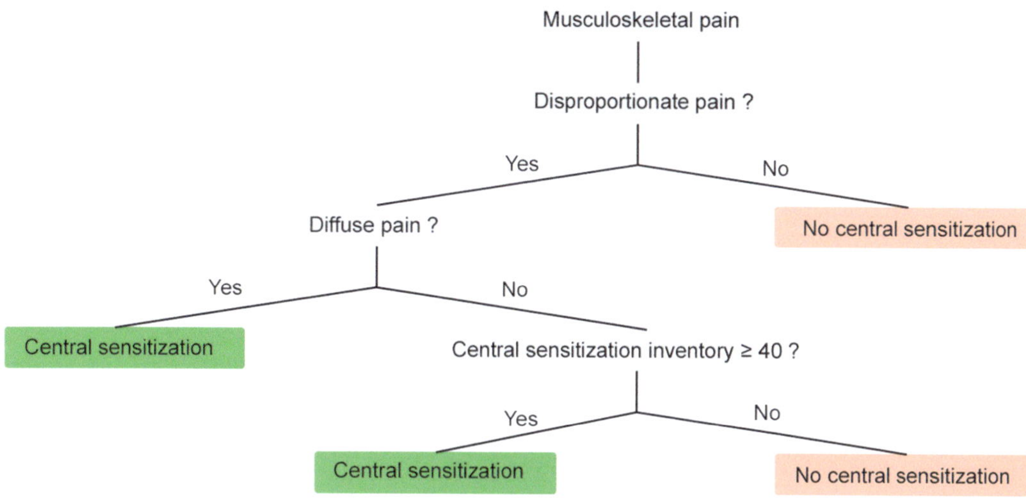

Fig. 14.47 Algorithm for classifying central sensitization according to Nijs

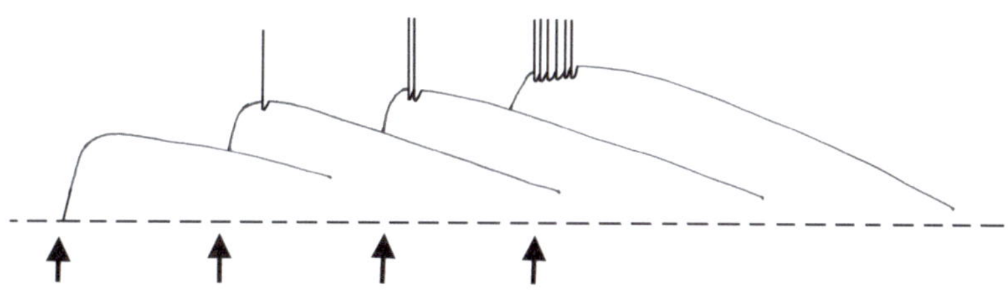

Fig. 14.48 Response amplification phenomenon according to Ru-Rong

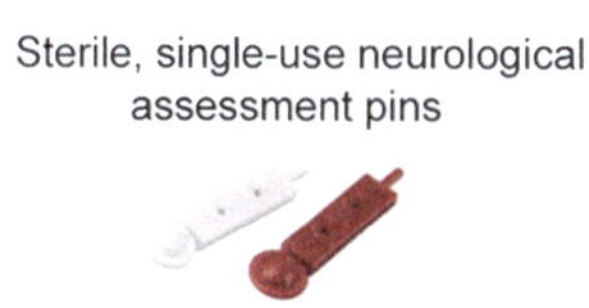

Fig. 14.49 Pin pricks

eral limb. As described by S. Acapo and T. Osinsky, this exercise not only tests but also participates in the rehabilitation of body mapping disorders (Fig. 14.54).

- ***Is there a disturbance in spatial perception?***

Here, the clinical disorders are spatially dependent, as we saw earlier. There is a delay in the integration of the information from the painful area. This increases disturbances in gesture and proprioception in this hemispace [85, 87, 90, 107].

➔ Assessing Peripheral Disorders

Our listening and observation will focus first and foremost on the cutaneous and fascial planes: whether signs and symptoms that could lead to cerebral or neuropathic pain are present.

- **Presence of disorders of the cutaneous and fascial planes**

  We will carefully observe the skin and its mobility over the entire affected limb, looking for:
  - Whitening of the skin on movement (the result of local hypoxia)
  - Or, on the contrary, redness indicating inflammation
  - Depression of the cutaneous plane
  - Adherences, even old ones (Fig. 14.55)
  - Edema

Fig. 14.50 Mc Gill pain questionnaire (QDSA in French)

What Does Your Pain Feel Like?
Some of the following words below describe your present pain. Circle ONLY those words that best describe it. Leave out any category that is not suitable. Use only a single word in each appropriate category - the one that applies best.

Group	Descriptor	Points	Descriptor	Points	Descriptor	Points
1 (temporal)	Flickering	1	Quivering	2	Pulsing	3
	Throbbing	4	Beating	5	Pounding	6
2 (spatial)	Jumping	1	Flashing	2	Shooting	3
3 (punctate pressure)	Pricking	1	Boring	2	Drilling	3
	Stabbing	4	Lancinating	5		
4 (incisive pressure)	Sharp	1	Cutting	2	Lacerating	3
5 (constrictive pressure)	Pinching	1	Pressing	2	Gnawing	3
	Cramping	4	Crushing	5		
6 (traction pressure)	Tugging	1	Pulling	2	Wrenching	3
7 (thermal)	Hot	1	Boring	2	Scalding	3
	Searing	4				
8 (brightness)	Tingling	1	Itchy	2	Smarting	3
	Stinging	4				
9 (dulness)	Dull	1	Sore	2	Hurting	3
	Aching	4	Heavy	5		
10 (sensory : miscellaneous)	Tender	1	Taut	2	Rasping	3
	Splitting	4				
11 (tension)	Tiring	1	Exhausting	2		
12 (autonomic)	Sickening	4	Suffocating	2		
13 (fear)	Fearful	1	Frightful	2	Terrifying	3
14 (punishment)	Punishing	1	Grueling	2	Cruel	3
	Vicious	4	Killing	5		
15 (affective-evaluative sensory : miscellaneous)	Wretched	1	Blinding	2		
16 (evaluative)	Annoying	1	Troublesome	2	Miserable	3
	Intense	4	Unbearable	5		
17 (sensory : miscellaneous)	Spreading	1	Radiating	2	Penetrating	3
	Piercing	4				
18 (sensory : miscellaneous)	Tight	1	Numb	2	Drawing	3
	Squeezing	4	Tearing	5		
19 (sensory)	Cool	1	Cold	2	Freezing	3
20 (affective evaluative : miscellaneous)	Nagging	1	Nauseating	2	Agonizing	3
	Dreadful	4	Torturing	5		

How Does Your Pain Change with Time?

Which word or words would you use to describe the pattern of your pain?	Continuous Steady Constant 1	Rhythmic Periodic Intermittent 2	Brief Momentary Transient 3

Do the following items increase or decrease your pain?
(1) liquor (2) stimulants such as coffee (3) eating (4) heat (5) cold (6) damp (7) weather changes (8) massage or use of a vibrator (9) pressure (10) no movement (11) movement (12) sleep or rest (13) lying down (14) distraction (TV reading etc.) (15) urination or defecation (16) tension (17) bright lights (18) loud noises (19) going to work (20) intercourse (21) mild exercise (22) fatigue.

How Strong is Your Pain?
People agree that the following 5 words (mild / discomforting / distressing / horrible / excruciating) represent pain of increasing intensity. To answer each question below write the number of the most appropriate word in the space beside the question.

Which word describes your pain right now?	Mild 1	Discomforting 2	Distressing 3	Horrible 4	Excruciating 5
Which word describes it at its worst?	Mild 1	Discomforting 2	Distressing 3	Horrible 4	Excruciating 5
Which word describes it when it is least?	Mild 1	Discomforting 2	Distressing 3	Horrible 4	Excruciating 5
Which word describes the worst toothache you ever had?	Mild 1	Discomforting 2	Distressing 3	Horrible 4	Excruciating 5
Which word describes the worst headache you ever had?	Mild 1	Discomforting 2	Distressing 3	Horrible 4	Excruciating 5
Which word describes the worst stomachache you ever had?	Mild 1	Discomforting 2	Distressing 3	Horrible 4	Excruciating 5

Interpretation: the higher the pain score, the greater the pain.
Minimum pain score: 0 (would not be seen in a person with true pain). Maximum pain score: 78.

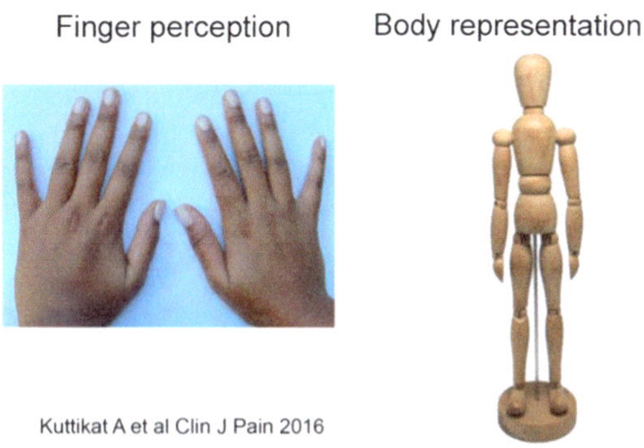

Fig. 14.51 Finger perception and body representation

- Antalgic, compensatory attitudes, or the consequences of an edema, for example, leading to cutaneous tension

This stage should not be neglected, as improving skin gliding planes has a beneficial effect on both neural pain and neuropathic pain [108].

- **Presence of dermo-mechanosensitivity**

The aim here is to determine whether we are in the presence of "neural" pain, which is not systematically concomitant with neuropathic pain; their management will differ.

Pain intensity in response to tactile stimuli can be significant, and these situations are sometimes confused with secondary static mechanical allodynia. The absence of prolonged aftereffects or symptom amplification after on-site work allows us to differentiate them.

The three following tests can be used to determine whether treatment of a mechanosensitive axon or nerve could bring relief to our patient.

- ***Manual Direction Test (MDT)***

Will a mild tension in the skin and superficial fascia reduce or eliminate mechanosensitivity, tremors, and paresthesia?

- ***The clock test***

After identifying the area of pain with the patient, perform light skin glidings in the cardinal directions (12 h–6 h; 9 h–3 h) to observe whether symptoms are improved or increased. When one direction improves, refine its direction (in our example, 3 h improved, but 2 h is more effective).

To be validated, this improvement evaluated by VAS must be over 50% (A. Taylor) (Fig. 14.56).

- ***Dermo-neuromodulation***

As we saw earlier, neural pain or mechanosensitivity may be linked to a malfunction of the hemato-perineurial barrier [48, 49] and/or to entrapment syndromes at the level of sensory axons [40, 53, 109]. According to the principles of Diane Jacobs, it is possible to test, by circular skin glidings around the limb, if the patient feels an improvement in pain symptoms. A favorable response will direct our management towards a "neuro-cutaneous" mobilization treatment (Fig. 14.57).

- ***Neurodynamic tests***
A. Schmid [41, 45] proposes the use of neurodynamic tests to distinguish C-fiber damage, more specifically to the nervi nervorum. They are not used to diagnose a neuropathy, but rather an increased mechanosensitivity of a nerve.

  Three situations may be encountered:

  - Positive Upper Limb Neurodynamic Tests (ULNT) without any neurological symptoms: situation of mechanosensitivity, classified as "nociceptive pain." The sensory assessment of C-fibers will be negative (thermal and algesic), indicating involvement of the nervi nervorum alone.
  - Positive ULNT with neurological symptoms, such as mild hypoesthesia or loss of strength and the presence of hyperalgesia, paresthesia, or allodynia. Classified as "gains in neurological function."
  - Negative ULNT with damaged nerves: in this situation, the greater the damage, the lower the chances of a positive ULNT test! The proposed classification for this group is that of "loss of neurological function," especially hypoesthesia or anesthesia.

The Bath CRPS Body Perception Distrubance Scale

Developed by Jennifer S.Lewis, The Royal National Hospital for Rheumatic Diseases
Bath, England.v2 G2008 All rights reserved

Patient name Date Assessement n° 12345

Diagnosis Date of symptom onset

Body part affected : 1)
2)
3)

1) On a scale of 0-10 how much a part of your body does the affected part feel ?
Very much a part = 0 - 1 - 2 - 3 - 4 - 5 - 6 - 7 - 8 - 9 - 10 = Completely detached

2) On a scale of 0-10 how aware are you of the physical position of your limb ?
Very aware = 0 - 1 - 2 - 3 - 4 - 5 - 6 - 7 - 8 - 9 - 10 = Completely anaware

3) On a scale of 0-10 how much attention do you pay to your limb in terms of looking at it and thinking about it ?
Full attention = 0 - 1 - 2 - 3 - 4 - 5 - 6 - 7 - 8 - 9 - 10 = No attention

4) On a scale of 0-10 how strong are the emotional feelings that you have about your limb ?
strongly positive = 0 - 1 - 2 - 3 - 4 - 5 - 6 - 7 - 8 - 9 - 10 = Strongly negative

5) Is there a difference between how your affected limb looks or is on touch compared to how it feels to you in terms of the following :

Size	yes ☐	no ☐	Comment
Temperature	yes ☐	no ☐	Comment
Pressure	yes ☐	no ☐	Comment
Weight	yes ☐	no ☐	Comment

6a) Have you ever had a desire to amputate the limb ? yes ☐ no ☐
6b) If yes, how strong is that desire now ?
Not at all =0 - 1 - 2 - 3 - 4 - 5 - 6 - 7 - 8 - 9 - 10 = Very strong
Desire amputate site :

7) With eyes closed describe a mental image of your affected and unaffected body parts
(drawn by assessor during patient description then verified by the patient

This is a accurate account of my image of my affected body part
Signature Date

Fig. 14.52 The Bath CRPS perception disturbance scale

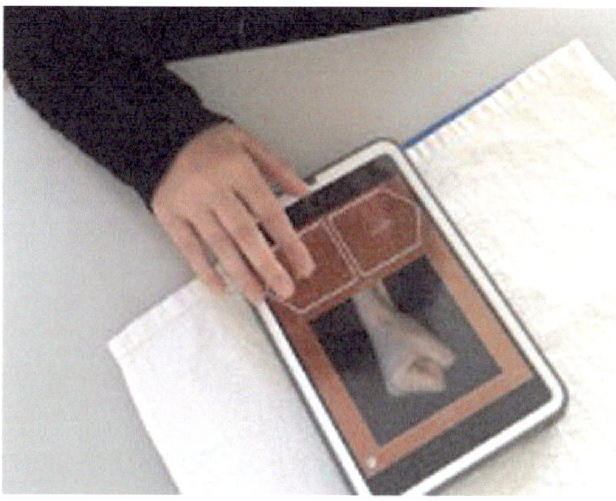

Fig. 14.53 Laterality recognition

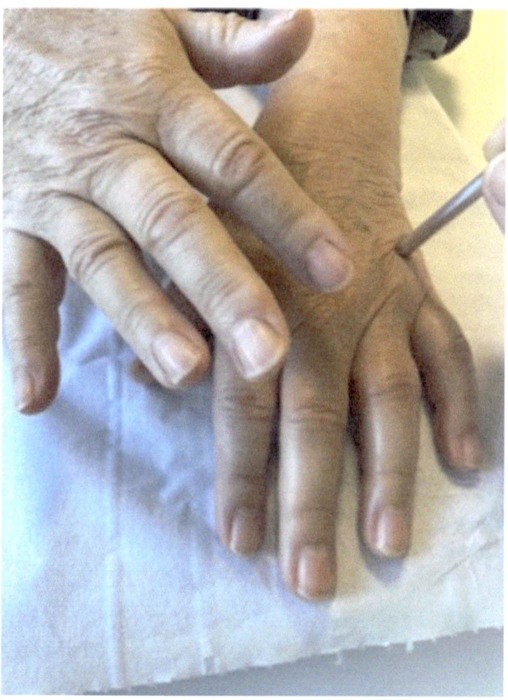

Fig. 14.54 Localization exercise

Let's not forget that paraclinical examinations (ENMG) essentially test the large fibers, i.e., 20% of the fibers in a peripheral nerve.

Presence of Axonal Lesions

The aim here is to determine whether we are in the presence of neuropathic pain (Fig. 14.58) by

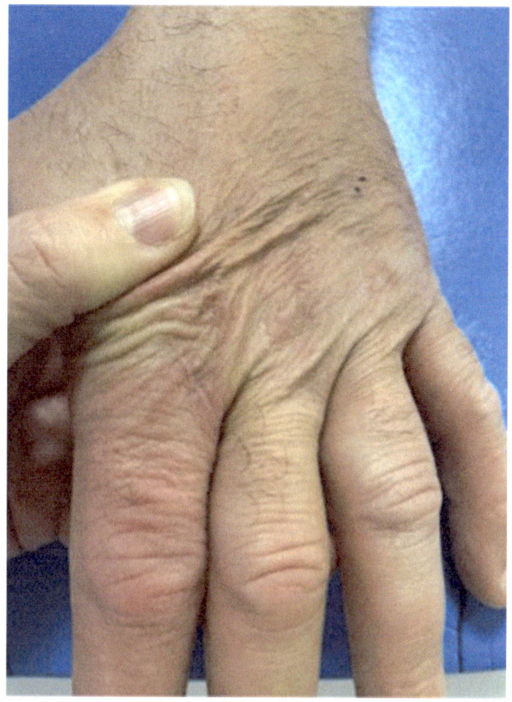

Fig. 14.55 Looking for scar adherences

assessing signs, symptoms, and severity. In this situation, the Aβ-fibers are damaged. The results will condition further treatment.

➔ Assessment of Neuropathic Symptoms and Signs in the Context of Hypoesthesia

In the context of CRPS, according to Spicher et al. and T. Packham, it is possible to encounter different situations: CRPS with hypoesthesia, with mechanic and static allodynia, with intermittent or intractable neuralgia, etc.

As developed in Volume 1 [110] by G. Mesplié, clinical reasoning is based on the decision algorithm established by C. Spicher and his team [111, 112] (Fig. 14.59). He shows us that, depending on the detected symptoms, the therapeutic strategy can diverge completely, so as not to become "therapeugenic."

The search for neuropathic pain is carried out by means of a diagnostic assessment for axonal injuries, using four tests:

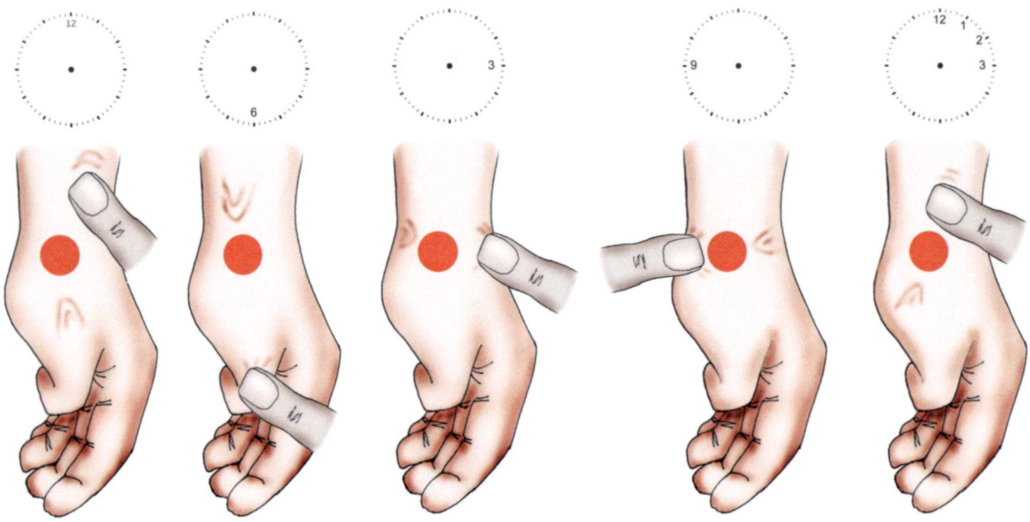

Fig. 14.56 Clock test

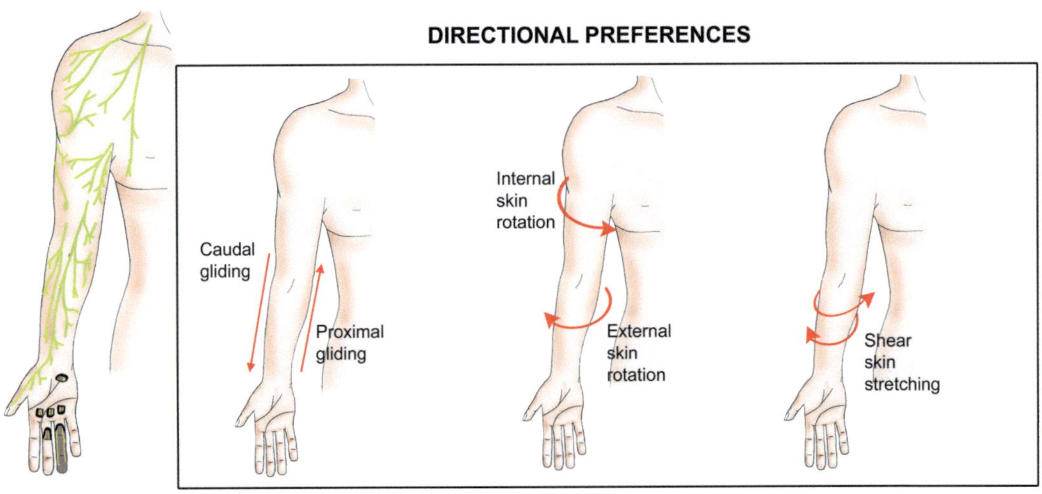

Fig. 14.57 Dermo-neuromodulation according to D. Jacobs

- Qualitative/NP4 (Fig. 14.60)
- Esthesiography
- Two-point static discrimination test (Fig. 14.61)
- Search for signs of "tingling"

➔ Assessment of Neuropathic Symptoms and Signs in the Context of Allodynia

In an allodynic situation: "hypoesthesia is paradoxically painful to the touch." The assessment will diverge:

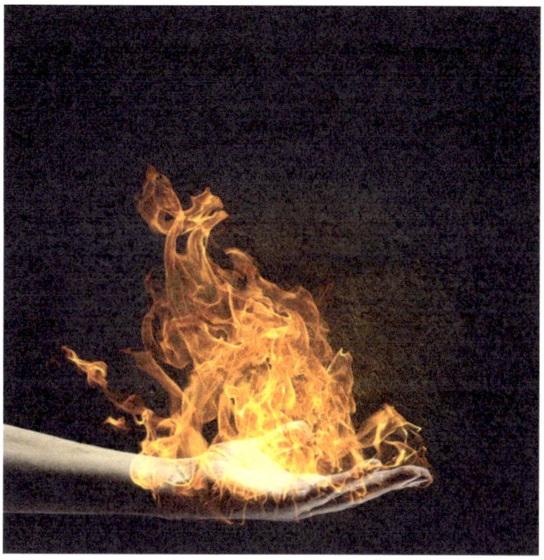

Fig. 14.58 The fire of neuropathic pain

- By redefining with the patient, the pain threshold not to be exceeded during the allodynography (VAS)
- By realizing an allodynography
- By assessing the fifth point, determining the severity of allodynia (Fig. 14.62)

Allodynia in CRPS is not insignificant, with a significant prevalence, ranging from more than half of patients [11, 15] to 70.3% for Harden et al. in 2010 [16].

In the book "Rééducation des douleurs neuropathiques" (*Rehabilitation of Neuropathic Pain*), it is described as burning sensations "in" the joint, with a vesperal character that prompts the limitation of activity at the end of the day, due to the increase of pain in 98% of cases ($n = 681$) after activity [113, 114]. This can have the effect of exacerbating feelings of anxiety.

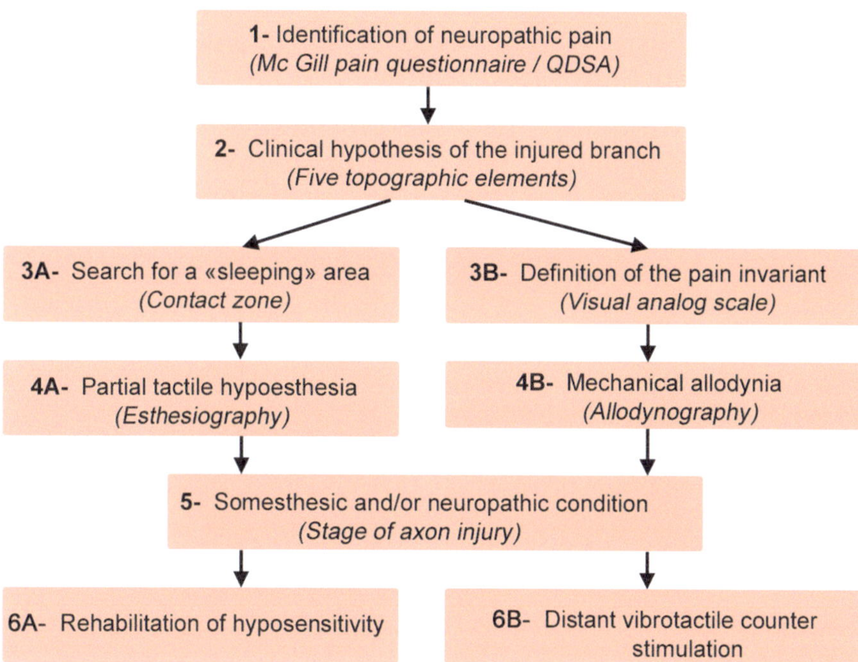

Fig. 14.59 Decision-making algorithm in axonal injury situations according to C. Spicher et al

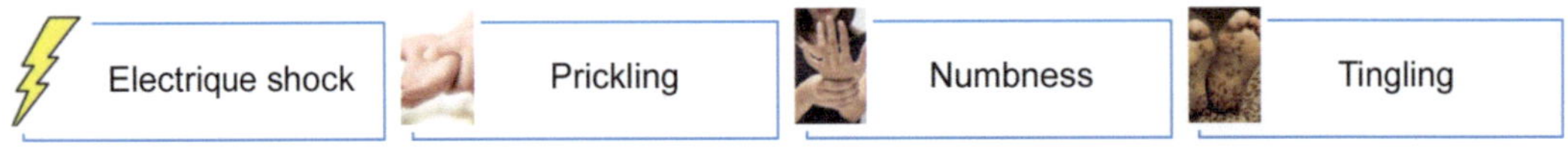

Fig. 14.60 Qualifiers for neuropathic pain

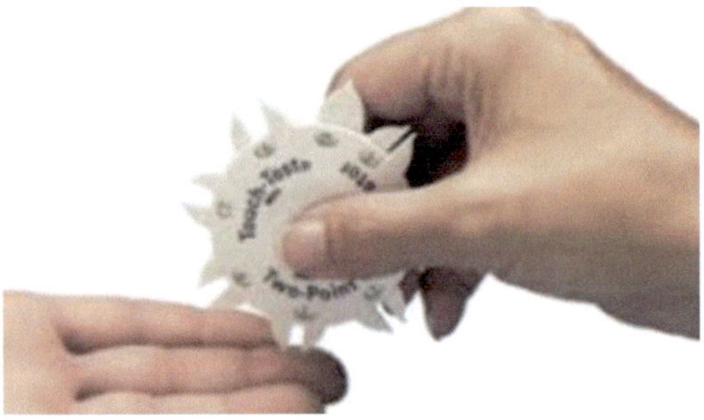

Fig. 14.61 Two-point static discrimination test

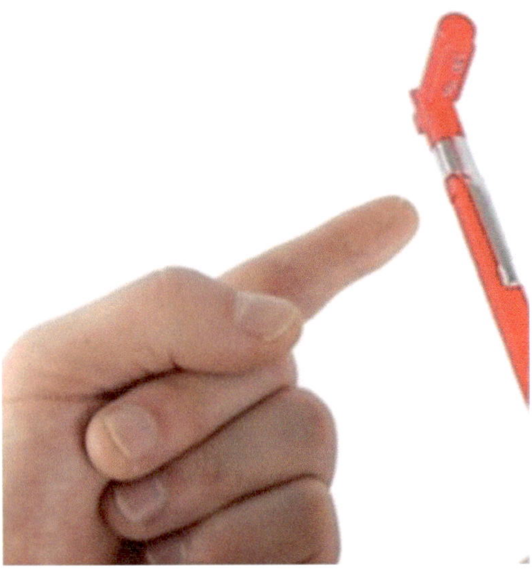

Fig. 14.62 Assessment of the fifth point

Therapeutic Strategies

What Do Anglo-Saxon Recommendations Tell Us?

We have 4 weeks to lift the irritative thorn; to fight against pain, inflammatory aspects, sweating, mottled skin, and edema; and to correct central phenomena if they are already present. Beyond this period, symptoms will be more difficult to manage [21] (Fig. 14.2).

To fight against pain and sensory-motor dysfunctions of the CRPS, there are two complementary strategies: a "top-down" approach aimed at correcting central phenomena that will lead to an improvement in peripheral symptoms, and a "bottom-up" approach aimed at training and correcting peripheral phenomena that will have an effect on the central phenomena—especially in terms of cortical re-expansion [69, 94, 95] (Fig. 14.63).

Rehabilitation Targeting Central Phenomena, Cortical Functional Reorganization, Top-Down Techniques

"Targeting maladaptive plasticity in higher functions to treat CRPS."

Several therapies, such as mirror therapy, graded motor imagery, and prismatic adaptation, appear to have beneficial effects on the neuropsychological and clinical symptoms of CRPS [66].

Graded Motor Imagery (GMI)

The protocol consists of three parts: laterality testing, motor imagery, and mirror therapy [78, 115]. It has been extensively developed in Volume 1 (Figs. 14.64 and 14.65).

F. Delaquaize recommends 5 daily 10-min sessions, progressing according to the patient's feelings and abilities [110]. Do not hesitate to go back if necessary. When there is no longer any benefit, the therapy can be stopped.

Prism

Drawing on the apparent analogy between CRPS and spatial neglect, Sumitani et al. [116] have proposed the use of the prismatic adaptation to restore the visual egocentric reference mismatch. Prisms are glasses with beveled lenses that induce an optical deviation (Fig. 14.66).

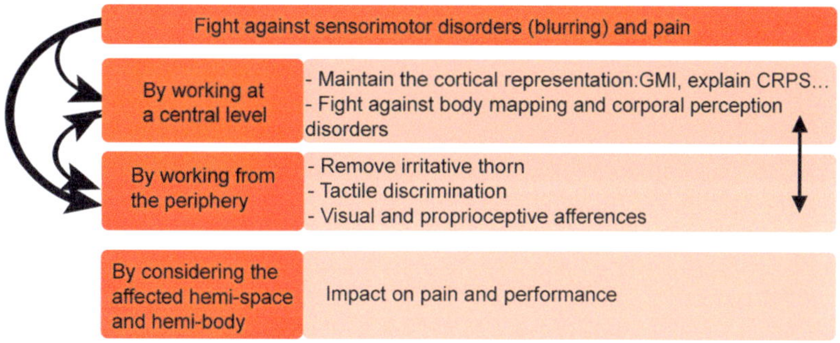

Fig. 14.63 Therapeutic strategies

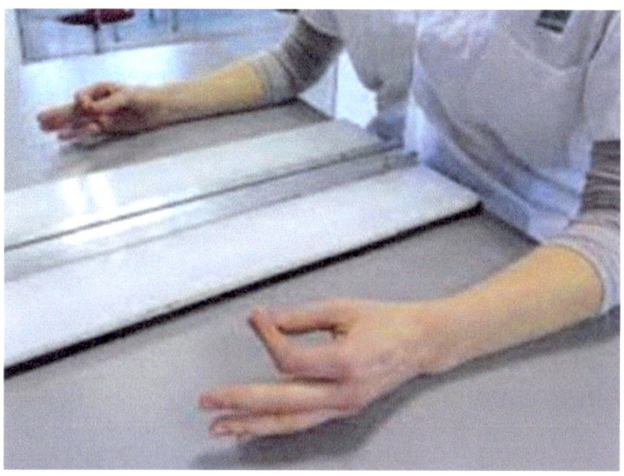

Fig. 14.64 Mirror therapy

In this example (Fig. 14.67), our patient has a left-sided CRPS, so we fit him with prismatic glasses with a right-sided deviation in the perception of the true location of objects: when he tries to point at an element located in front of him (second diagram), the finger will target the right side of it (deviation to the healthy side). The proprioceptive compensation causes a deviation to the left, while the visual compensation causes a deviation to the right. These two compensations enable a realignment, measurable after the prisms have been removed: the patient will then show a pointing shift towards the CRPS side (in this example to the left). This is referred to as prismatic adaptation [117]. It "corrects" the perception of the midline and has a significant therapeutic effect [118]. Rossetti obtained benefits in visuo-manual tasks (line bisection, drawing copying) but also in hypoesthesia, mental imagery, and postural balance [71].

At the end of the prism wearing, the visual egocentric reference is shifted to the side of the prismatic deviation, i.e., to the CRPS side, and the proprioceptive egocentric reference is shifted to the opposite side [71].

At 2 weeks, the results in terms of improvement in pain, mobility, and vegetative manifestations are in line with those found in the short-term period with mirror rehabilitation [119]. However, a recent RCT study showed inconclusive results [120].

Couldn't the sensation of finding this CRPS hand in the "healthy" hemispace also explain these beneficial effects [89, 116, 119]? This same question could also be raised when using the mirror [119].

> Protocol: In the context of CRPS, prisms require angles of 15° to 30° of orientation towards the healthy side. On the contrary, orienting them towards the CRPS side exacerbates pain. Neutral or weak angles have no effect.

> Christophe et al. [121] performed, with significant results (90% to 100% improvement in pain phenomena):
>
> - Two prismatic adaptation sessions per day for 8 days, spaced 5 h apart.
> - 15° prisms with deviation to the healthy side.
> - 80 pointing movements with targets located 10° on either side of the midline, in random order (every 3 s).

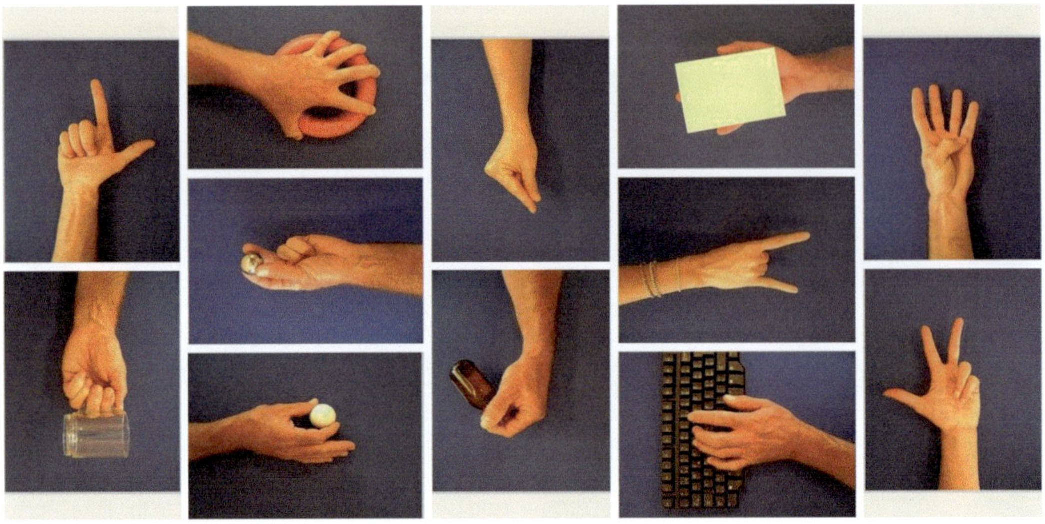

Fig. 14.65 Laterality recognition

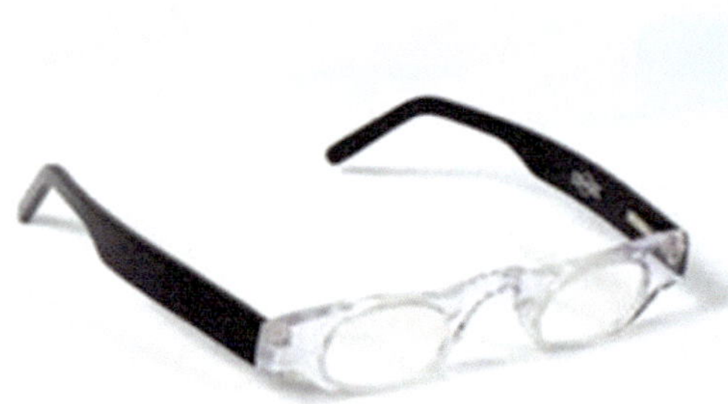

Fig. 14.66 Prismatic glasses

Fight Against Neuropathic Sensory Phenomena

➔ Management of Hypoesthesia

This will follow the procedures described for non-CRPS hypoesthesia in G. Mesplié's Volume 1. Depending on the assessment (Fig. 14.68), appropriate cutaneous stimulation exercises will be used to stimulate neuroplasticity.

➔ Management of Static Mechanical Allodynia

The management of allodynia in the context of CRPS will follow the same protocol as for a simple allodynia. The patient will be asked to perform distant vibrotactile counter stimulations (DVCS) in an area determined with the rehabilitator, for 1 min or less.

These DVCS can also be done over a lidocaine patch (iontophoresis effect). These patches are highly recommended for CRPS. They are worn for 12 h. They first target restless nights, then days when sleep has improved.

When the allodynia disappears, the underlying hypoesthesia must be managed to avoid any relapse (Fig. 14.69).

Fight Against Disorders in Body Perception

➔ By Acting on the Size of the CRPS Limb

The size of the CRPS limb has an impact on pain but also on edema: when the limb is enlarged, symptoms worsen. On the contrary, when it is reduced, they improve. Why not play with glasses or a shrinking mirror [79] (Fig. 14.70)?

➔ By Increasing Visual Stimulations from the CRPS Limb

- Sessions in which the patient is in control and looks at the color of his/her hand (according to the work of J. Lewis et al.) help to reappropriate and reduce the pain phenomena (Fig. 14.71).
- Taping can help to fulfill this role, as can lightly compressive and colored gloves (Figs. 14.72 and 14.73).

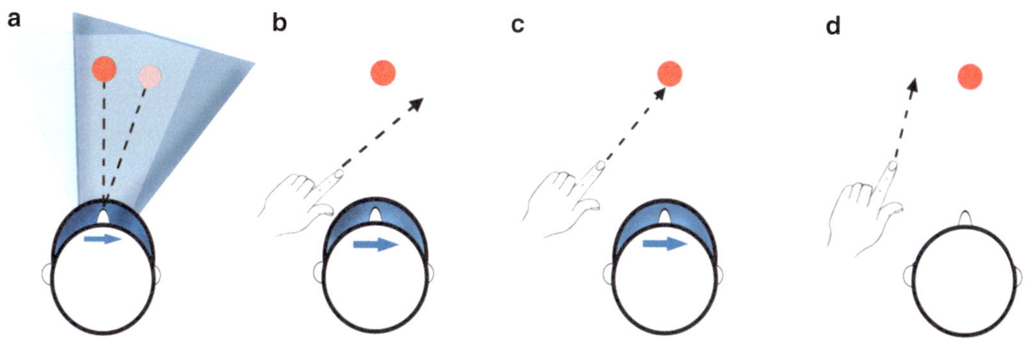

Fig. 14.67 Prismatic adaptation

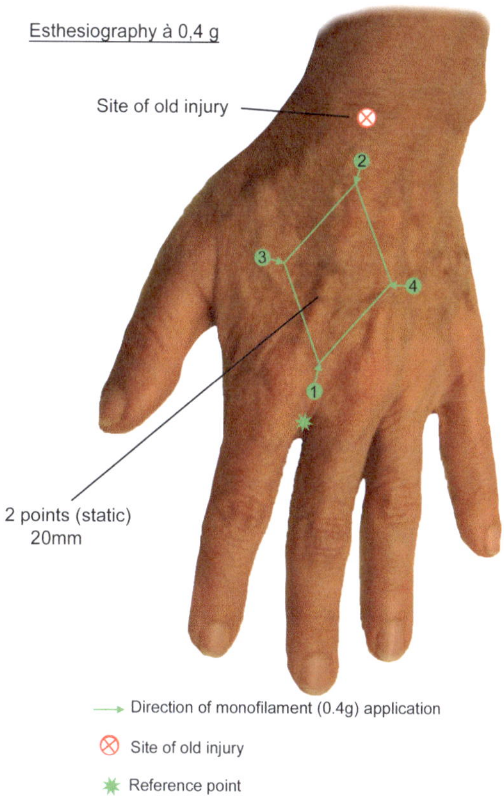

Fig. 14.68 Esthesiography

➔ By Identifying the Image of His/Her Hand

The patient should be able to recognize the photos of his hand that have been mixed with other hand images.

Fight Against Body Mapping Disorders

➔ Through Vision

Taping and compressive gloves have the dual advantage of providing an "enveloping" proprioceptive reminder, which is interesting in situations where the patient has difficulty locating and feeling the shape of the CRPS limb.

➔ Through Proprioception (Without Vision)

With stimulus-locating exercises, as we saw during the assessment. We can also play with the hemispace during this exercise (Fig. 14.74).

➔ Through Spatial Variables

Sensory-motor phenomena (edema, temperature, pain, blurring) are attenuated when a limb is in the healthy hemispace, so it may be interesting to simply cross the median line (Fig. 14.75) to take advantage of this, or to cross the two limbs during the exercises.

This opens many fields of simple self-rehabilitation exercises (Figs. 14.76, 14.77, and 14.78).

Pain Neuroscience Education

➔ Explain CRPS

The work of L. Moseley and D. Butler [122, 123] has shown that to answer the question "how can I get better?," especially when pain has been present for a long time, it is necessary to understand the painful experience of "why does it hurt?".

Fig. 14.69 Allodynography

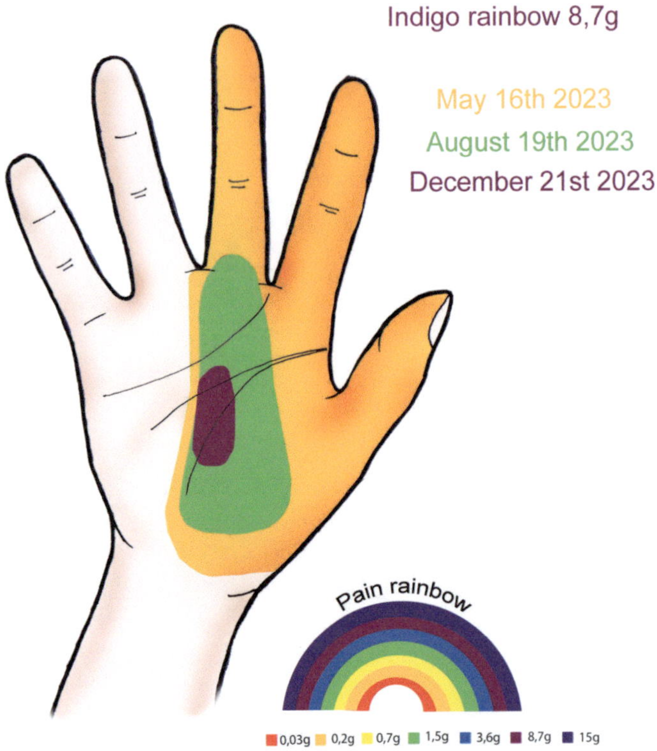

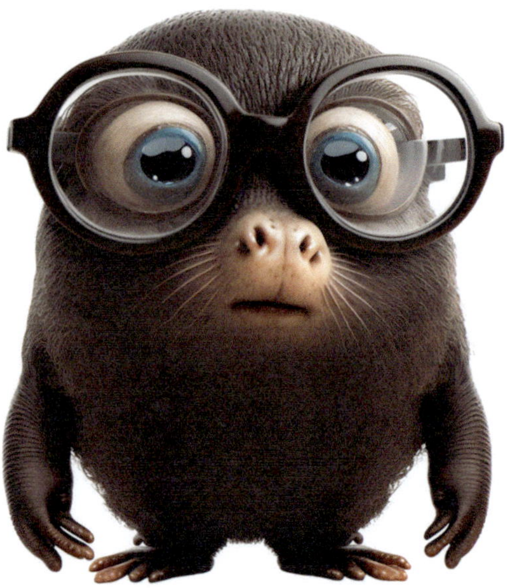

Fig. 14.70 Decrease the size of the limb with glasses

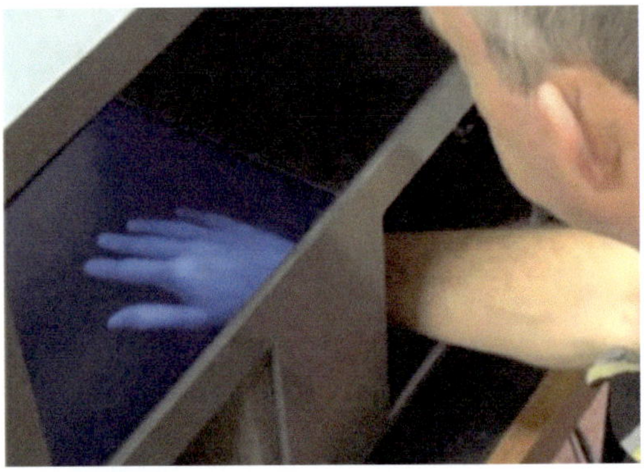

Fig. 14.71 Reclaim one's limb with color on demand according to J. Lewis

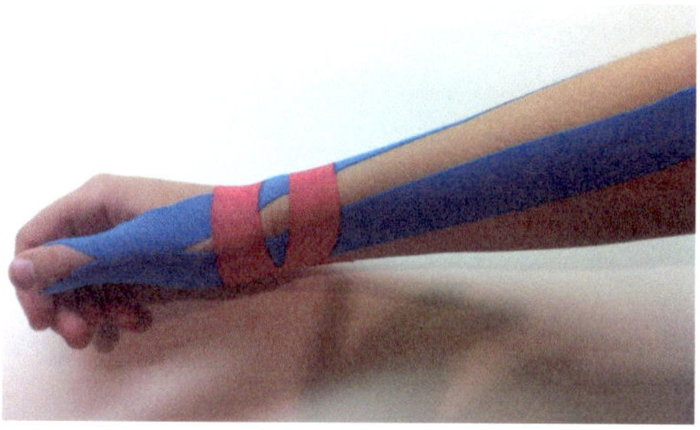

Fig. 14.72 Taping to reclaim one's limb

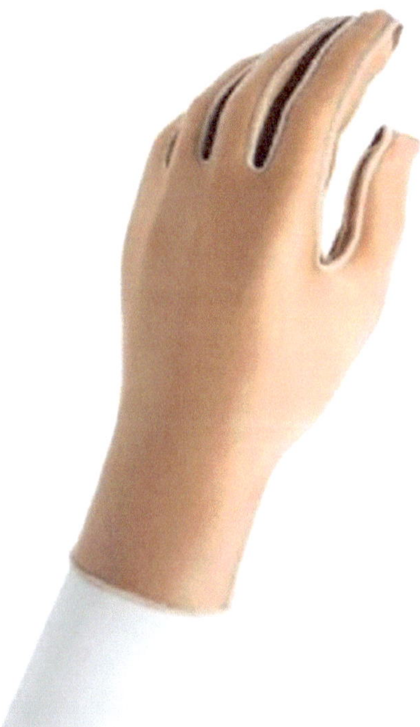

Fig. 14.73 Reclaim one's limb with proprioceptive feedback

It is more difficult than it may seem, as patients need to integrate notions of neuroscience to question their vision of pain, i.e., to dissociate it from the notion of injury and give it meaning (Fig. 14.79) [124].

Several studies have demonstrated significant results in terms of pain reduction, function recovery, reduction of fear-avoidance, and catastrophism when the patient understands "why it hurts" [122, 125, 126].

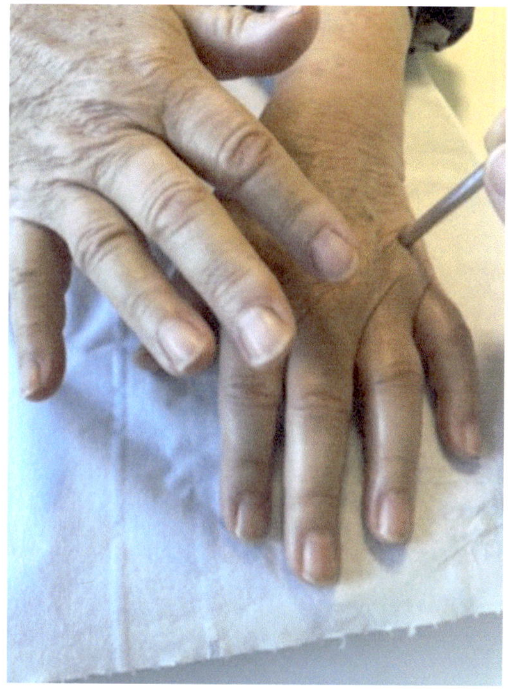

Fig. 14.74 Stimuli localization

Understanding is a medicine.

Following these principles, the aim is to explain to our patients with CRPS what this pathology is and what strategies are available to fight against its symptoms.

➔ SFETD Recommendations

Integrated into its recommendations, the SFETD (Société Française d'Étude et de Traitement de la Douleur) proposes a model of information to be given to the patients (Fig. 14.80).

➔ G. Lehman's Biopsychosocial Umbrella

G. Lehman, in his biopsychosocial approach, develops strategies which aim to create a change in transient perception, during which the patient feels that his body can get better. This reduces the sensitivity of the "alarm system."

He proposes a downloadable pain guide, containing several metaphors to explain the multifactorial aspect of pain, as well as a program that can be customized by therapists to best suit their patients (Fig. 14.81).

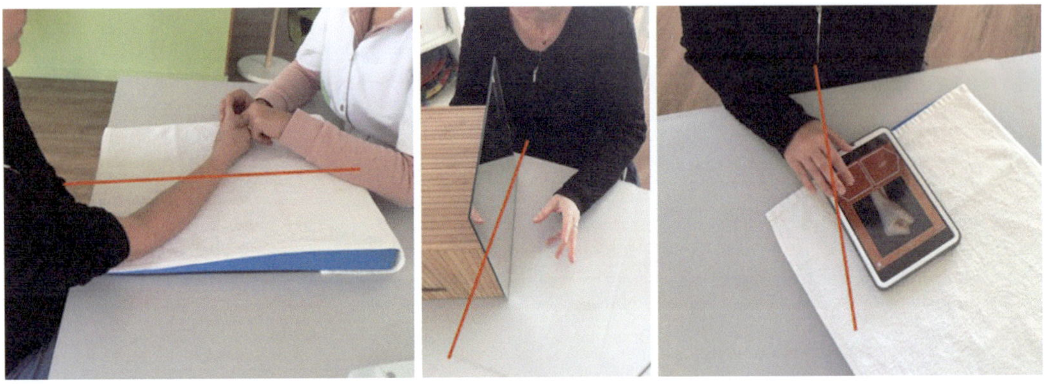

Fig. 14.75 Cross the midline

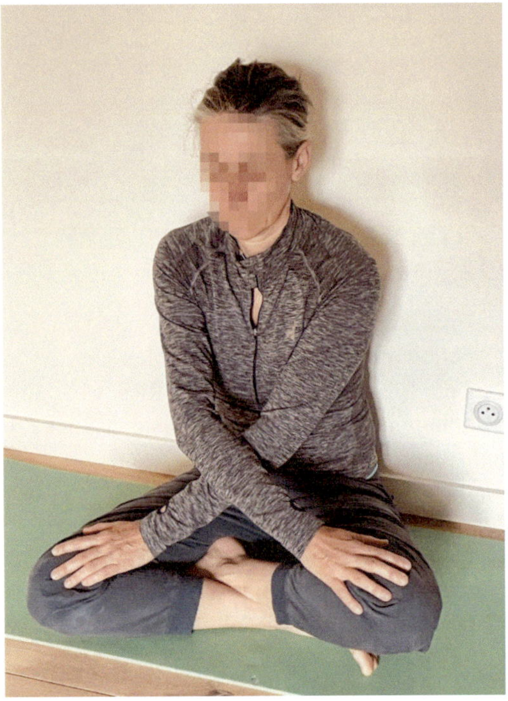

Fig. 14.76 Exercise idea with crossed hands (yoga)

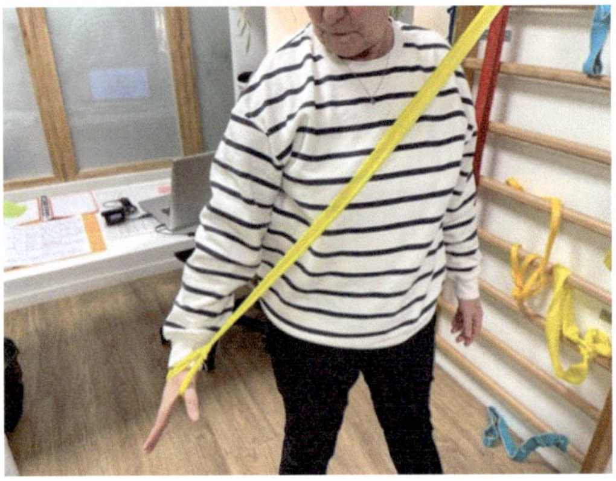

Fig. 14.77 Diagonal exercise 1

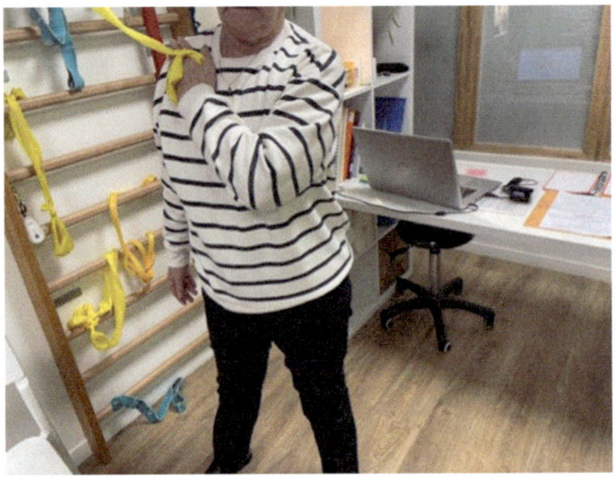

Fig. 14.78 Diagonal exercise 2

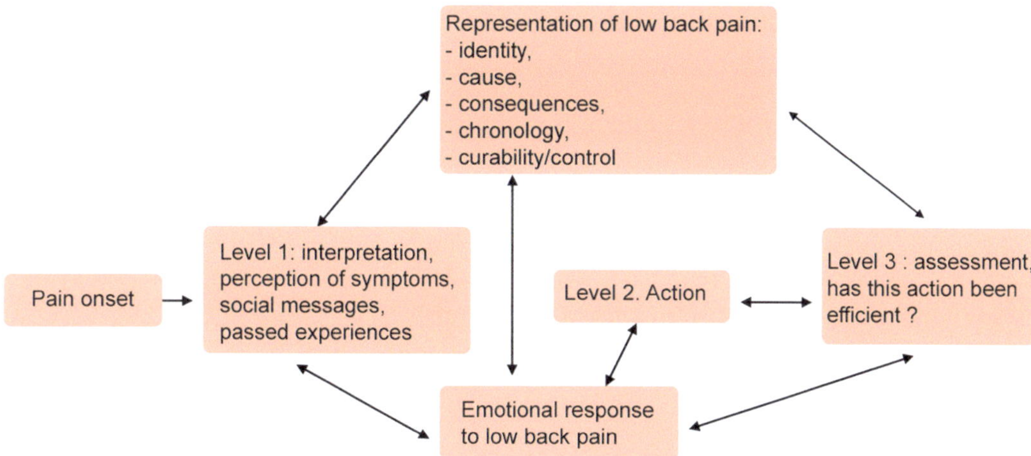

Fig. 14.79 How to give meaning to my pain, according to Bunzil

CRPS is a non-severe pathology with a favorable course, the duration of which is difficult to predict.
This pathology is linked to a dysfunction of the pain system (amplifying system) with no direct link to the surgical procedure or management of the initial trauma.
Several symptoms may potentially be present. Pain and reduced joint mobility are common.
Other symptoms may be associated: swelling, abnormal temperature in the painful area, sweating...
These symptoms can have repercussions on sleep, mood, concentration...
The intensity of symptoms may require medical, paramedical and psychological treatment.
Immobilization is to be avoided, as it aggravates the pathology.
It is important to continue mobilizing the affected joint to stimulate drainage and maintain mobility.
Imaging and additional tests: these are not always necessary and should be discussed with your doctor.
Concerning management:

- Pain may be provoked or increased by mobilizations.
  It should remain bearable and not last more than a few hours after the mobilization, this pain must be managed.
- While pain is being managed, it is important to continue with mobilization and physiotherapy.
- If pain changes, discuss it with your caregivers so that treatment can be re-evaluated.
- Medication management includes "classic" analgesics and/or drugs usually prescribed for other pathologies, but which also have an analgesic action (e.g. antidepressants).
- Non-drug treatment is essential. Several techniques can be proposed (physiotherapy, mind-body techniques, cutaneous neurostimulation, etc.).

Fig. 14.80 Information to be given to the patient according to the SFETD

➔ The Effects of the Therapeutic Alliance

In a long-term syndrome such as CRPS, we understand the importance of a good therapeutic alliance. This will not only maintain our patient's motivation to manage his/her own care and self-education but will also influence the results of the treatment for pain and disability, as well as for physical and mental health [127, 128] (Fig. 14.82).

This will require the establishment of a climate of trust, made possible by personalized care with listening, empathy, encouragement, and comforting therapeutic competence [128].

Fig. 14.81 G. Lehman's bio psychosocial umbrella

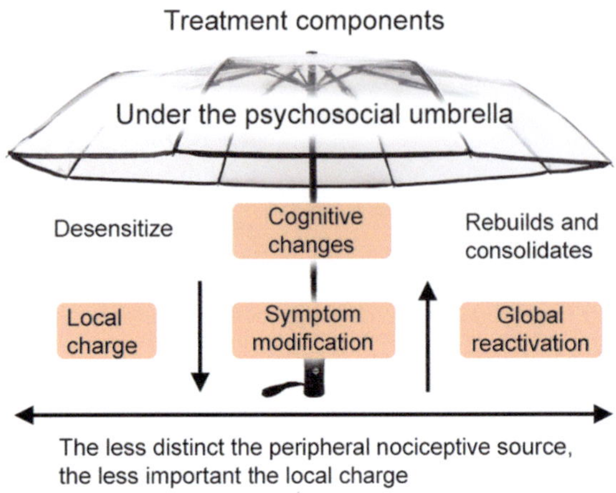

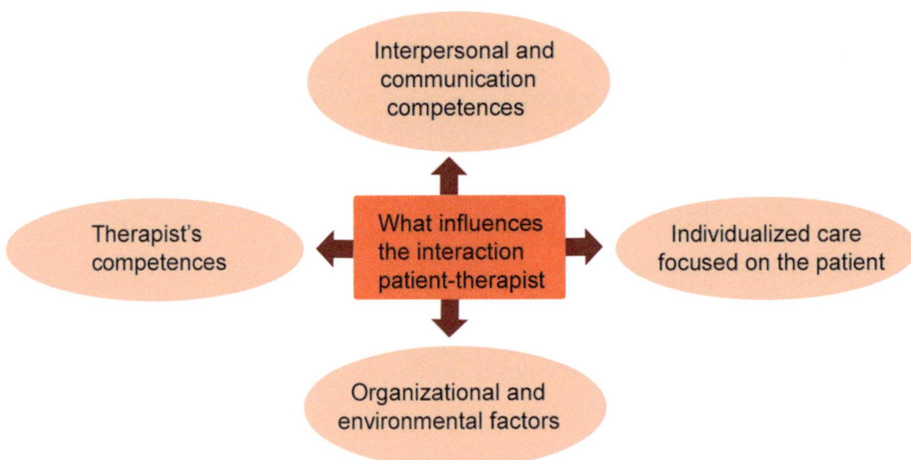

Fig. 14.82 The keys to the therapeutic alliance

Rehabilitation Targeting Peripheral Phenomena, Bottom-Up Techniques

Giving Back Space

"Giving back space in the skin" (Figs. 14.83 and 14.84).

Vibrations

➔ Proprioceptive Purpose

Vibrations with a frequency of between 60 and 80 Hz, via the neuromuscular bundles, create the illusion of movement of the antagonist muscle [129, 130]. For the joints immobilized by a plaster or an orthosis, windows can be provided to allow the vibration generator to be applied to the tendons affected by the immobilization.

From the outset of immobilization, this improves joint mobility, reduces apprehension, and facilitates movement.

➔ Analgesic Purpose

In his thesis, A. Gay obtained with these modalities a 30% gain in mobility and a 50% reduction in pain.

He justifies this gain by the effects of gate control: the stimulation by vibrations of Aβ-fibers through mechanoreceptors inhibits the C-fibers at a spinal level, as well as by the cortical reorganization through proprioceptive feedback, restoring adequacy between proprioception and motricity [131].

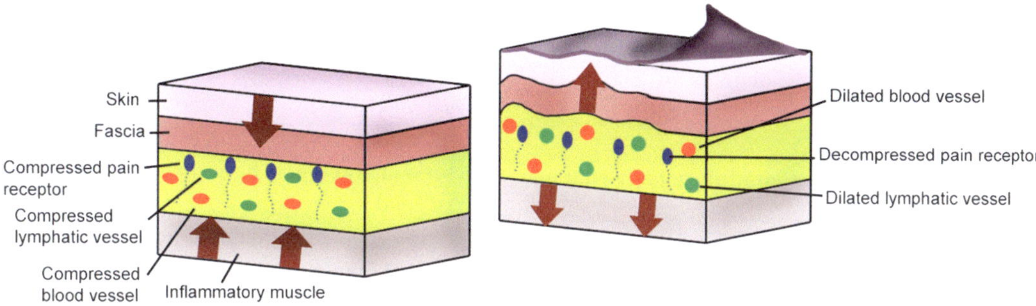

Fig. 14.83 Make the skin breathe

Techniques to restore space under the skin		
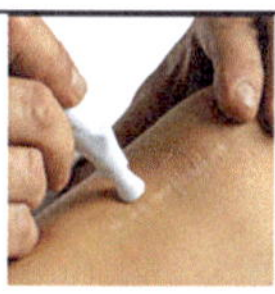		Vacuotherapy
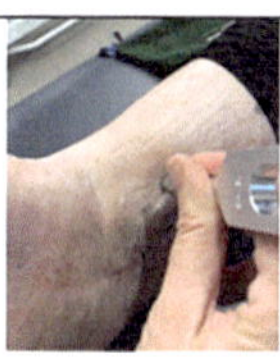	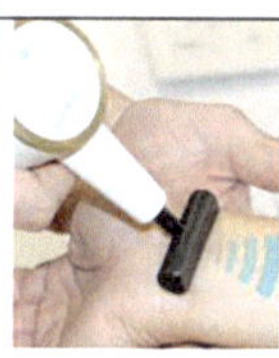	Mechanical or electrical vibrations. In these highly inflammatory situations, the patient will tolerate mechanical vibrations better (tuning fork).
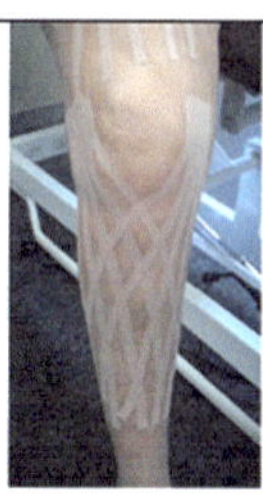	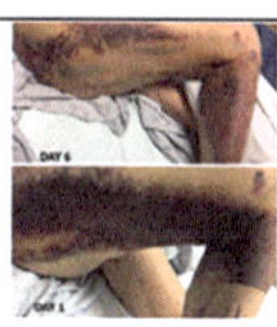	Taping: - Maintains cutaneous tensions in the desired direction - Slightly relaxes the skin by using its elastic properties - Drains
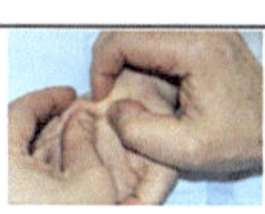		Various massage techniques.

Fig. 14.84 Techniques to restore space under the skin

"Dermo-Dynamics"

This term covers all the techniques used for the mobilization and neurodynamics of cutaneous nerves.

➔ DNM: Dermo-Neuromodulation by Diane Jacobs

Inside the perineurium, we have seen that the nerve is provided with several "vasa nervorum" to ensure its vascularization. They can undergo mechanical deformation, with torsion reducing or pinching their diameter (Fig. 14.85).

The nerve is connected by its vasa nervorum and is held in place by connective fibers that allow it to glide longitudinally in its neural envelope and deploy its vasa nervorum. This accordion-like mobility (extension-shortening) contributes to the venous drainage (Fig. 14.86). This presentation can be compared to the animated model of the flexor tendons with their extrinsic vascularization proposed by J.C. Guimberteau (Fig. 14.87).

D. Jacobs' dermo-dynamic techniques are based on two concepts:

- The twist (Fig. 14.86): by mobilizing the adjacent tissues, especially the skin, a torsion/detorsion force can be initiated between the nerve and its envelope.
- Acting on the envelope: by mobilizing a limb and its skin (e.g., an arm), which becomes the nerve's "container," it is also possible to "relax" a nerve along its entire path (Fig. 14.88).

➔ Taping

All skin mobilizations can be prolonged over time by applying tapes. We can imagine prolonging scar work but also a DNM mobilization.

Care must be taken, however, as there is a prestressing effect on the tape due to its elasticity, and its direction of application must be reversed if no tension is applied (Fig. 14.89).

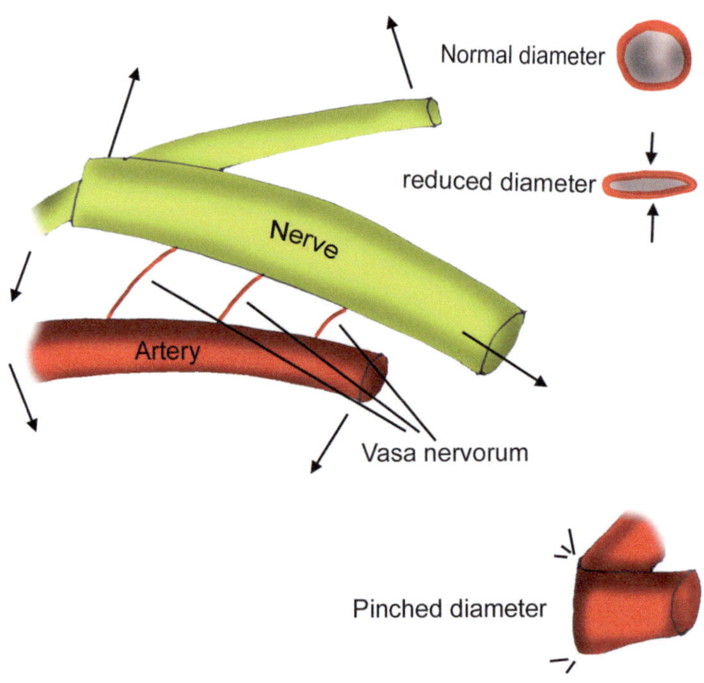

Fig. 14.85 Vasa nervorum according to D. Jacobs

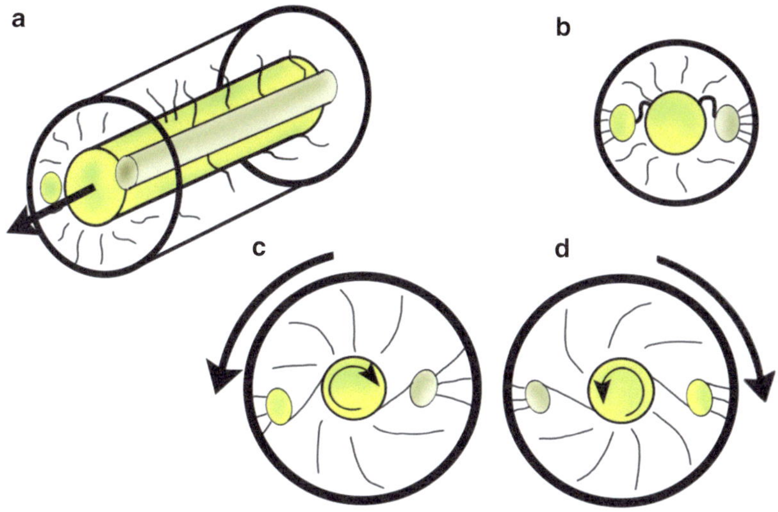

Fig. 14.86 Nerves and fascicles according to D. Jacobs. In (**a**), D. Jacobs presents a cross-section of a nerve connected through its vasa nervorum and held in place by fibers that allow it to glide longitudinally in its neural envelope and deploy its vasa nervorum. In (**b**), she proposes the principle of the twist which, by mobilizing the surrounding tissues, would initiate a torsion force between the nerve and its envelope (**c**)

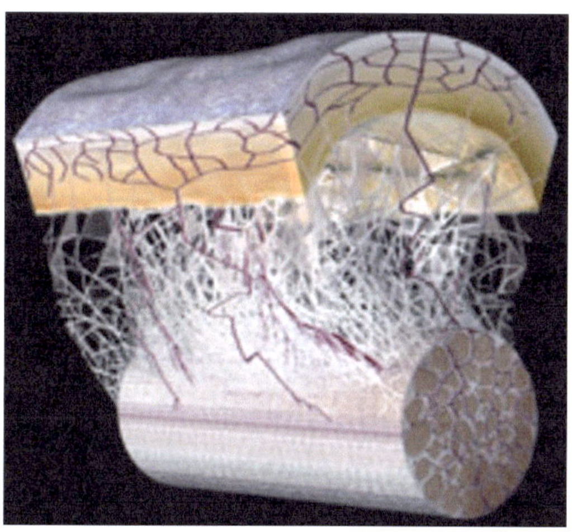

Fig. 14.87 Tendon and vascularization. (Reproduced with permission from the illustrator Jean-Claude Guimberteau)

We must also bear in mind the sensitivity of these patients, whose nerves have very low potentiation thresholds and are therefore highly reactive: tension in the application of the tape must always be "measured," at the risk of losing the analgesic effects at the expense of reactivating nociceptive discharges. To prevent this, the patient is instructed to remove the tape at the slightest unpleasant sensation.

Neurodynamic Mobilizations

They have an effect on:

- Mechanosensitivity, by dispersing endoneurial edema [132, 133]
- The longitudinal path of the nerve [55]
- Immediate hypoalgesia [134, 135]
- Anti-inflammatory at a distance from the site of injury (dorsal root ganglion and central nervous system) [41]
- Probable stimulation of endogenous opioids, which should also facilitate nerve repair [41]

Remember that these are mobilizations and not neurodynamic stretches (Fig. 14.90).

Examples of Sensory-Motor Retraining

➔ Graded Sensory Imagery by Milner et al. (Poster by Milner 2017)

Milner et al. propose a sensory rehabilitation program that follows the steps of the graded motor imagery program but concentrates on sensory aspects. This could be called graded sensory imagery (GSI) (the exercises, divided into five stages, propose a gradation of technique and aim to activate the central and then peripheral components of the syndrome). The patient performs the exercises alone, attentive and focused on his/her

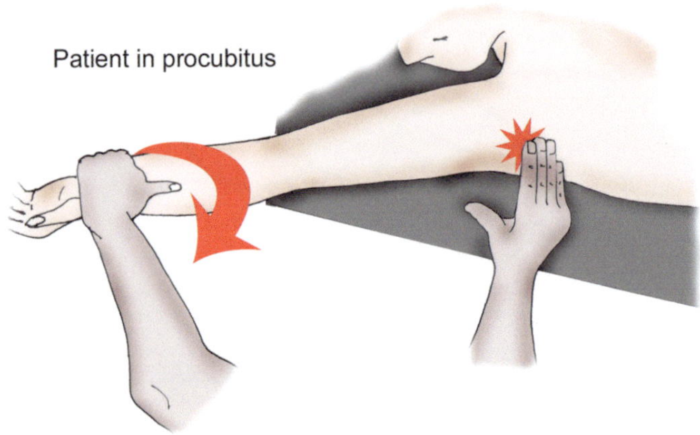

Fig. 14.88 Act on the envelope, according to D. Jacobs

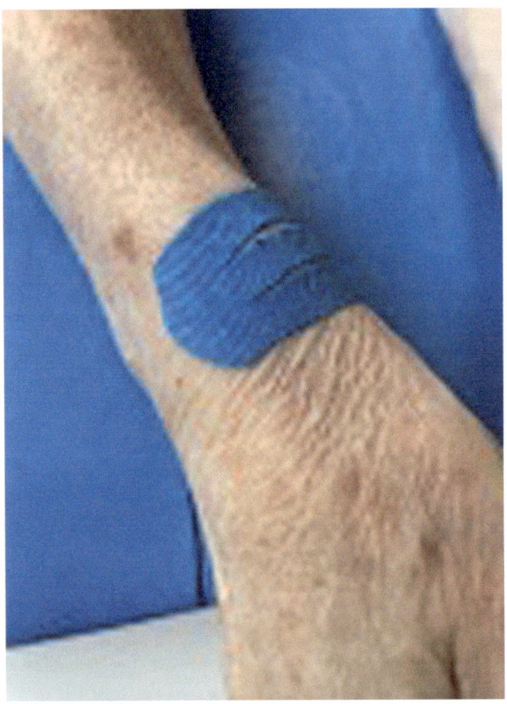

Fig. 14.89 Tapes

sensations, and the duration of each stage can be adapted [136] (Fig. 14.91).

- Step 1: sort materials according to sensations (cold, hot, hard, etc.).
- Step 2: imagine the sensations provided by the materials (cold steel, prickly, etc.).
- Step 3: the healthy hand explores and feels the materials; the CRPS hand recognizes, helped by vision.
- Step 4: CRPS hand in the mirror, texture recognition by the healthy hand while observing the reflection.
- Step 5: without looking, the CRPS hand will explore and feel materials, and the healthy hand will recognize them.

Lille SFETD Recommendations

Classic CRPS management is recommended, but some practices are refined, and others questioned [23].

➔ Rehabilitation

Functional rehabilitation is considered an essential part of CRPS treatment and should be started as early as possible. The intensity of treatment should be adjusted according to the severity of the syndrome, to avoid aggravating the pain over the long term (on the other hand, the no-pain rule is applied).

- **Skin desensitization combined with hypoesthesia rehabilitation is recommended** [14]

  It is the method of choice in the cases of neuroma, dysesthesia, and myofascial pain [14]. It should be pointed out that the recommendations on which the SFETD is based describe in their desensitization protocols that the discomfort felt post-effect will be short-lived [22]. It cannot therefore be a treatment targeting a proven static mechanical allodynia.

  In this case, the practice could prove therapeugenic, hence the importance of a well-conducted sensory assessment.

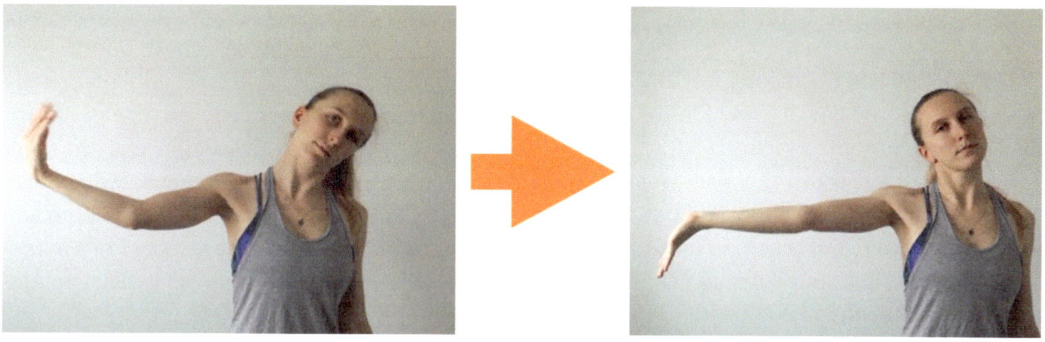

Fig. 14.90 Neurodynamic mobilizations

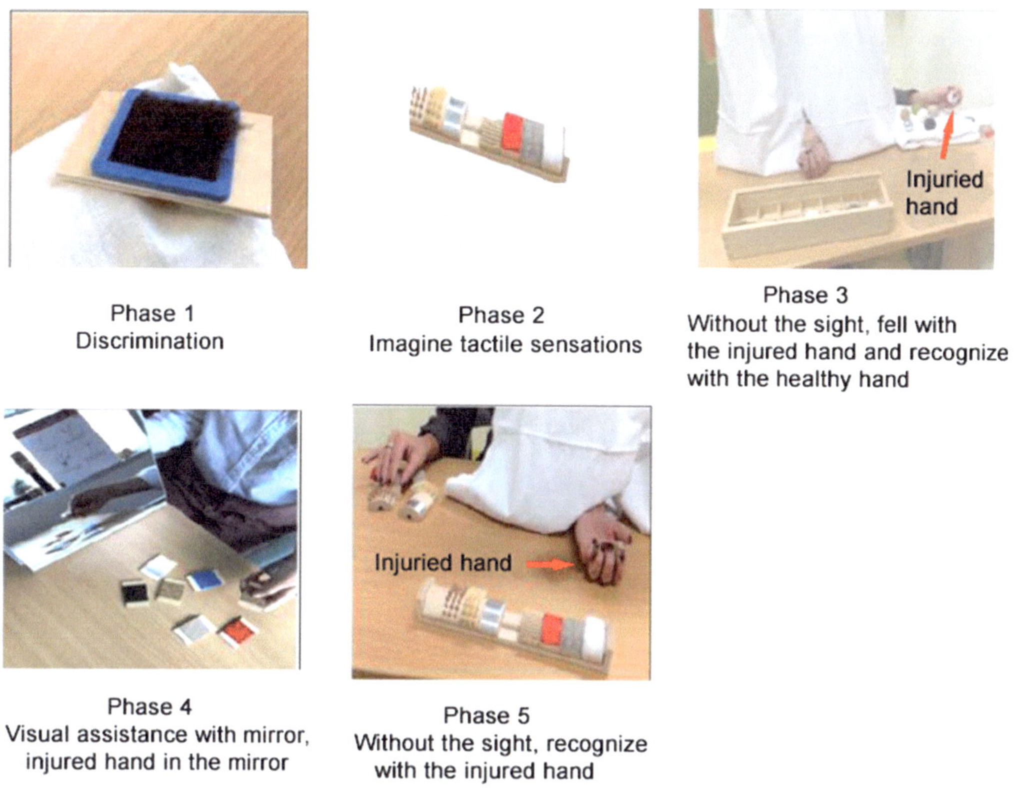

Fig. 14.91 Graded sensory imagery according to Milner

- **Scottish baths**

The use of Scottish baths for mild cases has been accepted by Harden et al. but is not recommended for the most severe CRPS, as immersion in cold water tends to increase pain [14].

The SFETD does not recommend this as a treatment for CRPS.

- **Manual lymphatic drainage**

Weak evidence suggests that manual lymphatic drainage is probably ineffective [137].

- **Immobilization**

Prolonged immobilization of the limb should be avoided, as should the use of orthoses covering the entire limb [14, 21–23].

- **Fight against kinesiophobia**

Behavioral and psychological factors can exacerbate the pain and dysfunction and maintain the syndrome in some patients [138].

Progressive exposure therapies suggest that "chronic" patients gradually confront activities they tend to avoid and mobilize limbs they tend to underuse by ignoring the pain [27]. They are recommended by the SFETD.

The concept is to subject the body to progressive stress to desensitize it in terms of threat perception and nervous system reaction. The idea is to rehabilitate and re-educate the nervous system (peripheral and central) through the dissociation of pain and movement.

Motivation and active participation on the part of the patient are decisive elements of this therapy [139].

"Start by moving at your own pace, being sure you don't feel any pain, then move a little more the next time."

This therapy is perfectly in line with the notions of therapeutic education and the fight against central pain phenomena, where the patient is an actor, reappropriating his limb and understanding his pain as the response of a hypersensitized alarm system, with no associated injuries (Fig. 14.92).

➔ Psychological Management of CRPS

It is necessary to consult a psychologist or psychiatrist to consider any psychological factors that may arise during CRPS.

➔ Drug Management

Corticosteroids, NSAIDs, and opioids are not recommended.

PEPT Protocol

Why ?
Pain is a false alarm signal.
Resume regular activity quickly, despite pain signals.

What ?
Exposure to painful movements and activities.
Without medication, TENS, orthoses or bandages.
Self-massage, forced use, exercises with progressive loads.
Muscle strengthening, joint amplitude exercises.
Information and education about CRPS, PEPT and the role of pain as a false alarm signal.

Who ?
2 rehabilitators
with a coaching role

How ?
Face to face, individually, with exercises to do at home and daily activities.

Where ?
At the practice, and in the daily life.

How much ?
5 sessions of 40 minutes maximum
Tailor-made to each individual's abilities and lifestyle.

Fig. 14.92 Pain exposure physical therapy (PEPT) by K.J. Barnhoorn

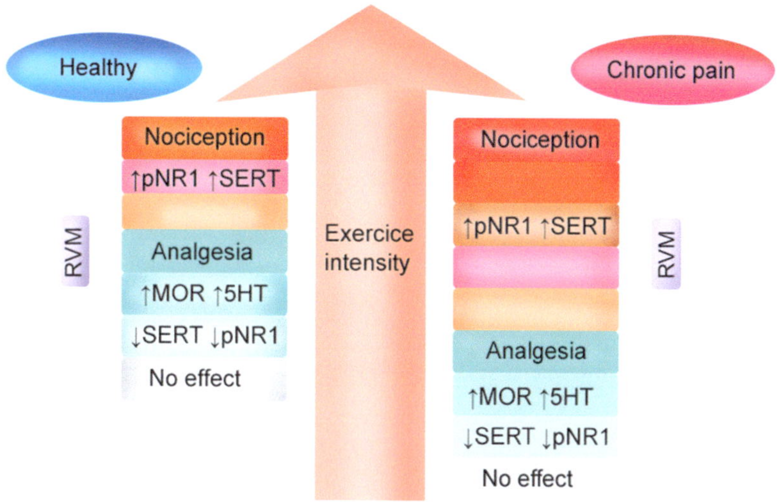

Fig. 14.93 Diagram summarizing the mechanisms involved in pain modulation sites, underlying the nociceptive and analgesic effects with increasing exercise intensity (Lima et al.)

Vitamin C is recommended for its possible action against free radicals in the interneurons of the posterior cornea.

The SFETD recommends 500 mg of vitamin C for 50 days following wrist fracture surgery.

TENS are recommended.

Despite the absence of studies on the efficacy or safety of lidocaine patches in CRPS, the SFETD recommends the application of a patch in the case of allodynia, over the area delimited by the allodynia.

➔ Regular Physical Activity

Exercise is an integral part of the therapeutic tools for patients suffering from central pain [140], including in CRPS [141]. Regular physical activity is recommended as a means of fighting against maladjustment and desocialization, reactivating general inhibition, and stimulating the feeling of "being able."

However, exercise can also increase algesic phenomena, making therapeutic adherence difficult [142] and promoting a sedentary lifestyle known to exacerbate the situation [143].

A single session of overly demanding exercise in a chronic situation can exacerbate pain, resulting in stimulation of NMDA receptors (pain facilitators) in the sites responsible for its modulation. However, regular exercise can have a beneficial effect, by reducing serotonin production and increasing opioid production (Fig. 14.93).

In their work, Lima et al. demonstrate that the intensity of exercise required to produce analgesic effects must be lower in patients with chronic pain, as nociceptive thresholds may be rapidly reached [144]. We must therefore take this into account and inform our patients.

In chronic pain patients, to be beneficial, exercise must be dosed at much lower intensities than in unaffected patients, at the risk of re-triggering nociceptive phenomena.

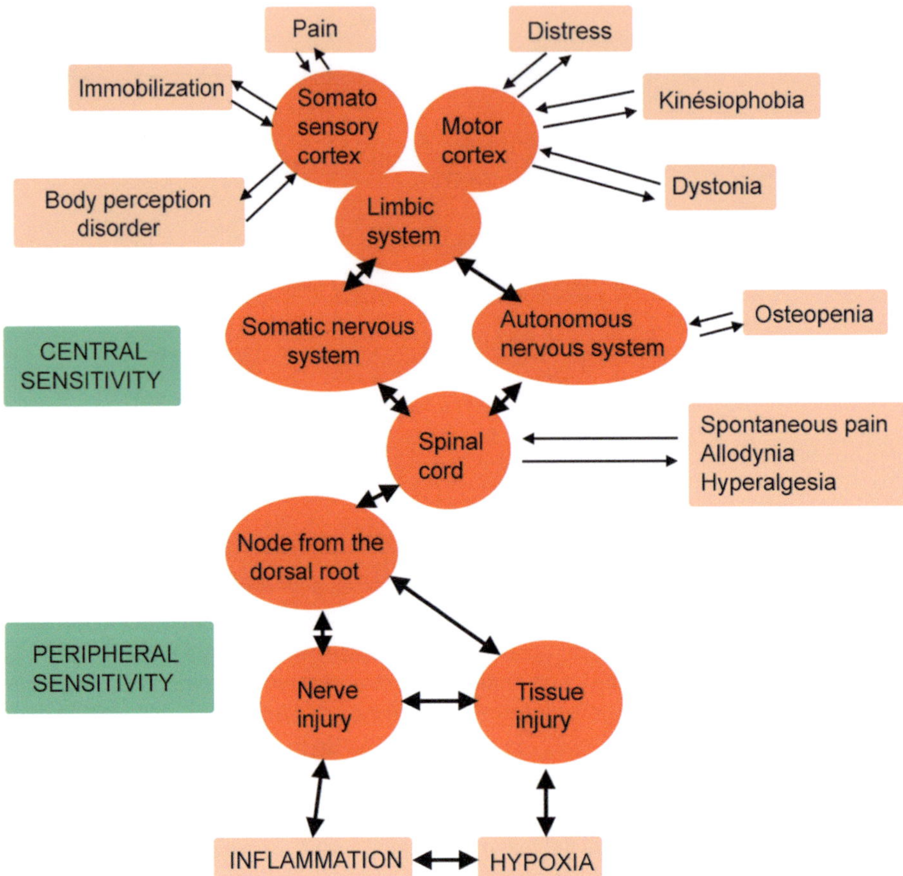

Fig. 14.94 Mechanisms and their interactions in CRPS (C. Maihöfner et al)

Conclusion

The best way to fight against CRPS is to prevent it. Should symptoms set in, it is essential to seek out the irritative thorn in the first few weeks, after which its management becomes more complex, requiring a multidisciplinary team to act on as many of the syndrome's active parameters as possible in a concomitant manner [23].

The advent of functional MRI has revealed the permanent interrelation between peripheral and central phenomena in CRPS patients. This active communication gives rise to maladaptive neuroplasticity phenomena, which are factors in the chronicity of the syndrome. But it is possible to reverse this phenomenon and use its neuroplastic abilities to bring the whole organism back to a more "serene" state, by reducing its sensitization.

Several mechanisms are at work, and if the irritative thorn has not been removed, recognizing and assessing them will allow a "tailor-made" management to optimize results [68, 93] (Fig. 14.94).

Therapeutic strategies can be either top-down or bottom-up; for example, by increasing discriminative sensitivity and cortical representation, algesic phenomena can be reduced. Let's not forget that pain, discriminative sensitivity, body mapping disorders, and cortical reorganization are interdependent [69, 77, 80].

Relearning through adjustments and corrections and an environment enriched with stimuli and new exposures will generate a change in transient, reassuring perceptions, leading to a desensitization of the body's vigilance system.

Complex regional Pain Syndrome		
Fight against sensori-motor (blurring) disorders and pain		
Tailor-made rehabilitation		
First prevention	**Work at a peripheral level**	**Work at a central level**
Goals: - Identify at-risk profiles: important pain, claustrophobia in the cast. - Remove irritative thorn as early as possible: is there an entrapment syndrome, an associated sprain, hurtful equipment ?	**Goals:** - Fight against mechanosensitivity: restore space under the skin (fight against edema, adherences, inflammation). - Remove irritative thorn if hypoesthesia or neuralgia. - Maintain mobility and function.	**Goals:** - Maintain cortical representation. - Fight against body mapping and body perception disorders. - Remove irritative thorn if allodynia. - Fight against kinesiophobia. - Favor therapeutic alliance
Techniques: - Adapt casts and orthoses: avoid points of pressure and flexed positions. -Reduce the orthosis if claustrophobia in the cast. - Favor the use of the affected limb even with a cast or orthosis (free healthy joints). - Treat pain: analgesics… - Preventative vitamin C.	**Techniques:** - Vibrations, taping, vacuotherapy, dermo-neuromodulation, neurodynamic glidings. - Sensory rehabilitation of hypoesthesia, discriminative work. - Desensitization in case of neuroma or dysesthesia. - Self-rehabilitation exercises for the mobility of the superior limb. - Self-rehabilitation exercises for neurodynamic gliding.	**Techniques:** - GMI, explain CRPS… - Prisms - Increase visual and proprioceptive stimulations coming from the CRPS limb (compressive glove, taping…). - Sensorimotor re-training. - Distant vibrotactile stimulations if allodynia. - Psychological support if necessary. - Avoid immobilization (orthoses…).
Risks: Evolution towards CRPS.	**Risks:** Maintain the cycle pain/stiffness/edema if maladapted constraints and/or physical agents.	**Risks:** Increase symptoms if maladapted protocol.
Do not forget:		
Allow transitory perception changes: if the body feels that it can move without pain, several protection systems disengage, and peripheral and central sensitizations decrease.		
Considering the affected hemi-space and hemi-body (midline) as they have an incidence on pain and performances.		
Practice a regular physical activity of moderate intensity in case of chronic pain, at the risk of becoming nocebo.		

Fig. 14.95 Summary table about CRPS

To optimize our results, the art of our therapy will lie in our ability to listen to and observe our patients, to constantly adapt our treatment (Fig. 14.95).

Bibliography

1. Crijns TJ, Van Der Gronde BATD, Ring D, Leung N. Complex regional pain syndrome after distal radius fracture is uncommon and is often associated with fibromyalgia. Clin Orthop. 2018;476(4):744–50. https://doi.org/10.1007/s11999.0000000000000070.
2. Merskey H, Bogduk N. IASP task force on taxonomy, classification of chronic pain, vol. 2. IASP Publ; 2011.
3. Ott S, Maihöfner C. Signs and symptoms in 1,043 patients with complex regional pain syndrome. J Pain. 2018;19(6):599–611. https://doi.org/10.1016/j.jpain.2018.01.004.
4. de Mos M, de Bruijn AGJ, Huygen FJPM, Dieleman JP, Stricker BHC, Sturkenboom MCJM. The incidence of complex regional

pain syndrome: a population-based study. Pain. 2007;129(1–2):12–20. https://doi.org/10.1016/j.pain.2006.09.008.
5. Velzen GAJ, Huygen FJPM, Kleef M, Eijs FV, Marinus J, Hilten JJ. Sex matters in complex regional pain syndrome. Eur J Pain. 2019;23(6):1108–16. https://doi.org/10.1002/ejp.1375.
6. Speck V, Schlereth T, Birklein F, Maihöfner C. Increased prevalence of posttraumatic stress disorder in CRPS. Eur J Pain. 2017;21(3):466–73. https://doi.org/10.1002/ejp.940.
7. Jo Y-H, Kim K, Lee B-G, Kim J-H, Lee C-H, Lee K-H. Incidence of and risk factors for complex regional pain syndrome type 1 after surgery for distal radius fractures: a population-based study. Sci Rep. 2019;9(1):4871. https://doi.org/10.1038/s41598-019-41152-x.
8. Rochlin DH, Sheckter CC, Satteson ES, Swan CC, Fox PM, Curtin C. Separating fact from fiction: a nationwide longitudinal examination of complex regional pain syndrome following treatment of Dupuytren contracture. Hand. 2022;17(5):825–32. https://doi.org/10.1177/1558944720963915.
9. Packham TL, Spicher CJ, MacDermid JC, Michlovitz S, Buckley DN. Somatosensory rehabilitation for allodynia in complex regional pain syndrome of the upper limb: a retrospective cohort study. J Hand Ther. 2018;31(1):10–9. https://doi.org/10.1016/j.jht.2017.02.007.
10. Beerthuizen A, et al. Demographic and medical parameters in the development of complex regional pain syndrome type 1 (CRPS1): prospective study on 596 patients with a fracture. Pain. 2012;153(6):1187–92. https://doi.org/10.1016/j.pain.2012.01.026.
11. Packham T, Holly J. Mechanism-specific rehabilitation management of complex regional pain syndrome: proposed recommendations from evidence synthesis. J Hand Ther. 2018;31(2):238–49. https://doi.org/10.1016/j.jht.2018.01.007.
12. Moseley GL, Herbert RD, Parsons T, Lucas S, Van Hilten JJ, Marinus J. Intense pain soon after wrist fracture strongly predicts who will develop complex regional pain syndrome: prospective cohort study. J Pain. 2014;15(1):16–23. https://doi.org/10.1016/j.jpain.2013.08.009.
13. Lipman MD, Hess DE, Werner BC, Deal DN. Fibromyalgia as a predictor of complex regional pain syndrome after distal radius fracture. Hand. 2019;14(4):516–22. https://doi.org/10.1177/1558944717735949.
14. Harden RN, et al. Complex regional pain syndrome: practical diagnostic and treatment guidelines., 4th ed. Pain Med. 2013;14(2):180–229. https://doi.org/10.1111/pme.12033.
15. Packham T. Complex regional pain syndrome: advancing rehabilitation through better evaluation and treatment [thesis]. Hamilton, Ontario: McMaster University; 2016. 146.
16. Harden NR, et al. Development of a severity score for CRPS. Pain. 2010;151(3):870–6. https://doi.org/10.1016/j.pain.2010.09.031.
17. Blumberg H, Hoffmann U, Mohadjer N, Scheremet R. Clinical phenomenology and mechanisms of reflex sympathetic dystrophy: emphasis on edema. In: Gebhart GF, Hammond DL, Jensen TS, editors. Proceedings of the 7th world congress on pain, progress in pain research and management, vol. 2. Seattle: IASP Press. p. 455.
18. Sinis N, Birbaumer N, Bredanger S, Schaller H-E, Haerle M. Memantine treatment of complex regional pain syndrome. Clin J Pain. 2007;23(3):7.
19. Bruehl S, Harden RN, Galer BS, Saltz S, Backonja M, Stanton-Hicks M. Complex regional pain syndrome: are there distinct subtypes and sequential stages of the syndrome? Pain. 2002;95(1–2):119–24.
20. De Rooij AM, et al. Spontaneous onset of complex regional pain syndrome. Eur J Pain. 2010;14(5):510–3. https://doi.org/10.1016/j.ejpain.2009.08.007.
21. Royal College of Physicians, Complex regional pain syndrome in adults UK guidelines for diagnosis, referral and management in primary and secondary care 2018; 2023.
22. Goebel A, Barker CH, Turner-Stokes L. Complex regional pain syndrome: UK guidelines for diagnosis, referral and management in primary and secondary care. London: Royal College of Physicians; 2012.
23. Groupe de projet spécifique (GPS) de la SFETD. Recommandations diagnostiques et de prise en charge thérapeutique des syndromes douloureux régionaux complexes: les recommandations de Lille. Douleur Analgésie. 2019;32(3):155–64. https://doi.org/10.3166/dea-2019-0074.
24. Mesaroli G, Hundert A, Birnie KA, Campbell F, Stinson J. Screening and diagnostic tools for complex regional pain syndrome: a systematic review. Pain. 2021;162(5):1295–304. https://doi.org/10.1097/j.pain.0000000000002146.
25. Goebel A, et al. The Valencia consensus-based adaptation of the IASP complex regional pain syndrome diagnostic criteria. Pain. 2021;162(9):2346–8. https://doi.org/10.1097/j.pain.0000000000002245.
26. Wertli MM, Brunner F, Steurer J, Held U. Usefulness of bone scintigraphy for the diagnosis of complex regional pain syndrome 1: a systematic review and Bayesian meta-analysis. PLOS One. 2017;12(3):e0173688. https://doi.org/10.1371/journal.pone.0173688.
27. Algorithme de prise en charge interdisciplinaire du syndrome de douleur régionale complexe (SDRC). Québec: Direction des communications du Ministère de la santé et des services sociaux; 2015.
28. Birklein F, Ajit SK, Goebel A, Perez RSGM, Sommer C. Complex regional pain syndrome — phenotypic characteristics and potential biomarkers. Nat Rev Neurol. 2018;14(5):272–84. https://doi.org/10.1038/nrneurol.2018.20.

29. Li W-W, et al. Neuropeptide regulation of adaptive immunity in the tibia fracture model of complex regional pain syndrome. J Neuroinflammation. 2018;15(1):105. https://doi.org/10.1186/s12974-018-1145-1.
30. Misidou C, Papagoras C. Complex regional pain syndrome: an update. Mediterr J Rheumatol. 2019;30(1):16–25. https://doi.org/10.31138/mjr.30.1.16.
31. Dirckx M, Stronks DL, van Bodegraven-Hof EAM, Wesseldijk F, Groeneweg JG, Huygen FJPM. Inflammation in cold complex regional pain syndrome. Acta Anaesthesiol Scand. 2015;59(6):733–9. https://doi.org/10.1111/aas.12465.
32. Sommer C, Leinders M, Üçeyler N. Inflammation in the pathophysiology of neuropathic pain. Pain. 2018;159(3):595–602. https://doi.org/10.1097/j.pain.0000000000001122.
33. Marinus J, et al. Clinical features and pathophysiology of complex regional pain syndrome. Lancet Neurol. 2011;10(7):637–48. https://doi.org/10.1016/S1474-4422(11)70106-5.
34. Baronio M, et al. Molecular aspects of regional pain syndrome. Pain Res Manag. 2020;2020:7697214. https://doi.org/10.1155/2020/7697214.
35. Wehmeyer C, Pap T, Buckley CD, Naylor AJ. The role of stromal cells in inflammatory bone loss. Clin Exp Immunol. 2017;189(1):1–11. https://doi.org/10.1111/cei.12979.
36. Barlow SJ. A non-surgical intervention for triangular fibrocartilage complex tears: triangular fibrocartilage tear intervention. Physiother Res Int. 2016;21(4):271–6. https://doi.org/10.1002/pri.1672.
37. Birklein F, et al. Activation of cutaneous immune responses in complex regional pain syndrome. J Pain. 2014;15(5):485–95. https://doi.org/10.1016/j.jpain.2014.01.490.
38. Bove GM, Light AR. The nervi nervorum. Pain Forum. 1997;6(3):181–90. https://doi.org/10.1016/S1082-3174(97)70011-4.
39. Jacobs D. Dermo neuro modulation. Éditions Louise Tremblay; 2018. p. 35.
40. Pećina MM, editor. Tunnel syndromes: peripheral nerve compression syndromes. 3rd ed. Boca Raton: CRC Press; 2001.
41. Schmid AB, Hailey L, Tampin B. Entrapment neuropathies: challenging common beliefs with novel evidence. J Orthop Sports Phys Ther. 2018;48(2):58–62. https://doi.org/10.2519/jospt.2018.0603.
42. Greening J, Dilley A, Lynn B. In vivo study of nerve movement and mechanosensitivity of the median nerve in whiplash and non-specific arm pain patients. Pain. 2005;115(3):248–53. https://doi.org/10.1016/j.pain.2005.02.023.
43. Teixeira MJ, Almeida DB, Yeng LT. Concept of acute neuropathic pain. The role of nervi nervorum in the distinction between acute nociceptive and neuropathic pain. Rev Dor. 2016;17. https://doi.org/10.5935/1806-0013.20160038.
44. Schmid AB, Fundaun J, Tampin B. Entrapment neuropathies: a contemporary approach to pathophysiology, clinical assessment, and management. Pain Rep. 2020;5(4):e829. https://doi.org/10.1097/PR9.0000000000000829.
45. Schmid A-C, Schwarz A, Gustin SM, Greenspan JD, Hummel FC, Birbaumer N. Pain reduction due to novel sensory-motor training in complex regional pain syndrome I – a pilot study. Scand J Pain. 2017;15:30–7. https://doi.org/10.1016/j.sjpain.2016.11.003.
46. Schmid AB, Bland JDP, Bhat MA, Bennett DLH. The relationship of nerve fibre pathology to sensory function in entrapment neuropathy. Brain. 2014;137(12):3186–99. https://doi.org/10.1093/brain/awu288.
47. Felten D, et al. Atlas de neurosciences humaines de Netter. 2nd ed. Issy-les-Moulineaux: Elsevier Masson; 2011.
48. Lim TKY, et al. Blood-nerve barrier dysfunction contributes to the generation of neuropathic pain and allows targeting of injured nerves for pain relief. Pain. 2014;155(5):954–67. https://doi.org/10.1016/j.pain.2014.01.026.
49. Lim TKY, et al. Peripheral nerve injury induces persistent vascular dysfunction and endoneurial hypoxia, contributing to the genesis of neuropathic pain. J Neurosci Off J Soc Neurosci. 2015;35(8):3346–59. https://doi.org/10.1523/JNEUROSCI.4040-14.2015.
50. Volpi N, Guarna M, Lorenzoni P, Franci D, Massai L, Grass G. Characterization of lymphatic vessels in human peripheral neuropathies. Ital J Anat Embryol. 2013;117:12. https://doi.org/10.13128/IJAE-11841.
51. Schmid AB, Coppieters MW, Ruitenberg MJ, McLachlan EM. Local and remote immune-mediated inflammation after mild peripheral nerve compression in rats. J Neuropathol Exp Neurol. 2013;72(7):662–80. https://doi.org/10.1097/NEN.0b013e318298de5b.
52. Lundborg G. Nerve injury and repair, 1. publ. Edinburgh: Churchill Livingstone; 1988.
53. Lundborg G. Intraneural microcirculation. Orthop Clin North Am. 1988;19(1):1–12.
54. Treede R-D, et al. Neuropathic pain: redefinition and a grading system for clinical and research purposes. Neurology. 2008;70(18):1630–5. https://doi.org/10.1212/01.wnl.0000282763.29778.59.
55. Shacklock MO. Clinical neurodynamics: a new system of musculoskeletal treatment, reprinted. Edinburgh: Elsevier Butterworth-Heinemann; 2007.
56. Goh EL, Chidambaram S, Ma D. Complex regional pain syndrome: a recent update, burns. Trauma. 2017;5:2. https://doi.org/10.1186/s41038-016-0066-4.
57. Kortekaas MC, Niehof SP, Stolker RJ, Huygen FJPM. Pathophysiological mechanisms involved

in vasomotor disturbances in complex regional pain syndrome and implications for therapy: a review. Pain Pract. 2016;16(7):905–14. https://doi.org/10.1111/papr.12403.
58. Tajerian M, Clark JD. New concepts in complex regional pain syndrome. Hand Clin. 2016;32(1):41–9. https://doi.org/10.1016/j.hcl.2015.08.003.
59. Cuhadar U, et al. Autoantibodies produce pain in complex regional pain syndrome by sensitizing nociceptors. Pain. 2019;160(12):2855–65. https://doi.org/10.1097/j.pain.0000000000001662.
60. Guimberteau JC. Promenades sous la peau = strolling under the skin. Paris: Elsevier; 2004.
61. Stecco C, Richard A. Atlas fonctionnel du système fascial humain. Paris: Tita éditions; 2020.
62. Colloca L, et al. Neuropathic pain. Nat Rev Dis Primers. 2017;3(1):17002. https://doi.org/10.1038/nrdp.2017.2.
63. Meacham K, Shepherd A, Mohapatra DP, Haroutounian S. Neuropathic pain: central vs. peripheral mechanisms. Curr Pain Headache Rep. 2017;21(6):28. https://doi.org/10.1007/s11916-017-0629-5.
64. Arendt-Nielsen L, et al. Assessment and manifestation of central sensitisation across different chronic pain conditions. Eur J Pain. 2018;22(2):216–41. https://doi.org/10.1002/ejp.1140.
65. Lévêque M. Chirurgie de la douleur. Paris: Springer Paris; 2014. https://doi.org/10.1007/978-2-8178-0509-2.
66. Halicka M, Vittersø AD, Proulx MJ, Bultitude JH. Neuropsychological changes in complex regional pain syndrome (CRPS). Behav Neurol. 2020;2020:1–30. https://doi.org/10.1155/2020/4561831.
67. Maihöfner C, Handwerker HO, Neundörfer B, Birklein F. Patterns of cortical reorganization in complex regional pain syndrome. Neurology. 2003;61(12):1707–15. https://doi.org/10.1212/01.wnl.0000098939.02752.8e.
68. Maihöfner C, Handwerker HO, Neundörfer B, Birklein F. Cortical reorganization during recovery from complex regional pain syndrome. Neurology. 2004;63(4):693–701.
69. Delaquaize F. Réorganisation corticale posttraumatique et plasticité cérébrale : rééducation par les techniques d'imagerie motrice. In: Gemmsor, editor. Rééducation de la main et du poignet ; Anatomie fonctionnelle et techniques. Paris: Elsevier Masson; 2013. p. 187–203.
70. Thomas O. Représentation du corps, fonctionnement du système nerveux central et douleur centrale : études chez le blessé médullaire, Recherche clinique innovation technologique, santé publique. Versailles Saint-Quentin-en-Yvelines: Université Paris-Saclay préparée à l'Université de Versailles Saint-Quentin-en-Yvelines; 2019.
71. Rossetti Y, Jacquin-Courtois S, Legrain V, Bultitude J, O'Shea J. Le syndrome douloureux régional complexe à la lumière des troubles de la cognition spatiale: des opportunités physiopathologiques et thérapeutiques? In: Syndromes douloureux chroniques en médecine physique et de réadaptation. Paris: Springer; 2013. p. 99–109. https://doi.org/10.1007/978-2-8178-0439-2_9.
72. Filbrich L, et al. Biased visuospatial perception in complex regional pain syndrome. Sci Rep. 2017;7(1):9712. https://doi.org/10.1038/s41598-017-10077-8.
73. Lewis J, McCabe C. Body perception disturbance (BPD) in CRPS. Pract Pain Manag. 2010;10:60–6.
74. Galer BS, Jensen M. Neglect-like symptoms in complex regional pain syndrome: results of a self-administered survey. J Pain Symptom Manage. 1999;18(3):213.
75. Förderreuther S, Sailer U, Straube A. Impaired self-perception of the hand in complex regional pain syndrome (CRPS). Pain. 2004;110(3):756–61. https://doi.org/10.1016/j.pain.2004.05.019.
76. Latremoliere A, Woolf CJ. Central sensitization: a generator of pain hypersensitivity by central neural plasticity. J Pain. 2009;10(9):895–926. https://doi.org/10.1016/j.jpain.2009.06.012.
77. Haggard P, Iannetti GD, Longo MR. Spatial sensory organization and body representation in pain perception. Curr Biol. 2013;23(4):R164–76. https://doi.org/10.1016/j.cub.2013.01.047.
78. Moseley GL, editor. The graded motor imagery handbook. Adelaide: Noigroup Publ; 2012.
79. Moseley GL, Parsons TJ, Spence C. Visual distortion of a limb modulates the pain and swelling evoked by movement. Curr Biol. 2008;18(22):R1047–8. https://doi.org/10.1016/j.cub.2008.09.031.
80. Lewis JS, Schweinhardt P. Perceptions of the painful body: the relationship between body perception disturbance, pain and tactile discrimination in complex regional pain syndrome. Eur J Pain. 2012;16(9):1320–30. https://doi.org/10.1002/j.1532-2149.2012.00120.x.
81. Lewis JS, Kersten P, McCabe CS, McPherson KM, Blake DR. Body perception disturbance: a contribution to pain in complex regional pain syndrome (CRPS). Pain. 2007;133(1–3):111–9. https://doi.org/10.1016/j.pain.2007.03.013.
82. Lewis J, Kellett S, McCullough R, Tapper A, Tyler C, Viner M. 269 a clinical evaluation of rehabilitation outcomes in complex regional pain syndrome. Rheumatology. 2018;57(suppl_3) https://doi.org/10.1093/rheumatology/key075.493.
83. Paillard J, editor. Brain and space. In: Oxford science publications. Oxford, New York: Oxford University Press; 1991.
84. Jeannerod M, Rossetti Y. Visuomotor coordination as a dissociable visual function: experimental and clinical evidence, Baillieres. Clin Neurol. 1993;2(2):439–60.
85. Sumitani M, et al. Pathologic pain distorts visuospatial perception. Neurology. 2007;68(2):152–4.

https://doi.org/10.1212/01.wnl.0000250335.56958.f0.
86. Uematsu H, et al. Complex regional pain syndrome (CRPS) impairs visuospatial perception,whereas postherpetic neuralgia does not: possible implications for supraspinal mechanism of CRPS. Ann Acad Med Singap. 2009;38(11):931–6.
87. Reid EJ, et al. Spatially-defined motor deficits in people with unilateral complex regional pain syndrome. Cortex. 2018;104:154–62. https://doi.org/10.1016/j.cortex.2017.06.024.
88. Gallace A, Torta DME, Moseley GL, Iannetti GD. The analgesic effect of crossing the arms. Pain. 2011;152(6):1418–23. https://doi.org/10.1016/j.pain.2011.02.029.
89. Moseley LG, Gallace A, Di Pietro F, Spence C, Iannetti GD. Limb-specific autonomic dysfunction in complex regional pain syndrome modulated by wearing prism glasses. Pain. 2013;154(11):2463–8. https://doi.org/10.1016/j.pain.2013.07.026.
90. Bultitude JH, Walker I, Spence C. Space based bias of covert visual attention in complex regional pain syndrome. Brain. 2017;140(9):2306–21. https://doi.org/10.1093/brain/awx152.
91. Bultitude JH, Petrini K. Altered visuomotor integration in complex regional pain syndrome. Behav Brain Res. 2021;397:112922. https://doi.org/10.1016/j.bbr.2020.112922.
92. Cowell F, Gillespie S, Cheung G, Brown D. Complex regional pain syndrome in distal radius fractures: how to implement changes to reduce incidence and facilitate early management. J Hand Ther. 2018;31(2):201–5. https://doi.org/10.1016/j.jht.2018.01.013.
93. Gillespie S, Cowell F, Cheung G, Brown D. Can we reduce the incidence of complex regional pain syndrome type I in distal radius fractures? The Liverpool experience. Hand Ther. 2016;21(4):123–30. https://doi.org/10.1177/1758998316659676.
94. Pleger B, et al. Patterns of cortical reorganization parallel impaired tactile discrimination and pain intensity in complex regional pain syndrome. NeuroImage. 2006;32(2):503–10. https://doi.org/10.1016/j.neuroimage.2006.03.045.
95. Pleger B, et al. Sensorimotor retuning corrected. In complex regional pain syndrome parallels pain reduction. Ann Neurol. 2005;57(3):425–9. https://doi.org/10.1002/ana.20394.
96. Parsons LM, Fox PT. The neural basis of implicit movements used in recognising hand shape. Cogn Neuropsychol. 1998;15:583–615.
97. Scerbo T, Colasurdo J, Dunn S, Unger J, Nijs J, Cook C. Measurement properties of the central sensitization inventory: a systematic review. Pain Pract. 2018;18(4):544–54. https://doi.org/10.1111/papr.12636.
98. Mayer TG, et al. The development and psychometric validation of the central sensitization inventory. Pain Pract. 2012;12(4):276–85. https://doi.org/10.1111/j.1533-2500.2011.00493.x.
99. Pitance L, et al. Cross cultural adaptation, reliability and validity of the French version of the central sensitization inventory. Man Ther. 2016;25:e83–4. https://doi.org/10.1016/j.math.2016.05.139.
100. Nijs J. Applying modern pain neuroscience in ClinicalPractice: criteria for the classification of central sensitization pain. Pain Physician. 2014;17(9):447–57. https://doi.org/10.36076/ppj.2014/17/447.
101. Neblett R, et al. The central sensitization inventory (CSI): establishing clinically significant values for identifying central sensitivity syndromes in an outpatient chronic pain sample. J Pain. 2013;14(5):438–45. https://doi.org/10.1016/j.jpain.2012.11.012.
102. Neblett R, Hartzell MM, Mayer TG, Cohen H, Gatchel RJ. Establishing clinically relevant severity levels for the central sensitization inventory. Pain Pract. 2017;17(2):166–75. https://doi.org/10.1111/papr.12440.
103. Ji R-R, Kohno T, Moore KA, Woolf CJ. Central sensitization and LTP: do pain and memory share similar mechanisms? Trends Neurosci. 2003;26(12):696–705. https://doi.org/10.1016/j.tins.2003.09.017.
104. Rolke R, et al. Quantitative sensory testing: a comprehensive protocol for clinical trials. Eur J Pain. 2006;10(1):77. https://doi.org/10.1016/j.ejpain.2005.02.003.
105. Kuttikat A, Shaikh M, Oomatia A, Parker R, Shenker N. Novel signs and their clinical utility in diagnosing complex regional pain syndrome (CRPS): a prospective observational cohort study. Clin J Pain. 2017;33(6):496–502. https://doi.org/10.1097/AJP.0000000000000434.
106. Moseley GL, Zalucki N, Birklein F, Marinus J, van Hilten JJ, Luomajoki H. Thinking about movement hurts: the effect of motor imagery on pain and swelling in people with chronic arm pain. Arthritis Rheum. 2008;59(5):623–31. https://doi.org/10.1002/art.23580.
107. Moseley GL, Gallace A, Spence C. Spacebased, but not arm-based, shift in tactile processing in complex regional pain syndrome and its relationship to cooling of the affected limb. Brain. 2009;132(11):3142–51. https://doi.org/10.1093/brain/awp224.
108. Taylor A. Rehab techniques in pain compression syndromes. ASPETAR. 2024;13:84–89.
109. Lundborg G. Nerve injury and repair regeneration, reconstruction, and cortical remodeling. Philadelphia: Elsevier/Churchill Livingstone; 2004. Consulté le: 19 mars 2016. En ligne. Disponible sur: http://www.sciencedirect.com/science/book/9780443067112.
110. Mesplié G. Examen clinique et outils de prise en charge rééducative avancée du poignet et de la main. In: Thérapie de la main, tome 1. Montpellier: Sauramps médical; 2021.
111. Spicher J, Fehlmann P, Maihöfner C. Management algorithm of spontaneous neuropathic pain and/

or touch-evoked neuropathic pain illustrated by prospective observations in clinical practice of 66 chronic neuropathic pain patients. E-News Somatosens Rehabil. 2016;13(1):4–28.
112. Spicher C, Quintal I, Vittaz M, Marchand S. Rééducation sensitive des douleurs neuropathiques: des troubles de base aux complications des troubles de la sensibilité cutanée lors de lésions neurologiques périphériques & cérébrales. Montpellier: Sauramps Médical; 2015.
113. de Boer RDH, et al. Distribution of signs and symptoms of complex regional pain syndrome type I in patients meeting the diagnostic criteria of the International Association for the Study of Pain. Eur J Pain Lond Engl. 2011;15(8):830.e1–8. https://doi.org/10.1016/j.ejpain.2011.01.012.
114. Perez RSGM, Collins S, Marinus J, Zuurmond WWA, de Lange JJ. Diagnostic criteria for CRPS I: differences between patient profiles using three different diagnostic sets. Eur J Pain Lond Eng. 2007;11(8):895–902. https://doi.org/10.1016/j.ejpain.2007.02.006.
115. Moseley GL. Graded motor imagery is effective for long-standing complex regional pain syndrome: a randomised controlled trial. Pain. 2004;108(1–2):192–8. https://doi.org/10.1016/j.pain.2004.01.006.
116. Sumitani M, et al. Prism adaptation to optical deviation alleviates pathologic pain. Neurology. 2007;68(2):128–33. https://doi.org/10.1212/01.wnl.0000250242.99683.57.
117. Rossetti Y. Des modalités sensorielles aux représentations spatiales en action: représentations multiples d'un espace unique. In: Proust J, editor. Perception et intermodalité : approches actuelles de la question de Molyneux. Paris: Presses Universitaires de France; 1997. p. 179–221.
118. Rossetti Y, et al. Prism adaptation to a rightward optical deviation rehabilitates left hemispatial neglect. Nature. 1998;395(6698):166–9. https://doi.org/10.1038/25988.
119. Bultitude JH, Rafal RD. Derangement of body representation in complex regional pain syndrome: report of a case treated with mirror and prisms. Exp Brain Res. 2010;204(3):409–18. https://doi.org/10.1007/s00221-009-2107-8.
120. Halicka M, et al. Prism adaptation treatment for upper-limb complex regional pain syndrome: a double-blind randomized controlled trial. Pain. 2021;162(2):471–89. https://doi.org/10.1097/j.pain.0000000000002053.
121. Christophe L, et al. Prisms to shift pain away: pathophysiological and therapeutic exploration of CRPS with prism adaptation. Neural Plast. 2016;2016:1–21. https://doi.org/10.1155/2016/1694256.
122. Moseley GL, Butler DS. Fifteen years of explaining pain: the past, present, and future. J Pain. 2015;16(9):807–13. https://doi.org/10.1016/j.jpain.2015.05.005.
123. Moseley GL, Butler DS. Explain pain supercharged: the clinician's manual. Noigroup Publications; 2017.
124. Bunzli S, Smith A, Schütze R, Lin I, O'Sullivan P. Making sense of low back pain and pain-related fear. J Orthop Sports Phys Ther. 2017;47(9):628–36. https://doi.org/10.2519/jospt.2017.7434.
125. Lee H, McAuley JH, Hübscher M, Kamper SJ, Traeger AC, Moseley GL. Does changing pain-related knowledge reduce pain and improve function through changes in catastrophizing? Pain. 2016;157(4):922–30. https://doi.org/10.1097/j.pain.0000000000000472.
126. Louw A, Zimney K, Puentedura EJ, Diener I. The efficacy of pain neuroscience education on musculoskeletal pain: a systematic review of the literature. Physiother Theory Pract. 2016;32(5):332–55. https://doi.org/10.1080/09593985.2016.1194646.
127. Hall AM, Ferreira PH, Maher CG, Latimer J, Ferreira ML. The influence of the therapist-patient relationship on treatment outcome in physical rehabilitation: a systematic review. Phys Ther. 2010;90(8):1099–110. https://doi.org/10.2522/ptj.20090245.
128. O'Keeffe M, et al. What influences patient-therapist interactions in musculoskeletal physical therapy? Qualitative systematic review and meta-synthesis. Phys Ther. 2016;96:609.
129. Roll J-P. 1.1. Physiologie de la kinesthèse. La proprioception musculaire : sixième sens, ou sens premier ? Intellectica Rev Assoc Pour Rech Cogn. 2003;36(1):49–66. https://doi.org/10.3406/intel.2003.1676.
130. Roll R, et al. Illusory movements prevent cortical disruption caused by immobilization. NeuroImage. 2012;62(1):510–9. https://doi.org/10.1016/j.neuroimage.2012.05.016.
131. Gay A. Proprioception musculaire et cutanée : implications dans le traitement de la douleur et de la mobilité articulaire du Syndrome Douloureux Régional Complexe de Type I; 2011.
132. Gilbert KK, Smith MP, Sobczak S, James CR, Sizer PS, Brismée J-M. Effects of lower limb neurodynamic mobilization on intraneural fluid dispersion of the fourth lumbar nerve root: an unembalmed cadaveric investigation. J Man Manip Ther. 2015;23(5):239–45. https://doi.org/10.1179/2042618615Y.0000000009.
133. Brown CL, Gilbert KK, Brismee J, Sizer PS, Roger James C, Smith MP. The effects of neurodynamic mobilization on fluid dispersion within the tibial nerve at the ankle: an unembalmed cadaveric study. J Man Manip Ther. 2011;19(1):26–34. https://doi.org/10.1179/2042618610Y.0000000003.
134. Beltran-Alacreu H, Jiménez-Sanz L, Fernández Carnero J, La Touche R. Comparison of hypoalgesic effects of neural stretching vs neural gliding: a randomized controlled trial. J Manipulative Physiol Ther. 2015;38(9):644–52. https://doi.org/10.1016/j.jmpt.2015.09.002.

135. Beneciuk JM, Bishop MD, George SZ. Effects of upper extremity neural mobilization on thermal pain sensitivity: a sham-controlled study in asymptomatic participants. J Orthop Sports Phys Ther. 2009;39(6):428–38. https://doi.org/10.2519/jospt.2009.2954.
136. Milner Z, Hogg M, O'Sullivan H, and White B. Sensory-motor Retraining Program: Part of a Clinical Pathway for Management of CRPS. Presented as part of: Specialist interest group of the IASP world conference on CRPS, Cork, 2017.
137. Cossins L, Okell RW, Cameron H, Simpson B, Poole HM, Goebel A. Treatment of complex regional pain syndrome in adults: a systematic review of randomized controlled trials published from June 2000 to February 2012. Eur J Pain Lond Engl. 2013;17(2):158–73. https://doi.org/10.1002/j.1532-2149.2012.00217.x.
138. Bruehl S, Chung OY. Psychological and behavioral aspects of complex regional pain syndrome management. Clin J Pain. 2006;22(5):430–7. https://doi.org/10.1097/01.ajp.0000194282.82002.79.
139. Barnhoorn KJ, et al. Pain exposure physical therapy (PEPT) compared to conventional treatment in complex regional pain syndrome type 1: a randomized controlled trial. BMJ Open. 2015;5(12):e008283. https://doi.org/10.1136/bmjopen-2015-008283.
140. Koltyn KF. Analgesia following exercise: a review. Sports Med. 2000;29(2):85–98. https://doi.org/10.2165/00007256-200029020-00002.
141. Topcuoglu A, Gokkaya NKO, Ucan H, Karakuş D. The effect of upper-extremity aerobic exercise on complex regional pain syndrome type I: a randomized controlled study on subacute stroke. Top Stroke Rehabil. 2015;22(4):253–61. https://doi.org/10.1179/1074935714Z.0000000025.
142. Dailey DL, Keffala VJ, Sluka KA. Do cognitive and physical fatigue tasks enhance pain, cognitive fatigue, and physical fatigue in people with fibromyalgia? Arthritis Care Res. 2015;67(2):288–96. https://doi.org/10.1002/acr.22417.
143. Damsgard E, Thrane G, Anke A, Fors T, Røe C. Activity-related pain in patients with chronic musculoskeletal disorders. Disabil Rehabil. 2010;32(17):1428–37. https://doi.org/10.3109/09638280903567877.
144. Lima LV, Abner TSS, Sluka KA. Does exercise increase or decrease pain? Central mechanisms underlying these two phenomena. J Physiol. 2017;595(13):4141–50. https://doi.org/10.1113/JP273355.

MIX
Papier aus verantwortungsvollen Quellen
Paper from responsible sources
FSC® C105338

If you have any concerns about our products,
you can contact us on
ProductSafety@springernature.com

In case Publisher is established outside the EU,
the EU authorized representative is:
Springer Nature Customer Service Center GmbH
Europaplatz 3, 69115 Heidelberg, Germany

Printed by Libri Plureos GmbH
in Hamburg, Germany